ERRATA

p. 25   Vit. B_{12} = 200–900 pg/ml
Folate, serum = 4–20 ng/ml
Folate, RBC = 100–400 ng/ml

p. 188   Somophyllin: strength = 21 mg/ml (*not* 18 mg/ml).

RESIDENTS' HANDBOOK OF PEDIATRICS

The Hospital for Sick Children, Toronto

SIXTH EDITION, 1979
REPRINTED WITH CORRECTIONS, 1980

Distributed through the University of Toronto Medical Bookstore, 63A St George St., Toronto, Canada M5S 1A6

Residents' Handbook of Pediatrics

THE HOSPITAL FOR SICK CHILDREN
TORONTO, CANADA

Editor-in-Chief
M. Rossi, M.D.

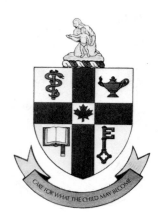

FOREWORD

This edition of our hospital's handbook takes on a new look, reflecting a different approach to its production. Unlike previous editions, this one was compiled by the medical residents and edited by the Chief Pediatric Resident, Dr Miriam Rossi. In this way it has been possible to present a more practical volume for trainees in pediatrics, for practising pediatricians, and for general practitioners who require a pocket-sized pediatric handbook.

Most of the sections have been rewritten, with contributions from many of the medical staff. The aim has been to replace much of the earlier descriptive material with tables and charts, and to add new trends in investigation and therapeutics. Of special note is the inclusion of a comprehensive glossary of age-related reference values in clinical chemistry, compiled by Dr Graham Ellis, and a contemporary version of the drug formulary. Lastly, it should be noted that the index has been completely redesigned, and the text contains handy cross-references to provide speedy access to related material in the book.

Neville J. Howard, M.B., F.R.C.P. (C)
Chairman, Education Committee
The Hospital for Sick Children
Toronto

July 1979

NOTICE

Every effort has been made to ensure that the drug dosage schedules are accurate and in accord with standards accepted at the time of printing. However, the reader is cautioned to check the product information sheet included in the package of each drug and to verify indications, contraindications, and recommended dosages.

HANDBOOK COMMITTEE   1979

INTRODUCTION

The Handbook is intended to give some practical, up-to-date information useful in the care of children, and this thorough revision represents the devoted work of many of the senior and house staff of The Hospital for Sick Children. I would like to thank and commend all of those involved, for their excellent work on this publication.

A great deal of effort has been expended on ensuring the accuracy of recommended drug dosages, and both the indications and contraindications for use. Even so, the rapid advancement of knowledge makes it absolutely mandatory to check the most recent authoritative source for this information.

David H. Carver, M.D., F.R.C.P. (C)
Paediatrician-in-Chief

CONTENTS

INVESTIGATION OF PATIENTS

In the interests of patient-care and for teaching purposes, the problem-oriented record* is recommended at this Hospital. (*Lawrence Weed: Medical Records, Medical Education, Patient Care. Cleveland, Ohio, Case Western Reserve & Univ. Press, 1969.)

DATA BASE
(history, physical examination, routine laboratory investigation)

Notes on Taking a Pediatric History
Objective: to delineate all the patient's problems – medical, social, emotional, and economic.
1. Careful documentation of this history helps both the history-taker and others in the assessment of the **PATIENT and his PROBLEMS.**
2. **Take a complete history.** Once the parents have left, it may be impossible to check details for several days. Also, it may be necessary to get further history from the referring physician or other agency. Interpreters are available if needed (Interpreter Service, ext 2422).

Chief Complaint (p 9)
1. One- or two-line summary of problem; note duration.
2. Ask parents: "Why have you brought your child to hospital?" or "Why did Dr X advise you to bring your child?" or "What seems to be the matter with your child?"

History of Present Illness (p 9)
(Name the informant and state your impression regarding reliability of the history given.)
1. Always start with: "When was your child last perfectly well, before the present symptoms started?"
2. "What happened then?"
3. Then: follow the story in logical sequence with the parents.
4. **Note.** Do not use day names – they have no meaning to anyone reading the history a month/year later.

History

1. POMR-21 (p 11) includes family history, neonatal history, feeding history, developmental history, past health, drug sensitivities, allergies. The back of the form (p 12) is a record of immunization, contagious disease.
2. Complete both sides on the first admission. The record is carried forward, and is reviewed/revised on each re-admission.

Functional Enquiry

1. POMR-24 (p 13-14) includes systems review, current developmental status, behavior, social conditions, diet.
2. Complete this form on **EACH** admission.

Physical Examination

1. Spend some time making friends.
2. a) *Infant:* remove all clothing for examination.
   b) *Older child:* though thorough, examination should respect the adolescent's privacy and sensitivity.
3. Spend a few minutes making further observations.
4. The order of examination will vary with:
   a) urgency of the situation
   b) age and co-operation
   c) suspected system involved
   Leave discomforting aspects to the end.

Suggested Order of Examination

1. Inspect patient: Does he look ill? Well developed and nourished? Note whether rash, birth marks, cyanosis, pallor, evidence of dehydration, respiratory distress or noisy breathing, forceful heart action, chest deformity, abdominal distention, visible gastric peristalsis, swollen joints, photophobia, neck retraction, etc.
2. Palpate anterior fontanelle: open or closed; bulging, flat, or depressed. Note whether neck stiffness.
3. Auscultate heart and lungs before doing percussion, etc., and femoral pulsations.
4. Palpate abdomen gently: tenderness, rigidity, organomegaly, masses. Follow with percussion, auscultation for bowel sounds. Check hernial orifices later.
5. Lymph nodes
6. Neck, back and spine, hips and other joints
7. External genitalia: ?abnormality. Tanner staging of sexual development

8. Motor system, reflexes, co-ordination; sensory if indicated
9. BP in arm
10. Eyes and optic fundi. If necessary, dilate pupils with 1% cyclopentolate or 2½% Neo-Synephrine. (If the room is darkened, this can usually be done without restraining the child.) Vision and fields; squint, nystagmus.
11. Ears (child being carefully restrained by parent/nurse).
12. Nose and mouth, including buccal mucosa, number of primary or secondary teeth (child being carefully restrained by parent/nurse)
13. Measurements: head, length, symphysis to heel
14. Rectal exam if indicated (e.g., intussusception)
15. Moro reflex and other special reflexes
16. Check for craniotabes and costochondral junction for rickets or scurvy.
17. Gait (if indicated)
18. Evaluate intelligence, development, behavior.

Routine Investigation

1. Tine test on all patients over 1 mo of age, unless known to be tuberculin positive or tested within the previous 3 mo
2. Hb, WBC, smear
3. Complete urinalysis
4. Urine metabolic screen in children under 2 yr of age
5. All neonates: do Guthrie test

List of Positive Findings

If *all problems* are to receive the attention of the hospital team, *all positive findings* should be summarized (including, for example, abnormal social situations, family difficulties, and incomplete immunization).

List these findings as groups of cues, so that problems can be formulated readily. See Master Problem List, p. 10.

A. Tentative Problem List
1. The record must be **PROBLEM-ORIENTED** rather than diagnosis-oriented.
   a) Identify and list *all* the patient's problems.
   b) Identify drug *sensitivities* and severe food *allergies* as problems.
2. Outline the differential diagnosis of each problem. The **TENTATIVE PROBLEM LIST** must be discussed with the senior resident and/or

ward chief, and then the **PERMANENT PROB-LEM LIST** is drawn up.

B. **Permanent Problem List**

The **PROBLEMS** form the **PIVOT** around which all patient care is planned.
1. The list must include **ALL** identified problems, numbered
2. All problems must be listed in the body of the notes
3. The Master Problem List (p 10) must be attached **in the FRONT of the chart within 24 hr of admission**
4. Enter the date at which each problem is:
    a) identified
    b) solved.

The problem list may be added to, but problems must not be removed:
– They may be solved; add date of solution to the list.
– They may merge with other problems as a complex becomes recognized as one problem; enter the date of the merger on the problem sheet, and give the new problem a new number.

The problem list is a **PERMANENT RECORD** which is continuously maintained and updated.

Patient's Careplan

Incorporate three facets:
1. Further data required to aid in diagnosis/therapy
2. Therapeutic plans
3. Patient/parent education

Each **PROBLEM, identified by its number** (taken from p 10), should be listed next to the plan directed at its solution; for example –

Problem No 2: Urinary tract infection
a) Midstream urine for culture and sensitivity
b) IVP with voiding cysto-urethrogram
c) BUN
d) Ampicillin (state dosage)
e) Child must not have "bubble bath"

Òrdering

1. When writing orders, **always list problem nos.**
2. Complete necessary requisitions at time of ordering. Include pertinent data on each form.
3. When prescribing drugs:
    a) Be specific about concentration, dose, frequency, mode of administration, and duration of therapy.

4

b) A qualified doctor must fill out and sign all pharmacy requisitions.
c) Familiarity with dosage, action, interaction and side effects of drugs used is mandatory.

Progress Notes

1. List **PROBLEM NUMBER** to which the note refers.
2. Progress notes should include, where applicable:
    a) Patient's subjective state (e.g., "I feel tired").
    b) Objective physical and laboratory findings — tachycardia; Hb, serum iron.
    c) Assessment — iron-deficiency anemia.
    d) Plan — bone marrow
        — ferrous sulfate tablets
        — dietary education
3. Write progress notes twice weekly for all patients; and daily for seriously ill patients, those having intensive therapy, and those who are terminally ill. Record date and time of note.
4. Time of death: record according to 24-hr clock.
5. All entries in chart must be signed (not just initialled).

Discharge of Patient

1. Discharge orders **must be PROBLEM-ORIENTED** and include:
    a) therapy
    b) follow-up plans
2. Transfer to another institution: a final note must accompany the patient.
3. Discharge to care of referring physician:
    a) A special form-letter (available on all wards) must be completed at time of discharge and given to parent. (This is to ensure that the referring physician understands the current status while awaiting the full report.)
    b) Final progress note (p 15), also, must be completed.
4. Write the *Discharge Diagnosis,* and name of doctor responsible for dictating final note, on the **ORDER SHEET.**

Discharge Report (see p 7)

1. A discharge report must be dictated at time of discharge.
2. The final note must be problem-oriented.
3. A telephone dictating system is available (p 8) — final notes can be completed quickly and easily on the ward.

4.   Summarize the **DATA BASE** (form [25] POMR), treatment, progress, and plans for the future. The final note is of immediate service to the referring physician, and in the event of further medical investigation here or elsewhere.

5.   **Format**
   a)   Discharge summaries should be dictated within 48 hr of discharge (charts remain on wards for 48 hr for this purpose). A yellow reminder is sent to the responsible doctor for every record not completed on the ward (these charts are held for dictation in Medical Records. A white slip clipped inside the record folder indicates what is needed.)
   b)   When you have dictated, write your name and the date on the face sheet where it says "Summary Dictated". (If this is not done, the history will be returned to you for dictation.)
   c)   The staff physician will complete the face sheet (diagnoses, operations, status at discharge).

Note. Each week the chiefs of all services and the Hospital Secretary are given a list of doctors with records incomplete 10 days after discharge. The Medical Advisory Committee staff regulation no. 15 states that: "Failure to comply with the final warning within 3 days will result in [action] and residents will be disciplined as the Chief of Service may determine."

Operation Report — see p 16

Outpatient Department, Surgical Clinic — see p 17

If you are in doubt about any of these procedures, the staff at Medical Records front counter (ext 1465) will be glad to help you. You are welcome to visit Medical Records at any time, day or night. However, it would help us if you would make any special arrangements during regular daytime hours.

IMPORTANT. In the event of a patient's death, Medical Records is responsible for release of the body. Please observe the instructions on p 18 — this is an area where any breakdown in communication must be avoided.

DISCHARGE REPORT

Please dictate as follows

1. Your name
2. Patient's name (spell the surname)
3. History no. (not the admitting no.)
4. Admission and discharge dates

A survey of referring doctors disclosed that they wish the ideal final note to contain:

1. **History**
   A brief outline covering major points.
2. **Physical Examination**
   A brief report confined to those areas having abnormal or surprisingly normal results.
3. **Tests and Investigations**
   A list, together with comments.
4. **Treatment and Results**
   A brief outline of major stages.
5. **Discharge Instructions**
   Including medication, dose and length of time.
6. **Suggestions for Future Treatment**
   Including follow-up appointments.
7. **Diagnoses**
8. **Your Name** (including initials)

DICTATING INSTRUCTIONS

1. **Discharge Reports**
    a) Dial 29 to connect tape recorder.
    b) Dial 1 to start tape running. (No dial tone after dialing "1")

2. **Operation Notes; Letters; Death Summaries**
    a) Dial 28 to connect tape recorder.
    b) Dial 1 to start tape running.

3. **Transfers** (0830 − 1700 hr only)
    a) Dial 1467 and request "stat" line.
    b) Dial 20 to connect tape recorder.
    c) Dial 1 to start tape running.

4. **To Stop the Tape while You Pause**
    a) Dial 4 (not necessary for a brief pause)
    b) Dial 1 to resume.

5. **To Play Back**
    a) Dial 3 to reverse, then 2 to stop tape.
    b) **Note. Always dial 1 to restart the tape** (this system is not voice-controlled).

6. Always replace receiver at end of dictation.

Note: Please spell new drugs
and rare diagnoses

THE HOSPITAL FOR SICK CHILDREN

HISTORY

INFORMANT_____

RELIABILITY_____

CHIEF COMPLAINT	DURATION
_____	_____
_____	_____
_____	_____
_____	_____
_____	_____

HISTORY OF PRESENT ILLNESS:

THE HOSPITAL FOR SICK CHILDREN

Master Problem List

PROBLEM NO.	DATE	PROBLEMS UNDER CONSIDERATION OR CURRENTLY ACTIVE	DATE	RESOLUTION OF PROBLEM
1.				
2.				
3.				
4.				
5.				
6.				
7.				
8.				
9.				
10.				
11.				

FORM 3300-2518-2   (11) POMR

THE HOSPITAL FOR SICK CHILDREN
Past History
(TO BE UPDATED ON EACH ADMISSION)

FAMILY HISTORY — state age, health, occupation

Mother _____

Father _____

Consanguinity _____

Children (in sequence, including miscarriages) _____

1. _____ 5. _____
2. _____ 6. _____
3. _____ 7. _____
4. _____ 8. _____

_____

FAMILY DISEASES (IF NOT POSITIVE, LEAVE BLANK FOR UPDATING)

Allergy	_____	Heart disease	_____	Congenital defects _____
Diabetes	_____	Bleeding tendency	_____	Mental retardation _____
Endocrine	_____	Convulsions	_____	Stroke _____
Psychiatric	_____	Migraine	_____	Other _____

_____

NEONATAL HISTORY

Pregnancy health _____ B.Wt. _____

Labor & delivery: type, duration _____

_____

Condition of infant: Resuscitation _____ Oxygen therapy _____

Exchange transfusions _____ I.V. _____ Cyanosis _____

Jaundice _____ Convulsions _____ Other _____

FEEDING:

Formula _____ Solids _____

Vitamins _____ Problems _____

_____

GROWTH & DEVELOPMENT

Sat alone _____ Walked alone _____

Single words _____ 2 – 3 Words together _____

Scheduled progress _____

School _____

_____

ILLNESS

	Type	Treatment	Date
Illnesses			
Injuries			
Operations			
Allergies			

FORM 33389   (21) POMR

11

Infectious Disease and Immunization Record

Infectious Diseases

	Yes	Date		Yes	Date		Yes	Date
Measles	☐	_____	Whooping cough	☐	_____	Scarlet fever	☐	_____
Rubella	☐	_____	Diphtheria	☐	_____	Tuberculosis	☐	_____
Mumps	☐	_____	Tetanus	☐	_____	Hepatitis A	☐	_____
Chickenpox	☐	_____	Polio	☐	_____	Hepatitis B	☐	_____
Zoster (shingles)	☐	_____	None	☐				

Other _____

IMMUNIZATION (Enter 'HSC' if given at this Hospital)

	Date	Result	Date	Result	Date	Result
TB Test	_____	_____	_____	_____	_____	_____

	Date	Date	Date	Date	Date
DPT & P	_____	_____	_____	_____	_____
DT & P	_____	_____	_____	_____	_____
Tetanus toxoid	_____	_____	_____	_____	_____
Polio, Salk	_____	_____	_____	_____	_____
Polio, Sabin	_____	_____	_____	_____	_____
Measles, live	_____	_____	_____	_____	_____
Measles, inactive	_____	_____	_____	_____	_____
Rubella (vacc.)	_____	_____	_____	_____	_____
Mumps (vacc.)	_____	_____	_____	_____	_____
Smallpox	_____	_____	_____	_____	_____
Primary revacc.	_____	_____	_____	_____	_____
Influenza	_____	_____	_____	_____	_____
Immune serum Gl (gamma glob)	_____	_____	_____	_____	_____
Hyperimmune serum	_____	_____	_____	_____	_____
Horse serum	_____	_____	_____	_____	_____

COMMENTS

_____

Initial history given by: _____

Initial history taken by: _____

THE HOSPITAL FOR SICK CHILDREN

Functional Enquiry

SYSTEMS REVIEW:

Eyes

Ears

Nose & throat

Respiratory systems

Cardiovascular

Alimentary

Hematology

G-U system

Locomotor

Skin

Gynecology

Endocrine

SOCIAL CONDITIONS:

CURRENT DIET:

BEHAVIOR:

Toilet training

Sociability

Problem areas

FORM 3300-2527-1 **(24) POMR**

Physical Examination

GENERAL DESCRIPTION:_____

_____

_____

_____

_____

DECIMAL AGE:_____

MEASUREMENTS: _____

Height _____ Centile _____ Head Circum._____ Centile _____

Weight _____ Centile _____ Other _____

B.P. _____ Pulse _____ Resp. _____ Temp. _____

GENERAL:_____

_____

_____

_____

_____

_____

_____

_____

_____

_____

_____

_____

_____

_____

_____

_____

_____

_____

_____

_____

THE HOSPITAL FOR SICK CHILDREN

Final Progress Note

CONDITION OF CHILD ON DISCHARGE

THE REFERRING DOCTOR OR FAMILY DOCTOR,
DR._____

    HAS BEEN TELEPHONED ☐
        OR
    HANDWRITTEN NOTE TO BE CARRIED BY PARENTS ☐

THE PROBLEM LIST HAS BEEN COMPLETED ☐

DATE _____ SIGNED _____

33394   **POMR**

THE HOSPITAL FOR SICK CHILDREN
OPERATION REPORT

Service of ....   No. ....

Surgeon ....

Assistants ....   NAME ....

....   WARD ....DATE ....

Anesthetist ....

PRE-OPERATIVE DIAGNOSIS ....

POST-OPERATIVE DIAGNOSIS ....

OPERATION (Standard Nomenclature) ....

---

1. **Begin** by telling the typist who you are and what you are about to dictate; e.g., "Dr John Jones, dictating an operation report on Sam Sober (spelled SOBER)"

2. **Then** dictate according to the headings on the top of this form.

3. **Finish** by repeating your name, including initials.

THE HOSPITAL FOR SICK CHILDREN
OUT PATIENT DEPARTMENT
SURGICAL CLINIC

CLINIC					
SCHOOL					
REFERRING PHYSICIAN				ADDRESS	
DR.					
O P D	DAY	MONTH	YEAR		

Dictate the following:

1. Your name.

2. Name of clinic.

3. Date of attendance.

4. Patient's name (spell surname).

5. History no.

Then, dictate the clinic note.

Finally: your name, including initials.

WHEN A PATIENT DIES

1. **Check-lists** are available on all wards to remind you of the steps necessary after a patient's death. Completion of the list is essential: it contains information we need before we may release a body to the undertaker.

2. **Death certificates** must be completed, signed, and delivered to Medical Records as soon as possible after a death occurs, together with the patient's record, the consent for necropsy, and the check-list.

3. **Consent for necropsy,** given by the legal parent(s), must be in writing or by telegram. Telephoned consents are not acceptable, even if witnessed. Medical Records must know whether a consent is obtained, expected, or refused: its staff cannot give permission for initiation of burial arrangements until they have this information. Never tell the parent(s) that a body will be ready by a certain time — the undertaker will call Medical Records for this information (p 92).

4. **Burial Arrangements.** The parents have sole responsibility. Do make sure they understand that permission for necropsy does not include disposal of the body. Parents should always be advised to contact an undertaker. If they live out of town their local undertaker will arrange shipment. Medical Records staff (ext 1465) have information for parents who cannot afford burial, but the responsibility for making arrangements cannot be delegated. Unclaimed bodies are assigned to the City Morgue.

5. **Necropsy findings** are anxiously awaited by most parents who give consent. When you obtain permission, please follow through to ensure that the parents will be informed, by the pediatrician, the family doctor, or you.

6. **Donations of bodies** are not accepted by or through this hospital.

For information not covered above, telephone ext 1465.

See also Support Services, pp 93, 95

TESTS

BLOOD TESTS & TRANSFUSION

See Specimens (p 21) *and* Values (p 24, 25)

Hemoglobin
1. Draw blood up to 20 mm³ mark of Hb pipet.
2. a) Wipe tip of pipet clean.
   b) Empty contents into exactly 5 ml of Drabkin's solution in a Fisher tube.
   c) Rinse all of blood out of pipet into the solution.
3. Read Hb level directly in Fisher hemophotometer after at least 5 min.
   - (The hemophotometer can be standardized, using the appropriate standards supplied with that machine. Very little alteration should be required.)

WBC Count
1. Using WBC-counting pipet, draw blood to 0.5 mark.
2. Add diluting fluid (3% acetic acid and stain) to 1.1 mark.
3. Shake; discard first 5 or 6 drops; allow 1 or 2 drops to saturate chamber.
4. Count 4 corner squares; multiply the sum by 50.

Blood Film
1. Spread blood in thin film.
2. Suggested staining technique: 2 min with Wright's stain.
3. Without removing stain, cover slide with distilled water. Allow to stand for further 3 min.
4. Rinse thoroughly and dry.

Apt Test
For detection of adult Hb (maternal blood) in neonate's vomitus or stool.
1. Mix grossly bloody stool or vomitus with water until supernatant fluid pink.
2. Centrifuge.
3. Add 5 parts of pink supernate to 1 part 1% NaOH.
   - Observe color in 1-2 min: yellow brown = adult blood: pink = fetal blood.

Screening for Bleeding Disorders

The following series will detect almost all bleeding disorders:

    a)   platelet count
    b)   Ivy bleeding time
    c)   prothrombin time (PT)
    d)   partial thromboplastin time (PTT)
    e)   factor-XIII screening test, if the bleeding disorder is thought to be inherited.

Ivy Bleeding Time

1. Apply BP cuff to 40 mm Hg.
2. Puncture forearm 3 times with no. 11 scalpel blade to depth of 2-3 mm.
3. Blot gently with filter paper at 15-sec intervals.
   a) Note times when bleeding ceases.
   b) Average the 3 results. (Normal: <10 min.)

BLOOD SPECIMENS FOR ROUTINE HEMATOLOGY TESTS

Test	Method	Container	Amount
CBC, platelets, reticulocytes, ESR	Fingerprick or EDTA	Pink-top vial	2.5 ml
PT, PTT, factor assays, fibrinogen	3.8% Na citrate	Special tube from coagulation lab	fill tube to 2 ml line
LE preparation	Defibrinated	Glass-bead flask	5 ml
Osmotic fragility	Defibrinated	Glass-bead flask	5 ml
Sickle-cell preparation	Fingerprick		
G-6-PD screen or assay; or PK screen or assay	Heparinized or in Alsever's soln	From Blood Bank	5 ml 5 ml in 5 ml Alsever's soln
Hb electrophoresis	EDTA	Pink-top vial	2.5 ml

CORD-BLOOD VALUES IN PREMATURE INFANTS AT BIRTH

Gestation (wk)	Hb (g/dl)	Hct (%)	RBC ($10^6/mm^3$)	MCV (μ^3)	Retics (%)	Nucleated RBC /100 WBC
28	11 – 17	30 – 40	3.0 – 4.5	120	5.0 – 20	100 – 200
34	12 – 18	35 – 50	3.0 – 5.0	118	5.0 – 10	50 – 100
38	14 – 20	40 – 55	3.5 – 5.5	110	1.0 – 7	10 – 40

BLOOD COUNT AND TOTAL & DIFFERENTIAL WBC COUNT IN RELATION TO AGE

	Birth	2 days	2 wk	3 mo	6 mo	1 yr	2 to 5 yr	6 to 14 yr
RBC count (x 10^6)	3.5 – 6.0	3.5 – 6.0	3.5 – 6.0	3.5 – 4.5	4.0 – 5.0	4.0 – 5.0	4.0 – 5.0	4.5 – 5.5
Hb (g/dl)	15 – 25	15 – 25	14 – 20	10 – 14	10 – 14	11 – 14	12 – 14	13 – 16
Hematocrit (%)	52 – 79	46 – 73	40 – 74	30 – 42	31 – 39	31 – 40	34 – 40	37 – 46
WBC (x 10^3)	20 – 40	10 – 40	5 – 25	5 – 15	5 – 15	5 – 15	5 – 12	4 – 10
Platelets (x 10^3)			150 – 400					
Differential smear (%)								
Polymorphonuclear neutrophils	50 – 80	30 – 70	15 – 50	15 – 40	15 – 40	15 – 60	25 – 65	25 – 65
Eosinophils	0 – 40	0 – 7	0 – 10	0 – 10	0 – 10	0 – 15	0 – 15	0 – 15
Lymphocytes	10 – 40	20 – 60	20 – 75	40 – 80	40 – 80	30 – 75	20 – 65	20 – 65
Monocytes	0 – 10	0 – 15	0 – 20	0 – 10	0 – 10	0 – 10	0 – 10	0 – 10
Reticulocytes	2 – 10	2 – 10	0.1 – 1	0.1 – 5	0.1 – 2	0.1 – 2	0.1 – 2	0.1 – 2
Metamyelocytes	0 – 2	0 – 2	-	-	-	-	-	-
Nucleated RBC/100 WBC	0 – 5	0 – 5	-	-	-	-	-	-

Note. Many of these figures were obtained from a 'normal population' in Toronto schools and well-baby clinics. Eosinophilia in 'normal' schoolchildren is very common, especially during 'allergy season'; however, the upper limit for an absolute eosinophil count is 500/mm³.

23

REFERENCE BLOOD VALUES
(see also Nuclear Medicine, p 84)

Ivy bleeding time	2 – 9 min
Prothrombin time (PT)	10 – 12 sec
Partial thromboplastin time (PTT)	25 – 40 sec
Thrombin time	within 4 sec of control
Factor VIII, IX, XI	50 – 150%
Fibrin split products	<5 μg/ml
Fibrogen	200 – 400 mg/dl
Euglobulin lysis time	>2 hr
Glucose-6-phosphate dehydrogenase (G-6-PD)	newborn, >160 U; >2 yr, 120–180 U.
Pyruvate kinase	newborn, 1.2– 2.1 U; older, 1.0–1.4 U.
2,3-Diphosphoglycerate (2,3-DPG)	4.2 – 5.7 μmol/ml RBC

Hb electrophoresis:
Hb A$_2$	1.5 – 3.1%
Hb F	premature, 90 – 95%; term, 80 – 90%; 6 mo, 2 – 5%; 1 yr, <2%.
Haptoglobin	absent at birth; 50 – 200 mg/dl by 6 mo
Mean cell vol (MCV)	birth – 1 wk 100 – 110 μm^3
	1 mo 90 μm^3
	2 mo 80 μm^3
	6 mo 70 μm^3
	older 80 – 94 μm^3
Mean cell Hb (MCH)	27 – 31 $\mu\mu g$
Mean cell Hb concn (MCHC)	32 – 36%
ESR (modified Westergren)	<10 mm in 1 hr
Serum iron	50 – 150 $\mu g/dl$
Total iron-binding capacity (TIBC)	250 – 400 $\mu g/dl$

BLOOD BANK AND TRANSFUSIONS

1. Blood Bank requisition must be completed in full, and carry the names of
   a) the ordering physician,
   b) the person who labels the tube, and
   c) the person who draws the blood sample.

No specimen will be accepted without a requisition.

2. Routine tests, including cross-matching, direct and indirect Coombs' tests, and RBC-antibody studies: 3-5 ml clotted blood.

3. Detection of cold agglutinins: check with Blood Bank. The clotted specimen must be kept at 37°C.

Urgent Blood Transfusions

1. Check parental permission.

2. Complete cross-match takes 2 hr.

3. Blood required urgently to protect life can be prepared sooner, but this carries increased hazard. The responsibility rests with the physician submitting the request.

4. Three types of 'urgent' preparations are released for use only in an emergency:
   a) Half-hour cross-match: detects most but not all significant incompatibilities.
   b) Unmatched blood of same group: ABO and Rh group-specific, but not cross-matched.
   c) Unmatched O, Rh-negative blood: use only when patient's blood is unobtainable for grouping.

Also, AB-type plasma is available for use as an emergency volume-expander in untyped patient.

Blood-component Therapy

Whole Blood

To maintain or restore blood volume; Hct = approx. 30 – 35%. Whole blood is not used to correct anemia (see Packed red cells, below).

1. Stored whole blood is collected in ACD and is stored at 4°C for up to 21 days. Satisfactory for most patients requiring whole blood.

2. Fresh whole blood (24 – 48 hr old) provides certain labile coagulation factors missing in stored blood. When less than 72 hr old, can be used for exchange transfusion.

Packed Red Cells

Preferred for most elective transfusions and anemia; useful when there is danger of circulatory overload in chronic anemia. Hct = about 70%. The usual dose (10 ml/kg body wt) should raise the Hb concentration $2 - 3$ g/dl.

Buffy-coat-poor Blood

Packed red cells with the buffy coat (leukocytes and platelets) removed. Prevents febrile reactions due to WBC or platelet antibodies. Used mainly in cases of thalassemia major.

Platelet Concentrates

One unit = the amount of platelets concentrated from 1 unit (500 ml) of whole blood and suspended in about 20 ml of plasma. Ideal preparation in cases of thrombocytopenia due to decreased production.

Platelet-rich Plasma and Platelets from Fresh Whole Blood

Useful in thrombocytopenic patients only when plasma and red-cell components also are required. Its usefulness is limited by the volume required for effective platelet increment.

Buffy-coat WBC for Transfusion

The uppermost layer of cells in sedimented whole blood contains most of the leukocytes. Given to neutropenic patients. To raise the total WBC count in an adult by $1000/mm^3$ requires the buffy coat from about 20 liters of normal donor blood.

Fresh Frozen Plasma

Plasma removed from fresh blood and immediately frozen at $-20°C$. Preserves labile coagulation factors (see p 209).

Cryoprecipitate

Contains factor VIII and fibrinogen. Prepared from the precipitate that forms when rapidly frozen fresh plasma is thawed for 24 hr at $4°C$.

Zoster-immune Plasma (ZIP)

For passive immunization against varicella–zoster infection. Used especially for immuno-compromised patients.

1. It will modify the infection if given within 72 hr after the exposure to the virus. Dosage: 10 ml/kg iv.

2. Zoster-immune globulin (ZIG) is available in the U.S.A. through the USPHS.

3. Any queries re V-Z immunization should be directed to Infectious Disease division.

General Rules for Transfusion

1. **BEFORE TRANSFUSION, IDENTIFY BOTH PATIENT AND UNIT OF BLOOD**
   a) Compare donor's blood group on blood unit with patient's blood group on Transfusion Record.
   b) Compare the name and history number on patient's arm bracelet with those on unit and on Transfusion Record.
2. **Do not use** glucose solutions in iv tubing (they damage red cells).
3. Infusion of 1 unit of blood or packed cells should not exceed 4 hr. Blood kept at room temperature for >6 hr is unsuitable for transfusion.
4. If several blood units are given over a prolonged period, the blood-giving set should be changed regularly (at least q12h), as fibrin clots in the filter may become contaminated.
5. **Never add** any medication to the blood pack (possibility of contamination).

Transfusion Reactions

Febrile

Common and not dangerous.
1. Treat with antipyretics – **not ASA.**
2. If reaction is severe, persistent, or suggests a hemolytic reaction (see below):
   a) Stop transfusion.
   b) Investigate, including: send samples of blood from donor unit and patient for culture.

Allergic

Usually readily controlled with antihistamines (po or parenterally). Occasionally, epinephrine is required. It is rarely necessary to stop the transfusion.

Hemolytic

Characterized by chills, fever, loin or limb and/or chest pain, hemoglobinuria, and oliguria (which can progress to anuria).
1. **Stop transfusion immediately.** Substitute a dextrose–saline solution.
2. From a site other than the vein used for transfusion: obtain blood specimens immediately for repeat cross-

match, direct and indirect Coombs' test, Hb, plasma Hb (anticoagulated specimen), BUN, electrolytes, bilirubin.

Do not squirt specimens through needle into tube (causes hemolysis).

3. Notify Blood Bank of the problem and send specimens:
   a) Withdraw specimen from donor blood pack and send it for culture.
   b) Return donor pack to the Bank.

4. Set up urine rack:
   a) First available urine specimen: observe color; test with Hemastix; examine microscopically; measure.
   b) Subsequent specimens: continue investigation and compare findings. Record output.

5. If any results suggest a hemolytic reaction:
   a) Notify Hematology and Nephrology, and give:
   b) Solu-Cortef 10 mg/kg rapid iv infusion
   c) mannitol, 1.0 g/kg iv (5 ml/kg of 20% solution) over 15 min
   d) dextrose—saline solution with no K added, at 65 ml/kg/24 hr.

6. If urine is diminished (<40 ml/m^2/hr during 2nd hr of therapy): assume renal shutdown (p 230).

URINE

Routine

1. *Color*
   a) Endogenous —
      — yellow-brown: bilirubin
      — red: blood, porphyrins, urate
      — brown-black: blood, hemosiderin, homogentisic acid, melanin, myoglobin.
   b) Exogenous
      — yellow or red: antipyrine, anthracine derivatives (rhubarb, cascara), beetroot (pH-dependent), phenolphthalein (cathartic), pyridium (phenazopyridine HC1).

2. *pH:* nitrazine paper, pH meter.

3. *Protein*
   a) Albustix (may not detect Bence—Jones protein)
   b) Sulfosalicylic acid. Add either:
      — 8 drops of 10% sulfosalicylic acid to 1 ml urine; **or**
      — 7.5 ml of 3% sulfosalicylic acid to 2.5 ml urine.
      — Can be semiquantified with *standards.*

29

URINE SEDIMENT

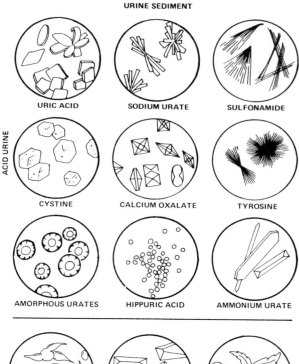

ACID URINE

URIC ACID | SODIUM URATE | SULFONAMIDE

CYSTINE | CALCIUM OXALATE | TYROSINE

AMORPHOUS URATES | HIPPURIC ACID | AMMONIUM URATE

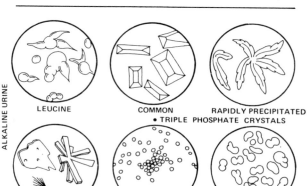

ALKALINE URINE

LEUCINE | COMMON | RAPIDLY PRECIPITATED

• TRIPLE PHOSPHATE CRYSTALS

CALCIUM PHOSPHATE | AMORPHOUS PHOSPHATES | CALCIUM CARBONATE

30

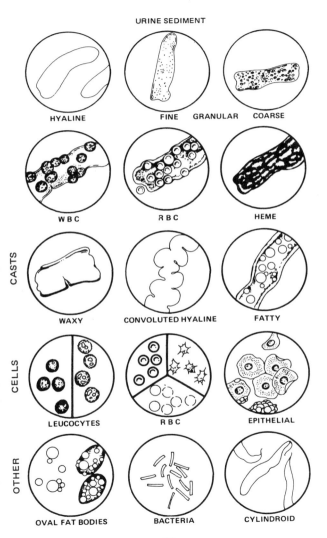

URINE SEDIMENT

HYALINE

FINE   GRANULAR   COARSE

WBC

RBC

HEME

CASTS

WAXY

CONVOLUTED HYALINE

FATTY

CELLS

LEUCOCYTES

RBC

EPITHELIAL

OTHER

OVAL FAT BODIES

BACTERIA

CYLINDROID

Protein Conc. (mg/dl)	Albustix	Sulfosal. acid
<5	0	Clear
5-10	trace	Faint turbidity
10-30	1+	Turbid: cannot read print through solution in test tube
30-100	2+	White cloud: cannot see black lines
100-500	3+	White cloud + precipitate
>500	4+	Flocculent precipitate: gel

c) Heat test for tubule protein:
   – Add sulfosalicylic acid to urine, to precipitate protein
   – Bring to boiling point; precipitate will disappear, and will return on cooling.

4. *Reducing substance*
    Non-glucose-reducing substances: ascorbic acid, fructose, galactose, homogentisic acid, lactose, pentose (xylose), tyrosine, chloramphenicol, chloral hydrate, sulfonamides, salicylate metabolites.
    i) **Clinitest** tablet (positive for all the above).
        Two-drop test = 2 drops urine, 10 drops water, add 1 tablet. Check color.

Color	Glucose	Color	Glucose
Blue	Negative	Yellow	2%
Blue-green	Trace	Yellow-orange	3%
Green	0.5%	Orange	5%
Green-brown	1%		

To detect glucose in the presence of other non-glucose reducing substances: boil specimen with equal volume 1 N HC1, then test with Clinitest tablet.
    ii) **Clinistix:** specific for glucose.
5. *Acetone:* Acetest tablet, Ketostix
6. *Hemoglobin:* Hemastix, Hematest tablet – both react with RBC, free Hb, myoglobin.
7. *Sediment* (see fig, p 30, 31).

Special
8. *Calcium* (Sulkowitch test)
    To 5 ml urine, add 2 ml reagent.
    Faint white cloud = normal. Clear fluid = low Ca.

9. *Lead (porphyrins)*
Acidify 5 ml urine with 2 or 3 drops glacial acetic acid; add 5 ml ether; shake; hold in front of Woods' or ultraviolet lamp.
Pink fluorescence = positive.

10. *Salicylates* (see Toxicology, p 485).
Boil 10 ml urine down to 5 ml (to remove ketone bodies); add 3 drops of 10% ferric chloride solution. Coca-cola brown indicates salicylates.

11. *Bilirubin:* Ictotest tablet.

12. *Urobilin* (see p 226)
a) Removal of bilirubin, if present.
To 10 ml urine, add 5 ml 10% aqueous BaCl soln; filter (use filtrate).
b) 5 ml urine filtrate   } Mix; filter; trans-
5 ml alkaline zinc   illuminate with
acetate solution   flashlight
3 drops Lugol's iodine soln }
Normal = slight green fluorescence. Abnormal = no fluorescence (no urobilin).
–   Increased fluorescence: proportionate to urobilinuria.

13. *Myoglobin*
a) Dissolve 2.8 g ammonium sulfate in 2 ml of urine. Hb is precipitated, whereas myoglobin stays in solution.
b) Repeat benzidine test (see 19c, below).
c) Spectroscopic techniques are more accurate.

14. *Phenylketones:* Phenistix.

15. *Ferric chloride reaction* (see Interpretation, p 34)
a) 1 ml Fe Cl_3 reagent in clean test tube.
b) Add 10 drops (0.5 ml) urine; mix well.
c) Observe color: disregard color appearing after 10-20 sec.

16. *Amino-acid or metabolic screen* (p 55).

17. *Specific sugar by chromatography* (p 59).

18. *Mucopolysaccharides:* spot screening test (to lab; see p 395).

19. *Hemoglobin:*
a) Urine microscopy for RBC.
b) Hemastix tablet.
c) Benzidine test. Centrifuge urine; to sediment, add 1 ml saturated benzidine soln (in glacial acetic acid) and 1 ml hydrogen peroxide. Blue = Hb.
d) Guaiac

20. *Dinitrophenyl hydrazine* (DNPH) test for keto acids (see Interpretation, p 55).

a) Dissolve 100 mg 2,4-DNPH in 100 ml 2 N HCl. Refrigerate this reagent.
b) Add 10 drops DNPH reagent to 1 ml urine (at room temp).
c) If yellow or chalky precipitate forms within 10 min, test is positive.

Interpretation of Positive Ferric Chloride ($FeCl_3$) Reaction.

Material responsible	Color of reaction	Clinical condition
Homogentisic acid	Blue-green; fades quickly	Alkaptonuria
Antipyrine; acetophenetidines	Cherry-red	Ingestion of anti-pyrine/acetophenetidine
Phenothiazine derivatives	Blue-purple	Ingestion of Compazine (prochlorperazine)/Thorazine (chlorpromazine)
Bilirubin	Green; moderately stable	Hepatitis, etc., in which direct reacting bilirubin is increased
Imidazolpyruvic acid	Brown-green; stable	Histidinemia
Acetoacetic acid	Red-purple; becomes negative when urine heated	Ketosis
Lysol	Green	Ingestion of Lysol (carbolic acid)
Branched-chain keto acids	Blue-black; present for several hours	Maple-syrup-urine disease (MSUD)
Phosphates; other anions	White to brown; **precipitates** *can* **obscure positive test**	Normal urine
p-Aminosalicylic acid (PAS)	Red-brown	Ingestion of PAS
Phenylpyruvic acid	Green; fades over hours	Phenylketonuria

RENAL FUNCTION

Glomerular Function
1. *Creatinine clearance* (C_{cr})

    A carefully timed urine collection is required (usually 24 hr).
    a) Urine collection, see p 388. *Note times accurately.*
    b) Take 2 ml blood for serum creatinine (p 363). Calculation:

    $$C_{cr} = \frac{UV}{P} \times \frac{1.73}{SA} \; ; \text{ where}$$

    U = urine concentration
    V = total vol of urine divided by no. of min in collection period (24 hr = 1440 min)
    P = serum creatinine, mg/dl
    SA = surface area, m^2 (nomogram is on p 340).
    c) Range of normal values for children, see p 364.
    d) Normal body production rate of creatinine:
        – female: 15-20 mg/kg/day.
        – male: 20-25 mg/kg/day.
2. *Isotopic method*, including differential GFR: see Nuclear Medicine, p 84.

Tubule Function
1. *Specific gravity*
    a) Urinometer
    b) Refractometer (requires 1 drop of urine)
2. *Osmolality;* freezing-point depression method (requires 0.5 ml of urine).
3. *Concentration.*
4. *Tubule maximum for glucose or bicarbonate.*
5. *Net acid excretion* (NAE)
    a) Measure titratable acidity, and excretion of HCO_3^- and NH_4^+ on 24-hr urine collection.
    b) During collection, measure blood pH, pCO_2, and HCO_3^-.
6. *Short urine-acidification test* (5 hr)
    a) Give NH_4Cl 5.5 mEq/kg (150 mEq/m^2) po.
    b) Hourly, for next 5 hr: measure urine pH and net acid.
    c) 3 hr after giving NH_4Cl: measure blood pH, pCO_2, and HCO_3^-.

NET ACID EXCRETION

A – After Acute Administration of NH_4Cl*		
Age	Urine	μEq/min/1.73 m²
(yr)	pH	TA[†]	NH_4+
<1	≤5.0	62 (43–111)	57 (42–79)
3–15	≤5.5	52 (33–71)	73 (46–100)

*After Strauss, M.B., and Welt. L.G. (eds): Diseases of the Kidney, 2nd ed. Boston, Little, Brown, 1971, p. 1360.

[†]TA = titratable acidity

7. *Long urine-acidification test* (3 days)
   a) Control period: 1-2 days.
      Collect 24-hr urine and measure NAE; also, blood pH, pCO_2, HCO_3⁻.
   b) For 3 days: give 2-3 mEq of NH_4Cl/kg/day in 4 divided doses. Then, collect 24-hr urine and measure NAE; also, blood pH, pCO_2, and HCO_3⁻.

NET ACID EXCRETION

B – Normal & After Prolonged Administration of NH_4Cl[‡]		
μEq/min/1.73 m²		
NH_4+	TA	NAE
Control		
2-11 mo	20.4 (7.3-34.0)	25.5 (3.6-41.7)	44.7 (8.4-73.2)
1-16 yr	20.9 (11.2-28.6)	11.9 (2.0-24.2)	29.2 (9.0-47.6)
After NH_4Cl		
2-11 mo	54.4 (26.3-100.0)	42.5 (20.6-72.0)	97.0 (67.1-172.0)
1-16 yr	64.5 (45.7-111.0)	30.2 (13.9-53.8)	95.1 (62.1-164.8)

[‡]After Peonides, A., Levin, B., and Young, W.F. The renal excretion of hydrogen ions in infants and children. Arch Dis Childh 40:33, 1965.

Miscellaneous

1. Total serum complement (normal 1/12 to 1/24).
2. $\beta_1 C$ globulin (normal, 100-150 mg/dl).
3. Renin: see Hypertension, p 238; and Biochemistry, p 379.
4. Renal biopsy: see Nephrology, p 241.

PULMONARY FUNCTION AND BLOOD-GAS DETERMINATIONS

Purpose
To detect disturbed pulmonary function and evaluate patient with respiratory complaint.

Ventilatory Function (Fig. 1 to 6)

Terminology

FEV_1	Forced expiratory volume in 1 sec
FRC	Functional residual capacity
FVC	Forced VC
MBC	Maximal breathing capacity
$FEF_{25-75\%}$	Forced expiratory flow rate
RV	Residual volume
TLC	Total lung capacity
$\dot{V}_{25}$	Flow rate at 25% VC
$\dot{V}_{50}$	Flow rate at 50% VC
VC	Vital capacity
PFR	Peak flow rate

Interpretation of Results
Compare observed values with normal standards* for corresponding height:

a) >80% of standard: normal ventilation
b) 65-80% of standard: mild impairment
c) 50-64% of standard: moderate impairment
d) 35-49% of standard: severe impairment
e) <35% of standard: very severe impairment

*Determined in 'healthy' children at The Hospital for Sick Children, Toronto.

LUNG VOLUME SUBDIVISIONS

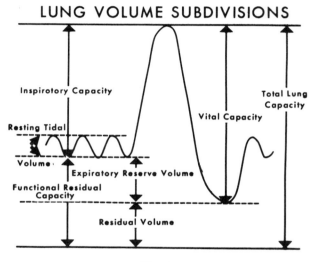

Fig. 1

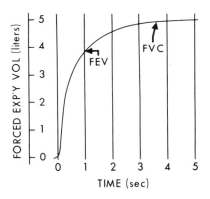

Fig. 2

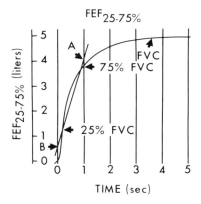

Fig. 3

Fig. 3. Spirometer tracing of forced expiratory flow (FEF). The $FEF_{25-75\%}$ is calculated from points representing 25% and 75% of total FVC. A line is drawn connecting the two points, and extended to intersect adjacent vertical time-lines at points A and B. The difference (in ml) is the volume/sec exhaled in the middle half of the FVC.

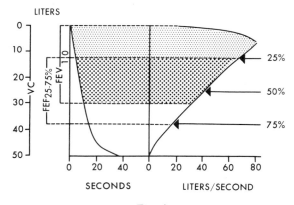

Fig. 4

Fig. 4. The forced vital capacity maneuver.

Left, timed VC; *right,* relationship between volume and flow. Arrows indicate maximal flow rates when 25%, 50%, and 75% of VC has been expired.

(After Cherniak, R.M., Naimark, A., and Cherniak, L.: Respiration in Health and Disease, 2nd ed. Philadelphia, Saunders, 1972. With permission.)

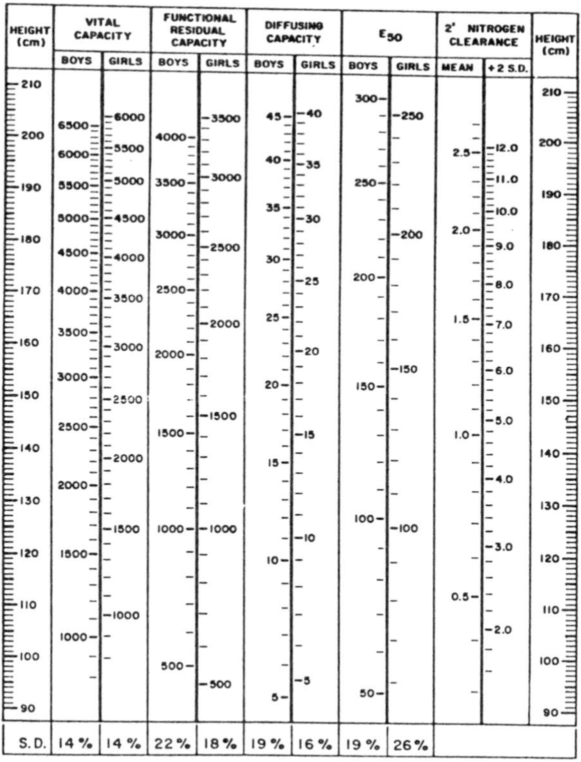

HEIGHT (cm)	VITAL CAPACITY		FUNCTIONAL RESIDUAL CAPACITY		DIFFUSING CAPACITY		E_{50}		2' NITROGEN CLEARANCE		HEIGHT (cm)
	BOYS	GIRLS	BOYS	GIRLS	BOYS	GIRLS	BOYS	GIRLS	MEAN	+2 S.D.	
S.D.	14 %	14 %	22 %	18 %	19 %	16 %	19 %	26 %			

Fig. 5

A nomograph relating the results of selected pulmonary function tests to standing height in centimeters.

DeMuth, G.R. and Arbor, A.: Prediction of lung function values in children. Am J Dis Child 109:444, 1965.

(With permission.)

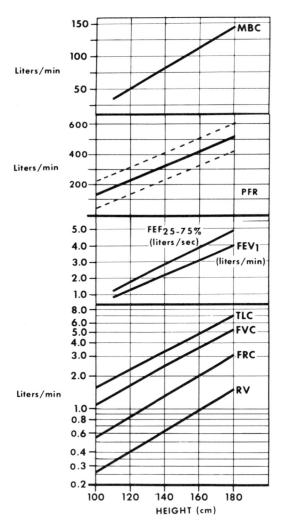

Fig. 6

42

PATTERNS OF IMPAIRED VENTILATORY FUNCTION

Test	Obstructive disease	Restrictive disease
FEV_1	Decreased	Unchanged *or* decreased
FRC	Increased	Decreased
FVC	Unchanged *or* decreased	Decreased
MBC	Decreased	Unchanged *or* decreased
$FEF_{25-75\%}$	Decreased	Unchanged *or* decreased
RV	Increased	Decreased
TLC	Increased	Decreased

Gas Exchange

1. From analysis of simultaneously collected samples of arterial blood (PaO_2, $PaCO_2$, pH) and expired air, one can calculate arterial gas tensions. minute ventilation, physiological dead space. and arterial–alveolar difference.

2. Heparinized arterialized samples are adequate for the analysis **if circulatory decompensation is not present.**

NORMAL MEAN PaO_2 AND $PaCO_2$ ($\pm$ 1 SD)

Age	PaO_2 (mm Hg)	$PaCO_2$ (mm Hg)
Birth to 1 wk	70 ± 7	30.5 ± 5.2
1-10 mo	85 ± 4	34.1 ± 1.9
1-9 yr	90 ± 5	35.3 ± 1.2
10-19 yr	96 ± 2	37.3 ± 1.4

Interpretation of Results

High $PaCO_2$ = hypoventilation

Low PaO_2 = hypoxia

Low PaO_2 with relatively normal spirometric values = peripheral-airway disease

Acid–Base Balance (see pp 124, 352)

Estimation of acid–base balance is essential:

1. Alterations in gas exchange can affect arterial pH and induce renal compensation.
2. Metabolic disturbances may lead to respiratory compensation.

GASTROINTESTINAL FUNCTION

D-xylose Absorption (p 387)

1. 1 day before test, notify Clin. Chemistry:
    – Advise patient's name, location, height, weight.
2. D-xylose (14.5 g/m^2) will be weighed, and delivered to ward.
3. Fast patient from midnight preceding test.
4. Give D-xylose po at 0800 hr (zero time).
5. At precisely 30 min and 60 min, take 0.6 ml blood (heparinized or clotted)
6. Deliver *promptly* to lab; specimen label should specify "Xylose Test".

Glucose Tolerance (p 53)

Disaccharide Tolerance

1. Prepare as for glucose tolerance test.
2. After taking sample for fasting blood sugar, give, in a drink, an oral load of the disaccharide to be tested (lactose, maltose, sucrose), 2 g/kg (maximum, 50 g).
3. Measure blood sugar at ½, 1, and 2 hr. Normal = rise of >20 mg/100 ml.

Collection of Duodenal Juice for Assay of Pancreatic Enzymes and Bicarbonate (p 179)

1. Under fluoroscopy, place a double-lumen tube in the duodenum with distal opening in fourth part.
2. Remove gastric juice by Gomco suction, using a separate tube placed at the greater curvature.
3. Infuse BSP 0.01% in the proximal port of the double-lumen tube, at 1.5 ml/min, throughout the study.
4. Aspirate duodenal juice from distal port intermittently by Gomco. Collect 4 consecutive 20-min specimens on ice.

5. After first 20 min, when steady state is reached, infuse pancreozymin (0.0125 U/kg/min) and secretin (0.0125 U/kg body wt/min) for 1 hr. Hormones are dissolved in 100 ml of "2/3:1/3" solution, given over 1 hr.

6. Analyze juice for BSP, amylase, lipase, trypsin, chymotrypsin and bicarbonate.

Sweat Chloride (p 404)

1. Pilocarpine iontophoresis as screening method.
2. Urecholine injection method (sweat collected in clean gauze and measured by titration).
    Note. Have atropine on hand in case systemic reaction develops.
    Intradermal injection:
    a) infants: 0.1 ml urecholine, 0.3 ml 5% glucose
    b) children: 0.2 ml urecholine, 0.2 ml 5% glucose.
    c) For repeats or when difficulty experienced: 0.3 ml urecholine plus 0.1 ml glucose or pure urecholine can be tried.

Stool Smear (p 80)

Stool Collection for Fat and Chymotrypsin Content (p 401)

1. Collect the feces for at least 4 days.
    a) infant: use a special liner in the diaper, or special collection frame.
    b) toilet-trained child: commode chair.
2. Store in airtight containers at 4°C.
3. Daily fat intake: must reach minimum of 30 g in infants and 60 g in older children.
4. Infants <3 mo: fecal-fat excretion >15% of fat intake = abnormal.
5. Older infants and children: fecal fat excretion >10% of fat intake, or average excretion >4 g/24 h, is considered abnormal.

Biopsy of Intestinal Mucosa (p 222)

1. *Resuscitative equipment must be at hand.*
2. Determine PT and PTT; smear for platelets.
3. Patient fasting 8 hr.
4. Sedation usually necessary: use CM3 (see Anesthesia, p 273).
    Give 0.05 ml/kg, up to maximum 1.5 ml, deep im, 1 hr before procedure.

5. Instrument now being used is the Crosby capsule.
6. Pass tube into stomach, and guide into small intestine under fluoroscopic control. Take mucosal specimen from distal duodenum or upper jejunum.
7. *Post-biopsy care.* Full fluids, bed rest; pulse and BP q1h until stable, then q2h for 18 hr.
    —   Hemorrhage and perforation are rare complications.
    Investigation
1. Distal duodenum:
    a) Microscopy
    b) Enzyme assay (disaccharidases).
        Normal values are: lactase >10 U/g protein; sucrase >40 U/g protein; maltase >150 U/g protein.
2. Rectum: microscopy.

Request GI consult if the following are required:
Endoscopy (esophagoscopy, gastroscopy)
Liver biopsy
Sigmoidoscopy (rectal biopsy often done at same time)
Colonoscopy.

ENDOCRINE FUNCTION

Posterior Pituitary

Water Deprivation
Indication: Suspected diabetes insipidus.
Preparation
1. Dangerous complication is hypernatremia with dehydration; therefore, supervise carefully throughout the test, with individual nurse. Monitor pulse rate, temperature, and behavioral status throughout.
2. Infants and young children may not be able to tolerate the full 7 hr of thirsting.
3. *Test should not be done if* significant hypernatremia, evidence of infection, dehydration, or renal function is severely impaired.
    Procedure
1. No restriction of fluid during preceding night.
2. At 0730 hr, normal breakfast. No food or fluid after this until test completed.
3. 0800 hr: weigh the patient.
4. 0900 hr: obtain urine specimen for osmolality, and serum for osmolality and electrolytes.

5. Older children: urine specimens may be collected hourly and measured for volume and SG (not essential).

6. Between 1500 and 1600 hr: obtain urine and serum specimens as in (4).

7. Weigh child, and calculate percentage weight loss.

8. If testing is to distinguish between nephrogenic and vasopressin-responsive diabetes insipidus:
   a) Inject aqueous vasopressin (Pitressin): 1 in 1000, 0.1 U/kg body wt, im (maximum, 5.0 U).
   b) Obtain at least 1 (preferably 2) urine samples for osmolality after injection of vasopressin.

9. Terminate test by 1700 hr.

Note

1. If patient evidences significant dehydration (weight loss of 3-5%, tachycardia, and/or fever) before 1500 hr: take specimens or urine and serum as in (4) and terminate test by giving fluids po.

2. If severe hypernatremia develops: do not give vasopressin with rapid infusions of hypotonic fluid (may result in water-intoxication, cerebral edema, and convulsions).

OSMOLALITY (m0sm/kg H_2O) – NORMAL VALUES*

	Initial		Final	
	Mean	Range	Mean	Range
Serum	290	282-299	289	283-295
Urine	676	241-1328	934	347-1282

*Ehrlich, R.M., and Kooh, S.W.: Pediatrics, 45:236, 1970.

Anterior Pituitary

Growth Hormone (HGH)

Random serum HGH levels are of little value except in hypersomatotropism and acromegaly. The exercise test is useful in screening for HGH deficiency. Arginine- and insulin-tolerance tests are required for the HGH Therapeutic Trial in Canada. Insulin-tolerance test may produce severe hypoglycemia; therefore, done only if no response to other tests.

Ideally, HGH tests are scheduled to start between 0800 and 0930 hr, after overnight fasting. Blunting of response to stimulation may occur with obesity, high dietary intake of CHO (>60% of total calories), hypothyroidism, and emotional deprivation.

All tests are carried out under direct supervision of Endocrine Service.

Exercise Test

1. Fast the patient from 2400 hr. (Fasting not mandatory. The test can be done as an office procedure later in the day).
2. Record baseline heart rate (HR) and respiratory rate (RR).
3. Baseline blood drawn for HGH at time 0.
4. 15 min vigorous exercise on bicycle.
5. Recheck HR and RR for significant increase.
6. Rest patient for 5 min after exercise; then repeat blood for HGH (time = 20 min).
7. Draw third blood for HGH at 40 min.

   Interpretation: normal response = rise in HGH to above 5 ng/ml with exercise.

Arginine Stimulation

Risks: Use with caution in patients with liver disease, renal disease, or acidosis.

1. Fast from 2400 hr. May have water up to 0800 hr.
2. Constant nursing care.
3. 0800 hr: start N saline iv; maintain rate just sufficient to keep needle open.
4. Take baseline fasting blood samples for HGH, insulin, and glucose, at 15 and 30 min after iv started.
5. Arginine infusion should be supervised by a dr.
   a) Arginine solution is slightly acidic; must be buffered before administration. Add 12.0 ml of 7.5% Na bicarbonate solution to a 50-ml bottle of 25% 1-arginine monochloride. Bring to total volume 100 ml with N saline (final concentration of arginine = 12.5%).
   b) Infuse 0.5 g arginine (4.0 ml of above solution)/kg body wt over 30 min. Max. dose = 30 g.
   c) Time zero is the moment the arginine infusion begins.
6. Collect blood samples for HGH, insulin, and glucose: at 30, 60, 90 and 120 min after time zero.
7. Vomiting, headache, and mild hypoglycemia may develop. If so, discontinue infusion and give glucose iv.

48

Interpretation: Glucose, insulin, and HGH levels should rise with arginine infusion. HGH response should be >5 ng/ml, but may be blunted if basal levels are elevated.

Insulin Tolerance

Lack of HGH response to this test is strong evidence of hypopituitarism.

a) **Severe hypoglycemic reactions may occur.** Limit to patients suspected of HGH deficiency who do not respond to other stimulatory tests.

b) Dose of regular (Toronto) insulin: 0.05 U/kg iv — but if history of spontaneous or documented hypoglycemia, give 0.025 U/kg. If blood glucose fails to fall more than 50% or to below 40 mg/dl, repeat insulin: give 0.1 U/kg.

1. Fast from 2400 hr. May have water until 0800 hr.

2. Constant nursing care.

3. Have 50-ml syringe of 50% dextrose solution available throughout.

4. 0800 hr: start iv just sufficient to keep needle open.

5. Take baseline blood samples for HGH and glucose at 15 and 30 min after iv started. At 30 min, take extra blood for serum cortisol.

6. Must be done by dr. Give regular (Toronto) insulin, 0.05 U/kg body wt, iv; record zero time at injection. Monitor patient closely for next 60 min.

7. Hunger, weakness, sweating or headache due to hypoglycemia usually occurs 20-40 min after insulin injection. Usually transient, but hypoglycemia is more severe in some patients, especially those with hypopituitarism.
   — *If any disturbance of the sensorium, terminate test immediately* by giving 50% glucose iv.

8. Collect blood for HGH and glucose at 10, 20, 30, 60, 90 and 120 min after insulin injection.
   At 40 min, take extra for serum cortisol.

9. Deliver samples promptly to the laboratory.
   Interpretation:
   — Glucose should fall to <40 mg/dl, or 50% of basal level, whichever is less.
   — HGH level should rise 2-3 fold from basal levels, with increase to >5 ng/ml — but rise may be blunted if basal levels elevated. Cortisol level should rise >15 ng/dl.

Thyrotropin (thyroid-stimulating hormone, TSH)
TRH Stimulation
Thyrotropin-releasing hormone (TRH) is used to test the pituitary reserve of TSH. This test can be done concurrently with LHRH stimulation.

1. Start iv with N saline (no fasting required).
2. Take baseline blood for TSH, T_3RIA, and T_4.
3. Infuse over 60 sec – 200 μg TRH per 1.73 m^2 surface area (or 400 μg per 1.73 m^2 for Graves' disease).
   – Time zero is start of infusion.
4. Take blood for TSH at 20, 30, and 60 min.

   Interpretation:
   – Normal children: TSH should rise 2- to 3-fold. Those on replacement thyroxine or who have hyperthyroidism: usually no response.
   – Primary hypothyroidism: excessive response.
   – Primary hypopituitarism: low values throughout test.
   – Hypothalamic hypopituitarism: subnormal response.

Gonadotropins (LH and FSH) See pp 367, 373
LHRH Stimulation
Luteinising-hormone-releasing hormone (LHRH) is used to test the pituitary reserve of gonadotropins. This test can be done concurrently with TRH stimulation.

1. Start iv with N saline (no fasting required).
2. Take baseline blood for LH and FSH.
3. Infuse over 60 sec – 50 μg of LHRH if surface area <1.0 m^2, or 100 μg of LHRH if surface area >1.0 m^2. Time zero is start of infusion.
4. Take blood for LH and FSH at 30, 60, and 90 min.

   Interpretation:
1. Normal results relate to age and pubertal rating.

		LH	FSH
A.	Prepubertal	Little if any change	Increase 50-100%
B.	Perinatal	Increase 100-200%	Increase 50% or more
C.	Adult Male	Increase 400-1000%	Increase 50-200%
D.	Adolescence	Values intermediate between A and C	

2. Altered response:
    — Gonadal hypogonadism and precocious puberty: hyperresponsiveness.
    — Primary hypopituitarism: low values and no response.
    — Hypothalamic hypopituitarism and delayed adolescence: response subnormal for age.

Adrenocorticotropin (ACTH): see p 353

ACTH can be measured in single samples of large volume (10-20 ml) collected in appropriately prepared tubes and transported quickly to laboratory. Make special arrangements with Endocrine Service.

Normal range: at 0800-0900 hr, 0-100 pg/ml

1. *Plasma cortisols* at 0800 and 2000 hr, or during insulin tolerance test, give indirect measurement of ACTH stimulation.
2. *Metyrapone test* — seldom used now, and difficult to interpret in children (see J Clin Endocr Metab 37:540, 1973).

Adrenal Cortex

Whenever possible, blood estimations of adrenal hormones should displace urine collections with tedious methodologies for urine steroids.

Short ACTH-stimulation Test

1. At 0800 hr, after 8-hr fast, take serum for cortisol estimation.
2. Inject 0.25 mg of β 1-24 ACTH (Cortrosyn or Synacthen), im or iv, diluted to 5.0 ml with N saline, over 2 min. Record time zero..
3. Take blood at 30 and 60 min.
    Interpretation:
A normal response = a peak cortisol level of >18 μg/dl or increase of 15 μg/dl from basal value (whichever is greater).

Dexamethasone Suppression

This test is used to distinguish adrenal hyperplasia from adenoma or carcinoma of the adrenal cortex and to test for Cushing's syndrome.

1. Days 1 and 2 (control days):
    a) Collect 24-hr urine for 17 0H-CS, 17-ketosteroids (and other intermediary metabolites, such as pregnanetriol, as indicated).

    b)   Take blood at 0800 hr for serum levels of adrenal hormones (e.g., androstenedione, 17 OHP) as indicated.

2. Days 3 and 4:
    a)   Give dexamethasone po, 0.5 mg q6h **or** 20 μg/kg body wt/day.
    b)   Repeat collections as in (1).

3. Days 5 and 6:
    a)   Give dexamethasone 2.0 mg po q6h
    b)   Repeat collections as in (1).

Interpretation:
- In normal subjects, the lower dose of dexamethasone will suppress, 50% or more, secretion of the urine and serum hormones.
- The higher dosage will suppress secretion in cases of congenital adrenal hyperplasia and (usually) Cushing's syndrome from hyperplasia, but usually not in cases of tumors of the adrenal cortex.

Adrenal Medulla

For measurement of urine catecholamines, see pp 390, 393, 395, 400.

Rogitine Test

    Indication: To counteract catecholamine secretion where pheochromocytoma is suspected. Rogitine (phentolamine) is a potent α-adrenergic blocking agent.

    Procedure

1. Proceed with test when systolic BP >160 mm Hg.

2. Start iv N saline and allow BP to stabilize.

3. Inject Rogitine 1.0 mg iv or 3.0 mg im. Check BP q30 sec for 3 min then q60 sec for another 7 min (longer if drug given im).

    Interpretation: A drop in BP of 60 mm Hg systolic and/or 25 mm Hg diastolic *within 2.0 min of iv* or *20 min of im injection* is a positive test and strongly suggests pheochromocytoma.

Endocrine Pancreas

For investigation of hypoglycemia, see p 56. The leucine-tolerance test is seldom an appropriate investigation (described in Arch Int Med 131:864, 1973).

Oral Glucose-tolerance Test

Indications

1. To confirm suspected cases of mild diabetes mellitus.
2. To detect the renal threshold for glucose in renal glycosuria.
3. To confirm the diagnosis of hypersomatotropism, acromegaly, or HGH deficiency.
4. To study carbohydrate tolerance in various metabolic states (e.g., obesity, hyperlipidemia).

Procedure

1. Patient fasts from 2400 hr. Water may be given until test begins, then not for 2 hr.
2. Give glucose 1.75 g/kg body weight, po, to maximum of 75 g.
3. Take samples for serum glucose, by capillary or venipuncture, at time zero (immediately before the glucose drink) and at precisely 30, 60, 120, and 180 min after the glucose.
4. If HGH measurements are required: the test can be prolonged to 6 hr, in which case an iv line for sampling is advisable.
5. Blood for insulin and HGH levels can be taken simultaneously with sampling for glucose.
6. If renal threshold for glucose to be judged: collect urine sample for glucose before the test and at each hour for the 3 hr.

Interpretation: Fasting glucose values are age-dependent (see p 369) but a peak rise of at least 50 mg/dl usually occurs at 30 or 60 min.

1. Values >200 mg/dl and <50 mg/dl are abnormal.
2. The fasting level should be regained by 3 hr.
3. Renal threshold for glucose is usually 180 ± 15 mg/dl.
4. Serum insulin should rise and fall with the glucose values (normal ranges, p 371).
5. HGH:
   a) Normal: usually elevated in the fasting sample, decreases with glucose ingestion, and rises again at about the fourth hr.
   b) HGH deficiency: the hormone = <5 ng/ml.
   c) Hypersomatotropism and acromegaly: high level of HGH, and the glucose load usually does not suppress this.

Testes

Normal testicular function is dependent on a negative feedback system between testosterone and pituitary gonadotropins. These hormones can be measured in blood (see p 370).

Human Chorionic Gonadotropin (HCG) Stimulation

HCG has LH-like activity and stimulated Leydig-cell production of testosterone.

Indications: To detect testes that are not palpable, and to judge testicular secretory capacity in hypogonadal states.

Procedure: No preparation of the patient is required.

1. Obtain a baseline serum testosterone (T) level on the first day.
2. Give HCG (Ayerst APL, or Parke-Davis Antuitrin-S) im for 3 days:
   a) <10 yr: 1000 U im daily
   b) >10 yr: 2000 U im daily.
3. Obtain 2nd blood sample for T on 4th day.

Interpretation: Normal testes produce a 3-fold increase in serum T with HCG. No response is seen in anorchia, and a subnormal response suggests gonadal hypogonadism.

Vaginal Cytology for Maturation Index

Useful for determining estrogen activity.

Collect specimen as directed (Tissue Pathology, p 91).

Interpretation

1. Superficial cornified cells: after the immediate neonatal period, none until late childhood when estrogen production increases.
2. Intermediate cell type: production increases as girl matures.
3. Marked increase in intermediate cells with little estrogen effect may indicate abnormal androgen production, or greatly diminished estrogen production, or pregnancy.
4. Maturation index is reported as percentages of basal cells/intermediate cells/superficial cells (e.g., normal 6-yr-old girl, 80%/20%/0). Interpret results in regard to clinical and other laboratory findings.

METABOLIC FUNCTION

Therapy, see Metabolic Disorders (p 254)

Diagnosis of Metabolic Disease

1. The *mass screening approach* is restricted to neonates.
2. In all sick neonates, as well as older children, the *diagnostic work-up approach* is applied — correlation of appropriate analyses based upon the individual patient's signs and symptoms. See Neonatology, p 172.

1. NEONATAL MASS SCREENING

1. On admission, take blood samples for:
   a) RBC galactosemia screening test
   b) hypothyroidism screening test, using T_4 and TSH.
2. After 2 days on milk formula po, **or** 4 days after admission irrespective of nutrient intake: take samples for:
   a) Guthrie PKU screening test (*blood*)
   b) qualitative thin-layer amino-acid chromatograms, *in blood* (1 dimension) *and urine* (2 dimens)
   c) the DNPH test, *in urine*, for α-keto acids (especially branched-chain keto acids of maple-syrup-urine disease) and the cyanide nitroprusside test for sulfur-containing compounds (e.g., cystinuria and homocystinuria).

2. DIAGNOSTIC WORK-UP APPROACH

A clinical approach to disorders of intermediary metabolism (glucose and amino acids) and lysosomal metabolism is proposed. Immemorable lists of individually rare disorders are avoided wherever possible, being replaced by an approach to diagnosis based upon presenting symptom(s).

Carbohydrate Metabolism

A. GLUCOSE

Hypoglycemia

Arbitrary definition: a blood glucose value <40 mg/dl, irrespective of age. Thus, the aim of treatment is to maintain blood glucose above this level.

The key to diagnosis is analysis of a blood sample obtained during hypoglycemia — a spontaneous episode or induced by starvation.

Starvation Tolerance Study

Indication: To differentiate the type of hypoglycemia — whether hyperketotic (ketotic hypoglycemia syndrome) or hypoketotic (hyperinsulinism).

Procedure
1. Last Supper at 1800 hr; then nil orally except water.
2. Next day: Take blood sample (0.5 ml heparinized) at 0900, 1200, and 1500 hr.
   Note. Glucose and 3-hydroxybutyrate (3HOB) must be measured within 30 min of venipuncture.

Interpretation

Diagnosis	Blood Glucose	Blood 3HOB
Normal adult	↓	↑
Normal child	↓↓	↑↑
*Ketotic hypoglycemia	↓↓↓	↑↑↑
Hyperinsulinism	↓↓↓	N or ↑

*In this test, ketotic hypoglycemia syndrome (exaggeration of normal response to starvation during childhood) is mimicked by (a) the growing child with intercurrent infection and (b) hormonal deficiency (cortisol, ACTH, HGH, catecholamines).

Metabolic Acidosis

Key to diagnosis: identification of anions responsible for an increased anion gap; i.e., $Na^+ - [Cl^- + HCO_3^-]$ >18mM. See p 126.

Procedure
Measurement of lactate and 3 hydroxybutyrate (3HOB) in a plasma sample.

Interpretation
1. If accounted for by lactate and/or 3HOB, likely diagnoses are:
   a) cytosolic gluconeogenic defects*
      – glucose-6-phosphatase
      – fructose 1.6 diphosphatase
   b) mitochondrial gluconeogenic defects
      – phosphoenolpyruvate carboxykinase
      – pyruvate carboxylase
   c) defect of pyruvate dehydrogenase complex.

*Cytosolic gluconeogenic defects are characterized by severe hypoglycemia with hepatomegaly, hyperlipidemia, and hyperuricemia. The two enzyme defects are differentiated by the glycemic response to gluconeogenic substrates (Table A, p 58) administered during hypoglycemia.

2. If anion gap is *not* accounted for by lactate or 3HOB: *organic acidurias* must be considered. (These are diagnosed by analysis of random urine sample by gas chromatography and mass spectrometry.) Organic acidurias are characterized by the accumulation of hydroxy- and/or keto-acids derived from catabolism of amino and fatty acids. Examples include methylmalonic aciduria, propionic acidemia, and thiolase deficiency.

Hepatomegaly in Metabolic Disorders

Disorders characterized by hepatomegaly, without significant hypoglycemia or lactic acidosis, occur in the degradative pathway of hepatic glycogen metabolism. These are differentiated as in Table B, p 58.

TABLE A.

Enzyme Defect	Test glycemic response to gluconeogenic substrates given iv		
	Galactose (0.5 g/kg)	Fructose* (0.5 g/kg)	Glucagon (100 µg/kg, to 1 mg)
Glucose-6-phosphatase	–	–	–
Fructose-1,6-diphosphatase	+	–	–

*Fructose-tolerance studies *MUST* be performed under very close supervision, as precipitous falls in blood glucose levels are common.

TABLE B.

Defective Enzyme	Glycemic Respose to Glucagon (100 µg/kg, up to 1 mg, iv)		Lactate Response to Glucose (0.5 g/kg iv)
	Fed	Fasting	
Debrancher	+	–	+
Phosphorylase	–	–	+
Phosphorylase kinase	(+)	+	+++

58

B. GALACTOSE

Galactosemia

Galactose-1-phosphate uridyl transferase (gal-1-PUT) deficiency causes hepatomegaly with or without jaundice, failure to thrive, feeding difficulties with vomiting and the renal Fanconi syndrome — *plus cataracts*.

Key to diagnosis
1. Clinical suspicion — in this event: modify diet to CHO-free formula plus added glucose.
2. RBC galactosemia screening test.
   Note. Urinary reducing substances ARE NOT AN ACCURATE DIAGNOSTIC TEST, as urine may not always contain galactose.

Interpretation
1. If screening test positive, seek confirmation by quantification of gal-1-PUT in RBC (p 368).
2. If diagnosis confirmed, see Metabolic Disorders (p 255).
3. If negative, alternative diagnoses are hereditary fructose intolerance and tyrosinemia.

C. FRUCTOSE

Hereditary Fructose Intolerance

Fructose aldolase deficiency causes hepatic and renal changes identical to those in galactosemia. Hypoglycemia is more pronounced, serum phosphate may be low, serum uric acid level may be high, *but cataracts DO NOT DEVELOP.*

Key to diagnosis
1. Clinical suspicion — in this event: give CHO-free formula with added glucose.
2. Fructose tolerance study and/or liver needle biopsy for enzymatic analysis.

Interpretation
1. If positive, diagnosis confirmed (see Metabolic Disorders, p 255).

Lysosomal Storage

The basic defects are described in Metabolic Disorders, p 257. Specific assays available for differentiating the disorders are listed in the table overleaf.

Disease	Enzyme Assay	Source of Enzyme*
Gangliosidoses		
G_{M1}	β-galactosidase	w, f
G_{M2}	hexosaminidase A & B	s, w, f
Leukodystrophies		
Krabbe's	cerebroside-β-galactosidase	w, f
metachromatic	arylsulfatase A	s, w, f
Niemann–Pick A & B	sphingomyelinase	w, f
Gaucher's disease	β-glucosidase	w, f
Fabry's disease	α-galactosidase	w, f
Mucopolysaccharidoses		
I	α-iduronidase	w, f
II	iduronate sulfatase	f
IIIA	sulfamidase	f
IIIB	α-glucosaminidase	f
IV	GlcNAc-6-sulfatase	f
VI	GalNAc-6-sulfatase	f
VII	β-glucuronidase	w, f

60

Sialidosis	α-neuraminidase	f
I-cell disease	Diagnosed by high level of serum arylsulfatase but low WBC arylsulfatase, or with fibroblasts.	s, w, f
Mannosidosis	α-mannosidase	w, f
Fucosidosis	α-fucosidase	w, f

*Preferred source is in italics

s – serum; 1 ml clotted blood

w – leukocytes; 5 ml heparinized blood

f – fibroblasts; arrange skin biopsy with Genetics

Amino Acid Metabolism & Transport

Some of the most important amino-acid metabolic defects are listed in the table below.

Disease	Preferred Fluid for Amino-acid Screen	Other Urine Screening Tests
PKU & hyperphenylalaninemia	Blood	$FeCl_3$ test: green
Tyrosinemia	Blood	Nitrosonaphthol
MSUD & variants	Blood	DNPH (dinitrophenylhydrazine)
Nonketotic hyperglycinemia	CSF	—
Ketotic hyperglycinemia	Blood	Ketostix. Organic-acid screen (e.g., propionic acid, methylmalonic acid)
Homocystinuria: deficiency of		
a) cystathionine synthase	Blood – methionine increased Urine – homocystine increased	Nitroprusside
b) methylene tetrahydrofolate reductase, or B_{12} defects	Blood – methionine normal Urine – homocystine increased	Nitroprusside
Hyperalaninemia (secondary to lactic acidosis)	Blood	

SPECIFIC AMINOACIDURIAS

Transport System Deleted	Condition	Diagnosis by
1. *Neutral amino acids*	Hartnup disease (pellagra)	Urine screen
2. a) *Basic:* cystine, ornithine, arginine, lysine (COAL)	Cystinuria (renal stones)	Urine screen & urine nitroprusside test
b) *Basic:* mitochondrial	Lysinuric protein intolerance (NH_3^+)	Urine screen; blood NH_3
3. *Acidic*	Dicarboxylic aminoaciduria (benign)	Urine screen
4. *Iminoglycine*		
a) proline, hydroxyproline, glycine	Neonatal iminoglycinuria normally present up to 3-6 mo (benign)	Urine screen
b) proline, hydroxyproline, glycine	Familial iminoglycinuria (probably benign)	Urine screen

Ammonia Metabolism

Hyperammonemia (see also p 258)

   Definition. Blood ammonia level = $>250\ \mu$M

   Key to diagnosis

1. Blood ammonia level $>250\ \mu$M in any child is evidence of acute hepatic encephalopathy.

2. **Note. Any child with intermittent vomiting, semicoma, or migraine:** determine blood ammonia level (p 356) while symptoms present — **especially if the child is experiencing developmental delay.**

   Procedure

   Urgent — quantitative and qualitative analysis of:

1. amino acids in blood and urine (pp 355, 390)

2. organic acids (specifically orotic acid) in urine (p 395).

   Interpretation

1. Alanine, glutamine, lysine, and methionine: may be elevated nonspecifically in any case of hyperammonemia.

2. Cytosolic urea-cycle defects: accumulation of amino acids specific to each defect — citrullinemia, arginosuccinic aciduria, and argininemia.

3. Mitochondrial urea-cycle defects: no accumulation of specific amino acids. These disorders are differentiated by:
   a) massive accumulation of orotic acid in OTC deficiency
   b) absence of orotic acid in CPS deficiency.

4. Various organic acidurias and rarer disorders of ammonia metabolism are identifed by findings appropriate to each disorder.

VIROLOGY

(No *tests* in Virology — investigations)

Types of specimen(s) taken and test system(s) operated depend on:

1. Clinical presentation; duration of illness
2. Patient's age; previous illnesses; immunizations
3. Geographic location of domicile/recent visit
4. Season; viruses currently prevalent.

Note

1. Many of the syndromes outlined can be caused by bacteria or parasites, also.
2. Only *viral* etiologic agents are considered in this section.

Aseptic Meningitis
1. Send CSF and nasopharyngeal suction (NPS) for virus isolation.
2. Etiology — main contenders: enteroviruses (ECHO, Coxsackie A and B, poliomyelitis) and mumps.
3. Mumps serology is helpful; enteroviral serology is of limited value.

Encephalitis/Encephalopathy
1. Send NPS if signs and symptoms of a preceding URI.
2. Send CSF, vesicle fluid, and blood samples taken during acute stage and convalescence for serology.
3. Brain biopsy tissue must not be placed in formalin, as it is destined for virus isolation and immunofluorescence microscopy.
4. Note. In the late stage (4 wk from onset) of encephalitis (e.g., Herpes simplex, Epstein—Barr virus), the CSF may contain the corresponding antibody.

Paralytic Disease
1. Send CSF and NPS.
2. If symptoms present for >1 wk, send stool also.

Vesicular Skin Lesions
1. Select a small vesicle ('dew-drop' variety, if possible):
   a) Remove dome of skin, and scrape base of vesicle (use a disposable needle).
   b) Smear over small area of microscopy slide and apply Giemsa or H & E stain.
   c) Look for giant cells and intranuclear inclusions.
2. Vesicle fluid, plus scraping from base of vesicle, suitable for EM also.
3. Vesicle fluid suitable for virus isolation.

Congenital Defects/Disease: (T) ORCH
1. Take 5 ml blood from mother, and 3-4 ml from infant, into sterile test tubes.
2. Routine investigation includes rubella, cytomegalovirus, herpes, and other.
3. Virologists will order additional specimens prn.

Croup, Bronchiolitis, Pertussis-like Syndrome, Pneumonia (pp 181, 183)
1. Send NPS.

Myopericarditis
1.   If of recent onset: send NPS, stool sample (collected in screwtop test-container with glass beads).
2.   Send 5 ml clotted blood taken during acute stage and convalescence, for serology.
3.   If pericardial aspiration: send fluid to Virology.
4.   Constrictive pericarditis: send some unfixed tissue from the thickened pericardial sac.

Infectious Mononucleosis Syndrome
1.   First, serology for cytomegalovirus (CMV) and EBV.
2.   Depending on findings, specimens may be taken for virus isolation.

Measles (Rubeola), Rubella, and Mumps
1.   Serology (acute and convalescent phase) provides an accurate means of establishing a diagnosis.
2.   NPS for isolation of virus, and/or for immunofluorescence studies.
3.   Mumps involving the nervous system: CSF yields virus in many cases.
4.   Subacute sclerosing panencephalitis (SSPE): serum and CSF for measles-antibody studies.
5.   Mumps skin test not recommended.

Hepatitis
1.   Serum hepatitis (i.e., hepatitis B (HB) or Australia antigen):
     a)   Acute stage: 5 ml clotted blood for antigen in serum.
     b)   Convalescent or chronic stage: 5 ml clotted blood for either antigen or antibody.
2.   Other hepatitis: may be caused by CMV, EBV, rubella, Coxsackie B, especially in neonates.
     Telephone virologist to find out most appropriate specimens.

Antiviral Agents

Adenosine Arabinoside (Ara-A; Vidarabine)
Available only through consultation with Virology (still on investigational protocol).
   Used when following infections confirmed:
1.   Herpes simplex
     a)   generalized infection of newborn
     b)   encephalitis in immunologically normal/abnormal patients.

66

2. Varicella-zoster (V-Z)
   a) clinically severe chickenpox in immunosuppressed patients
   b) chickenpox pneumonia of life-threatening severity
   c) clinically severe herpes zoster in immunosuppressed patients which has disseminated beyond primary involved dermatomes.

Requirements for confirming diagnosis:
1. Cutaneous V-Z infections
   a) typical skin lesions
   b) Tzanck test of lesion-scrapings (by Virology)
   c) viral culture of lesions: must be obtained **before** start of treatment.
2. Generalized herpes simplex infection of newborn
   a) exposure to maternal infection
   b) typical skin lesions: scraped for Tzanck test and viral culture
   c) clinical signs consistent with generalized infection and/or encephalitis
   d) viral cultures — obtained **before** beginning treatments; appropriate cultures of CSF, skin lesions, throat swabs, stool, and bloody buffy coat
   e) CSF examined for fluorescent antibodies
   f) serology; acute and convalescent phases.
3. Herpes simplex encephalitis
   a) signs: fever, convulsions, focal neurological signs (especially temporal lobe), depressed level of consciousness with or without typical skin lesions
   b) diagnostic studies: CSF for viral culture and fluorescent antibodies; cultures of saliva, urine, and skin or mucosal lesions
   c) EEG, brain scan, CT scan (Neurology consultation)
   d) brain biopsy — preliminary results (must be known **before** start of therapy) should include histologic exam and viral culture.
4. Chickenpox pneumonia of life-threatening severity
   a) radiographic signs of pneumonitis plus varicelliform skin lesions
   b) viral cultures of skin lesions, obtained before start of therapy, for retrospective confirmation.

Inappropriate to use adenosine arabinoside:
1. If CNS already severely compromised.
2. Pregnant patients: consider comparative risks in each case individually.
3. Patient has received other antiviral agent or zoster-immune plasma within preceding week.

4. Severe liver or kidney disease that would alter rate of metabolism or secretion of adenosine arabinoside.

   Dosage of adenosine arabinoside (decided in consultation with Virology)

1. Varicella-zoster infections and herpes simplex encephalitis:
   10-15 mg/kg/day, infused iv over 12 hr, for 5-10 days.

2. Generalized herpes simplex of the newborn:
   20 mg/kg/day, infused iv over 12-24 hr, for 7-14 days.
   a) This is maximal dose at present.
   b) Not given to patients older than 3 mo.

   Special instructions

1. Because of risk of teratogenicity:
   a) contraceptive control *must* be maintained during therapy, with abstinence advised during and for 2 wk after therapy.
   b) when applicable, do pregnancy test before start of therapy.

2. Treatment/prophylaxis for ophthalmologic complications of herpes simplex or varicella-zoster:
   a) 3% adenosine arabinoside ophthalmic ointment is available (ophthalmology consultation required).
   b) Dosage: apply in both eyes qid.

N-Methylisatin β-Thiosemicarbazone
(Methisazone; Marboran)

1. Treatment of eczema vaccinatum, generalized vaccinia, progressive vaccinia, and vaccinia gangrenosa.

2. Give orally, 200 mg/kg body wt *stat*, then 50 mg/kg q6h for 8 doses. This dose may be halved for young children.

3. Nausea and vomiting are the most troublesome side-effects.

COMMON TECHNICAL PROCEDURES
General Points to Remember

1. The success of any procedure depends largely on adequate immobilization of the patient. ALWAYS have a nurse assist you: she usually will be more familiar than you are with the techniques.
2. Have ALL the necessary tapes, tubes, caps, etc, READY before beginning.
3. Before starting any dangerous procedure, have the senior resident in attendance.

BLOOD

Cubital Vein Puncture — Route of choice at all ages.
1. Insert a no. 23 or 25 scalp-vein iv needle.
2. Do not exert excess suction on the syringe barrel.

Scalp Vein — Insufficient flow for blood sampling.
1. Immobilize head and arms.
2. Insert a no. 23 or 25 scalp-vein iv needle.
3. Secure the needle with thin strips of adhesive tape.
4. Cut a plastic medicine cup in half longitudinally; cover the cut edge with adhesive tape.
5. Tape the half cup over the puncture site, to form a shield for the needle.

Heel or Finger Capillary Prick
1. 0.5 to 1 ml of capillary blood can be collected for microchemistry and hematology.
2. Hematocrit may be distorted by this method.
3. Tests for predominantly intracellular ions (e.g., K^+, Mg^{++}) are invalid by this technique.
4. In small infants the heel may become badly bruised.
5. For arterialized capillary blood gases, warm the heel or finger immediately before the prick, to ensure sufficient hyperemia.

External Jugular
1. Hyperextend the head and laterally flex it through $90°$.
2. Lower it to below level of shoulders, by placing a roll beneath the shoulder or hanging the head over the edge of the bed.

3. Make infant cry (to distend vein).
4. Use a no. 23 scalp vein needle or bend a long beveled sharp needle 90° from the line of the syringe, and insert into vein.
5. At completion: sit child up, and exert pressure over puncture site for at least 2 min.

Internal Jugular – Dangerous
1. Adequate mummying is essential; patient flat, with head extended and laterally rotated through 90°.
2. Select a point on posterior border of sternomastoid at the junction of its upper 1/3 and lower 2/3.
3. Place a finger on the sternal notch.
4. Insert needle at selected site, parallel to floor and aimed at finger in sternal notch.
5. Transfix vein; withdraw needle while exerting pressure on plunger.
6. At completion: sit child up, and apply firm pressure over puncture site for at least 2 min.

Femoral Venous Puncture – Least desirable (may produce septic arthritis of hip joint)
1. Flex hip; rotate it externally as far as possible.
2. Identify femoral pulse.
3. Insert needle just medial to femoral pulse, aiming vertically, slightly toward the head and slightly laterally, to transfix vein.
4. a) Withdraw needle gradually, exerting traction on plunger.
   b) When blood appears in syringe, stop withdrawing needle and remove appropriate quantity of blood.
5. At completion: maintain pressure on puncture site for at least 2 min.

Sagittal Sinus Puncture – There is NO indication for this procedure.

Saphenous Vein Cut-down
1. Make incision 0.5-1.0 cm through the skin, 0.5 cm above and anterior to border of medial malleolus.
2. Dissect subcutaneous tissue with a snap until the blue thin-walled vein is identified just superficial to the periosteum.

3. Pass a small curved snap under the vein, and pull through a doubled length of catgut under the vein. Cut the folded end of the catgut.

4. Tie distal piece of gut, to halt venous return. Use proximal piece of gut to elevate vein. With vein scissors, make a small nick in vein wall until the lumen is exposed.

5. Open the vein orifice with a small vein-guide.

6. Use an Intramedic catheter of appropriate size and with a dull point, or the inner cannula from an Intracath previously filled with saline. (Or a small feeding tube, no. 3 1/2, 5, 8, can be used.) Insert it into the vein and advance proximally.

7. Tie the upper catgut stay around the catheter, to keep it in place.

8. Close the skin with 4-0 silk or nylon, passing it through the skin and around the catheter.

9. Splint the limb if necessary.

Radial Artery Puncture — for determining blood gas.

1. Palpate radial artery over distal end of radius.

2. Place your thumb over the thenar eminence, and your fingers behind the wrist. Hyperextend the wrist.

3. Use a no. 25 needle in infant *or* no. 23 needle in older child, and heparinized syringe.

4. Transfix the artery, holding needle and syringe at 60° angle to the arm.

5. Withdraw needle slowly until blood spurts into syringe.

6. After completion: exert pressure over artery for at least 2 min.

7. Remove all air bubbles from syringe. Place syringe in ice and send immediately to lab.

Umbilical Catheterization

1. Obtain appropriate pack from CSR.

2. Immobilize infant in frog position, with hands also immobilized. A syrup-coated pacifier makes the procedure more pleasant for the patient.

3. Measure distance from shoulder tip to umbilicus.

4. Glove, mask, and gown.

5. Clean umbilical area with iodine. Wash off with 70% alcohol, and dry carefully. Place the center-hole towel over the abdomen.

6. Prepare radio-opaque end-hold catheters.
   a) For arterial line: attach a 2.5 FR catheter via a two-way stopcock to a syringe filled with normal saline.
   b) For venous line: attach a 5 FR catheter, similarly prepared.
7. Grasp the umbilicus by its clamp. Using a scalpel, amputate it approx. 0.5 cm above skin.
8. To halt bleeding, apply a gauze square and elevate the stump.
9. Place a loosely tied circumferential stitch around the skin margin of the umbilicus.
10. Probe the orifice of the vein and of one artery.
11. a) Using blunt, cupped, tissue forceps, grasp edge of vessel.
    b) Insert catheter:
       — Venous catheter: approx. half shoulder—umbilicus length.
       — Arterial catheter: approx. two-thirds shoulder—umbilicus length.
       — If catheter fails to progress, rotate it through 180°.
12. Check position of catheter radiographically:
    a) Tip of arterial catheter should lie between the bodies of L_3 and L_4.
    b) Tip of venous catheter should lie in the IVC, above the diaphragm but below the atrium.
13. Suture the umbilicus with a purse-string suture, including the catheters in separate knots.
14. Bridge with clear adhesive tape, ensnaring both catheters in the horizontal piece.
15. Connect the infusions to each catheter. Use Millipore filters and constant-infusion pump.

Note. Some color change in feet, due to arterial spasm, is common after insertion of umbilical catheter. This usually resolves quickly; if effect is unilateral, resolution can be hastened by applying warmth to other leg. **No improvement in color for 45 min is an ABSOLUTE INDICATION for removal of catheter.**

CEREBROSPINAL FLUID

Lumbar Puncture
1. Check eye grounds and BP for evidence of raised ICP.
   — If ICP is raised, consult Neurology or Neurosurgery.

2. Before gloving:
   a) Check equipment, decide on number of specimens needed.
   b) Place patient with back fully flexed and sitting up or lying on one side. Child must be held securely in this position.
3. Mask and glove.
4. Scrub patient's back with iodine and wipe off with alcohol, avoiding fecal contamination. Place 1 towel under patient and 1 over patient's back.
5. Identify L_{4-5} interspace below an imaginary line joining the iliac crests. In infants *(not neonates)* and older children, infiltrate skin and sc tissue with 1% lidocaine (Xylocaine).
6. Use a short, sharp-beveled LP needle, no. 22 or 23 in infant *or* no. 18 or 20 in older child.
   Insert horizontally, parallel to floor, with point slightly angled toward head.
   Note. In children, a click is not usually felt when the dura is penetrated.
7. Take pressure reading when child is not crying and preferably with legs straightened.
8. *Assistant must do this step:*
   a) Open chocolate-agar slant bottle
   b) Hold it near hub of spinal tap needle, to collect 2-3 drops of CSF on agar.
   c) Close the bottle aseptically.
   Remember: outside of bottle is not sterile.
9. Collect 1.0-1.5 ml CSF in round-bottomed tube for chemistry (sugar and protein), and 1 ml in each of 2 centrifuge tubes for bacteriology (culture, cell count, smear, Gram stain) and for virology culture.
   Note. Wait for fluid to emerge — **DO NOT ASPIRATE.**
10. Additional CSF may be needed for counterimmune electrophoresis (CIE), cytology, etc.
11. Take off a few drops of CSF for resident's cell count and smear.

Traumatic Tap
1. If unsure, allow fluid to drip and see if it clears.
2. To be sure: centrifuge, and check supernatant fluid for xanthochromia.
   - RBC:WBC ratio should not exceed 240:1 in bloody tap.
3. If tap bloody, sit patient up and insert needle 1 interspace higher.

Xanthochromia: Indicates hemolyzed blood that was in CSF before LP. This may be acceptable in a neonate.

Subdural Tap

1. Mummy patient and place supine. Place rolled diaper under neck, to extend it.
2. Shave vertex thoroughly from just behind the ears forward.
3. Identify point on coronal suture in midpupillary line. At this point, insert a sharp, *short* beveled subdural needle, at right angle to skull surface.
   - Just before the needle passes through the dura, a resistance will be felt.

   Note. Do not insert needle more than 0.5 cm.
4. **Wait for fluid to emerge: DO NOT ASPIRATE.**
5. Closing the puncture hole: apply a dab of collodion, or run a single silk suture through the puncture site.

Ventricular Tap

1. Is done in an emergency in a baby who has a non-communicating hydrocephalus or blocked shunt. If at all possible, consult Neurosurgery first; but if medullary signs are present, ventricular tap is urgently necessary.
2. Proceed as for subdural tap above.
   When the dura has been pierced: advance toward the feet, aiming at a vertical line projected posteriorly from the inner canthus of the patient's ipsilateral eye.
3. Remove the stylet frequently until there is a rush of fluid.
4. When no further fluid flows, remove needle.
5. Closing puncture hole: see Subdural Tap, point 5, above.

Examination of CSF

A. Cell Count

1. Gently mix CSF well.
2. Flood one side of clean, dry Fuchs–Rosenthal counting chamber (with coverslip in place) with undiluted CSF.
3. Count WBC and RBC in 5 large squares (= 80 small squares = 1 mm^3).
4. If >5 cells/mm^3:
   a) in separate test tube, mix 3 drops CSF and 1 drop acetic-acid/ gentian violet stain.
   b) flood other side of counting chamber with mixture.
   c) repeat cell count after 3 min (any RBC present will be lysed).

B. *Gram Stain* (to identify micro-organisms)

Reagents
1. 0.5% crystal violet
2. Lugol's iodine.
3. 95% alcohol.
4. For CSF, safranin — (otherwise, use dilute carbol fuchsin).

Procedure
1. Prepare a thin film of the material to be examined, allow to dry, and fix with gentle heat.
2. Flood the slide with crystal violet, stain for 30 sec, rinse gently with water.
3. Flood with iodine solution, and let sit 60 sec (2 min if there is any question whether the organism is Gram-positive or -negative).
4. Rinse with 95% alcohol until no further color flows from slide (usually 10-20 sec, depending on thickness of smear). *See also* Results, point 3.
5. Rinse with water.
6. Counterstain CSF smears with safranin for 1 min (other smears, use dilute carbol fuchsin for 30 sec). Rinse with water.
7. Blot carefully with clean blotting paper.

Results
1. Gram-positive organisms retain the violet–iodine complex and stain dark purple.
2. Gram-negative organisms stain red.
3. **Note.** If overdecolorized with alcohol, Gram-positive organisms may appear Gram-negative.

C. *Pandy test*
1. Place 1 ml Pandy solution in test tube.
2. Hold against black background and add 1 drop of CSF.
3. Positive test if fluid cloudy, indicating globulin in CSF.

Paracentesis

Peritoneal
1. Bladder must be empty. Percuss to check; if unsure, catheterize and drain.

2. Infiltrate skin, sc tissues, muscle, and peritoneum, with 1% lidocaine (Xylocaine), at a point midway between anterior superior iliac spine and umbilicus on left side.

3. a) Insert a no. 20 Medicut needle through skin, muscle, and peritoneum.

   b) A 0.5 cm incision with a scalpel may be necessary to penetrate skin.

   c) Fluid is visible, rising up the outer tube, when peritoneum is pierced. Remove needle; remove fluid as required.

Pleural

1. Older child: sit him up facing backrest of chair and with arms encircling it.
   Younger child: rest his head on pillow on feeding tray.

2. Identify point of maximal dullness, and check radiograph for position of fluid.

3. Sterilize skin and infiltrate skin, muscle and pleura with 1% lidocaine (Xylocaine).

4.A. Use a no. 18 needle attached via a two-way stopcock to a 20-ml syringe.

   a) Insert needle in posterior axillary line in 8th intercostal space, staying as close as possible to the upper border of the lower rib (to avoid intercostal vessels).

   b) Advance needle until a click and reduced resistance indicate penetration of pleura.

   c) Aspirate and expel fluid, using the two-way stopcock.

   Or

4.B. Alternatively (less chance of lung trauma), use a large Intercath. Withdraw the needle, leaving in the chest only the inner cannula connected to the two-way stopcock.

Pericardial – Dangerous

1. Must be supervised by experienced senior or cardiac fellow.

2. Have patient sit up.

3. Use a no. 20, long, beveled needle, attached to a two-way stopcock and syringe, and if possible attached with a bulldog clamp to an ECG electrode.

4. Insert needle at junction of left subcostal margin and xiphisternum. Aim it posteriorly, superiorly, and slightly laterally.

Examination of Paracentesis Fluid
1. Volume and gross appearance.
2. Total and differential cell-count, and smear.
3. Culture.
4. Protein and SG.
5. Look for tumor cells if indicated.

Pneumothorax

Emergency Treatment of Tension Pneumothorax
A. **In dire emergency:** insert large-bore cannula into chest, for rapid decompression.

B. **If less urgent:**
    1. Cut off the bottle end of an iv administration set.
    2. Connect a no. 18 needle through a two-way stopcock to the set.
    3. Place the cut-off end of the tube under water in a feeding bottle filled with water.
    4. Attach other outlet of 2-way stopcock to a 20-ml syringe.
    5. a) Turn stopcock to allow syringe aspiration.
        b) Insert needle in 3rd intercostal space in anterior axillary line.
    6. Once air has been aspirated, turn stopcock to allow drainage via the underwater seal.

Insertion of Intercostal Drain
Once the tension pneumothorax has been relieved there is no emergency, so get correct instrument pack from CSR.
1. Position patient on side, with arm held extended above head by assistant. Mask and glove.
2. Scrub the chest wall thoroughly with iodine, and wipe off with alcohol.
3. Use intercostal drain tube of appropriate size — usually no. 12 in neonate, no. 16-18 in older child.
    a) Grasp drainage tube with hemostat, as close to its end as possible and with hemostat as near parallel to the tube as possible.
    b) Apply another hemostat to cross-clamp tube at other end.
4. Infiltrate skin, muscle, and pleura, in 6th or 7th intercostal space, midway between the anterior and midaxillary lines.

5. a) Use a scalpel to make incision 1.0-1.5 cm long in 6th or 7th intercostal space, midway between anterior and midaxillary lines. Continue incision through skin and muscle until you encounter the gritty feeling of pleura, then:
    b) Push tip of drainage tube held by hemostat through the incision: continue pushing until hemostat enters the pleural space, indicated by sudden decrease in resistance and increasingly easy passage of tube. (The lung should be collapsed, and thus not damaged by this procedure.)

6. Remove the hemostat that is parallel to the tube. Continue to feed the drainage tube into the chest for approximately 2/3 of its length.

7. Connect a Heimlich value to the drainage tube, with the flat end pointing away from the chest. This is a one-way valve, allowing only the escape of free intrathoracic air; when valve is in place, the cross-clamp can be removed.

8. a) Close the incision with a purse-string suture.
    b) Place a separate holding suture through the skin and around the drain.
    c) Apply a gauze dressing around the wound, and tape drain in place.

9. Connect distal end of Heimlich valve to underwater seal, to which wall suction can be attached if desired.

URINE

Suprapubic Aspiration of Bladder

Done by experienced, specially trained residents only.

Indications

1. Suspected neonatal sepsis, etiology unknown.
2. Suspected urinary tract infection in infants (PUO, failure to thrive) from whom midstream urine cannot be obtained.
3. Midstream urine has $>10^4$ colonies/ml.

Note, before doing suprapubic aspiration:

1. If obstructive uropathy is suspected:
    a) The danger of extravasation of infected urine is great.
    b) Consult Urology re emergency IVP before aspiration, or leave urine culture until Urology does cystoscopy.

2. If obvious signs and symptoms of urinary-tract infection: Patient can safely be catheterized to obtain urine for culture before starting antibiotic therapy.
3. If catheter-voiding cystourethrogram is planned in the next day or two and the situation is not urgent: the catheter urine sample can be used for culture and sensitivities, and suprapubic aspiration may be unnecessary.

Preparation

1. Have the patient drink several glasses of water about 30 min before procedure. If patient has urinated within preceding 30 min, postpone procedure.
2. Get suprapubic bladder-puncture set: from treatment rooms of infants' wards, or from CSR if patient on older children's ward.
3. If necessary, sedate.

Procedure

1. Place patient on firm surface, supine in frog position. Have nurse hold the legs with her hands and steady the body with her elbows.
2. Palpate or percuss bladder to ensure that it is full.
3. a) Clean skin between symphysis pubis and umbilicus with antiseptic. Premature or newborn infants, use tincture of Zephiran (benzalkonium chloride) 1:1000; others, use 2 1/2% iodine in isopropyl alcohol.
    b) No local anesthetic required.
    c) Dry with sterile swab.
4. a) Make puncture in midline, 1-2 cm above symphysis.
    b) Pass needle quickly through skin, then downward into bladder at angle of 10-15° from vertical. (Necessary depth of penetration varies but in infants averages 2-3 cm. With experience, the sensation of penetrating the bladder is readily recognized.)
5. Aspirate urine gently, then withdraw needle.
6. Remove cotton plug from tube that contains a cork. Force point of needle (with syringe attached) into cork. Tape syringe to tube.
7. Remove all Zephiran or iodine from the skin, using 70% isopropyl alcohol.

8. a) Label the syringe and tube with its contained specimen.
    b) Send immediately to Bacteriology.
       If lab is closed, the specimen should be left in the night specimen refrigerator in Bacteriology reception area.
9. Warn parents (and child, if indicated) that transient minimal hematuria may follow and is no cause for alarm.

EXAMINATION OF FECES

Stool Smear
1. Place small drop of feces on glass slide.
2. Place single drop of normal saline on edge of cover slip and, using this edge, agitate the drop of stool and mix it with the saline.
3. Lower the cover slip over specimen and examine by microscope.
4. Look for fat, starch, meat fibers, WBC, RBC, yeast and parasites.
    a) Neutral fats: a drop of stool and 2 drops Sudan red stain on slide; mix with 2 drops saline, then place cover slip and examine slide under microscope. Red-stained droplets = fat globules.
    b) Fatty-acid crystals: best seen with polarizing attachment on microscope.
    c) Leukocytes suggest bacterial infection or inflammatory bowel disease.
    d) Erythrocytes suggest amebic colitis.
    e) Parasites: examine stool smear-slide under low power to locate and under high power to identify. Add 1 drop 1% potassium iodide stain to 1 drop of stool on slide, for easier species identification.

Examination for Pinworms (Oxyuriasis)
1. Cellophane-tape specimen should be obtained, before patient bathes, in am:
    a) Put piece of tape, sticky side out, on end of wooden tongue depressor.
    b) Gently apply taped end of stick to perianal area.
    c) On a glass slide, put 1 drop xylol, then apply the piece of tape (sticky side down), and search for ova under the microscope.

Reducing Substances in Stool
(to detect carbohydrate malabsorption)

1. a) Dilute small amount of liquid stool with twice its volume of water in a test tube; **or**
   b) *If to detect sucrose* (which is not a reducing sugar): add 1 N HCl, instead of H_2O, to stool; boil mixture very briefly.

2. In another tube, put 1 Clinitest tablet, add 15 drops of stool mixture, and compare color of resulting solution with Clinitest chart.

3. Value $<0.25\%$ is normal; $>0.5\%$ suggests carbohydrate malabsorption.

RADIOLOGY

Filling out Radiology Consultation Form
(see also Nuclear Medicine, p 84)

1. Circle part to be examined, and check appropriate box. (Remember to check R or L if applicable.)
2. State provisional diagnosis, suspected pathology, and reason for examination.
3. Dr must sign form.
4. Requisition must be addressographed on ward or in clinic *before* being sent to Radiology.

Note. If these are not done, the form will be returned to the ward.

Booking for GI, GU, and Tomographic Studies

1. Between 0800 and 1600 hr, call local 2323 and make booking.
2. After hours, call same local; state patient's name, ward, and examination required. A booking will be telephoned shortly after 0800 hr.
3. *Emergencies:* contact Radiology resident on call.

GI Studies: Preparation

1. Esophagus
2. Stomach and duodenum } at least 4 hr fasting
3. Colon (routine) – usually no preparation.
4. Colon (double contrast) – clear fluids only for 36 hr; *castor oil 1 ml/kg preceding afternoon, and saline or Fleet enema preceding evening and morning of examination.

   *Do not give castor oil if the patient has colitis.

5. Cholecystogram, oral – tablets and diet as instructed.
6. Cholangiogram, iv – at least 4 hr fasting.

Note. Patients from infectious disease ward: consult radiologist.

GU Studies: Preparation

1. None for IVP or cystogram unless specified by radiologist.
2. Catheter cystogram is the correct examination for assessing ureterovesical reflux in children with proven urinary tract infection.
3. Noncatheter cystogram is rarely indicated.

Arteriography, Venography, and Lymphography

Booking: make booking only after consultation with radiologist.

Preparation

1. Decision about anesthesia/sedation is made by radiologist and clinician (depends on patient's condition, urgency of need for examination, availability of anesthesia).
2. If local anesthesia and sedation to be used:
   a) Only clear liquids after midnight, and npo for the last 4 hr.
   b) Sedation, if necessary, will be given in Radiology.
3. *Exception.* Lymphangiography requires no preparation, but the patient *must return for radiographs the next day.*

Neuroradiology

1. Ventriculogram
2. Twist drill ventriculogram
3. Air study (AEG)
4. Cerebral angiography
5. Spinal angiography
6. Orbital venography
7. Positive contrast myelography
8. Air myelography
9. Computed tomogram (C.T.)

Booking

Made by Radiology in consultation with referring dr. Radiology will notify booking to ward the day before examination.

Preparation for Anesthesia/Sedation

Note. If problems arise, consult radiologist in charge. These rules are for guidance only and exceptional circumstances will be respected.

1. If *general anesthesia* is required:
   a) Radiology will notify Anaesthesia by 1300 hr the day before.
   b) If booking is made after 1300 hr, the dr ordering the study must call local 1601 to arrange for anesthetic services.
2. *Local anesthesia and sedation:*
   a) Only clear liquids after midnight, and npo for the last 4 hr.
   b) Sedation, if necessary, will be given in Radiology.

NUCLEAR MEDICINE

Filling out Nuclear Medicine Form
1. State requested study, provisional diagnosis, and patient's weight.
2. On reverse, summarize clinical findings briefly.
3. Dr must sign form.
4. Requisition must be addressographed on ward or in clinic *before* its receipt in Nuclear Medicine.

Note. If these are not done, the form will be returned to the ward.

Booking
A tentative booking may be given, but usually the patient is "on call".

Preparation
1. Schilling's test
2. Perchlorate flush test   } 8 hr fasting
3. Scan for Meckel's diverticulum
4. *Urine collection.* Unless it is part of the actual study, collection should be made before or 24 hr after a nuclear medicine procedure or injection with isotope. If this is not feasible, at least 6 hr must elapse before collection is started — **and the urine container(s) must be labelled "radioactive".**
5. *Sedation.* Children 3 mo to 5 yr of age may require sedation for some procedures. The Nuclear Medicine physician will order this (usually Nembutal, 5-6 mg/kg); the ward will be advised of the time to give it.

Routine Studies Available
1. Scans: brain, thyroid, lung, liver, spleen, bone, CSF, Meckel's diverticulum.
2. CSF-shunt patency.
3. Renal studies, including GFR measurement.
4. Pericardial effusion.
5. Radionuclide angiograms.

Normal Values
1. *Radioactive-iodine uptake* (RAIU): 2-hr uptake = 3 to 9%; 24-hour uptake = 6 to 26%.

2. *Perchlorate flush test:* >10% reduction in RAIU (p 84).
3. *T_3-suppression:* >50% reduction in RAIU.
4. *TSH-stimulation:* significant increase in uptake (varies with age, but usually 10% of RAIU; if original RAIU was <10%, a smaller increase may be significant) (p 50).
5. *Schilling's test:* >10% excretion in 24 hr.
6. *Protein-losing enteropathy:* <1% of isotope dose in stools in 96 hr.
7. *Rose Bengal study:* >85% of Rose Bengal dose in stool in 72 hr.
   <5% of dose = complete biliary obstruction.
   5-10%, result indefinite.
   <10% = ? congenital extrahepatic biliary atresia (surgical exploration needed).
   >10% = ? intrahepatic disease (needle biopsy of liver needed).
8. *Total blood volume:* in adult males, 73 ± 5 ml/kg; adult females, 67 ± 5 ml/kg.
9. *Red-cell volume:* in adult males, 30 ± 5 ml/kg; adult females, 24 ± 5 ml/kg.
10. *Plasma volume:* in adults, 43 ± 5 ml/kg.
11. *Erythrocyte survival* (^{51}Cr): T 1/2 = 25 ± 5 days.
12. *Ferrokinetics:* plasma clearance T 1/2 = 80-120 min; red-cell incorporation = 70-85% in 7-10 days.

GENETICS

Genetic Consultations

1. Diagnostic
2. Family history and pedigree analysis
3. Genetic counselling
   a) Inpatients: call Genetics Dept., preferably at least 2 days before patient is discharged.
   b) Outpatients: all appointments are made by Genetics.

Chromosomes: Routine Studies

Procedure
1. Send 1-3 ml heparinized blood, with requisition (completed by Resident) giving full details of indications for study.
2. Evenings/weekends: store blood in refrigerator; send to Genetics next day or Monday.

Main Indications
1. Suspected chromosomal syndromes; e.g., Down, trisomies 13 and 18.
2. Multiple congenital anomalies.
3. Suspected sex-chromosome anomalies.
4. Chromosome breakage syndromes; e.g., Fanconi anemia.

Note. In general, relatives of patients with chromosome problems are followed-up by Genetics Dept.

Special Procedures

1. **Skin biopsy for chromosome or biochemical studies**
   Order by arrangement with Genetics. In an emergency, when no arrangements have been made: take biopsy, and contact Genetics as soon as possible.

   IMPORTANT. Everything MUST be kept sterile.
   a) Clean area thoroughly with alcohol swabs.
   b) Inject 0.5 ml Xylocaine just below skin.
   c) With sterile forceps and scalpel, remove 2 mm of skin — must be deep enough to draw blood.
   d) Place skin biopsy in bottle of medium provided by Genetics (emergency supply in 7G) or a bottle of sterile saline.
   e) Refrigerate until delivery to Genetics.

2. **Philadelphia chromosome**

   Indication: chronic myeloid leukemia

   a) Send 0.5 ml of heparinized bone marrow, in vial of medium provided. (Before noon, Monday thru Friday)
   b) Also, send 2-3 ml of heparinized blood separately. (As early as possible, any day except Friday and weekends)

3. **Buccal smear:** taken by Genetics technician

   Indications:

   a) Suspected X-chromosome abnormalities; e.g., Turner, Klinefelter.
   b) Sex determination.

   Note. Anomaly in buccal smear, or finding of fluorescent Y body (below), must be confirmed with chromosome studies.

4. **Fluorescent Y body**

   Detects Y chromosome. Ordered only by Genetics, except in special circumstances to be discussed with geneticist.

5. **Dermatoglyphics**

   Indications:

   a) Routine if chromosome study ordered.
   b) Certain dysmorphic syndromes; e.g., Cornelia de Lange, Rubinstein–Taybi.
   c) Determination of twin zygosity.

IMMUNOLOGY

Recognition of Immunologic Problems

1. *Family history*
   - Early infant deaths
   - Frequent purulent infections
   - Collagen vascular disease

2. *Patient's history*
   a) Recurrent and/or persistent infection (bacterial, fungal, or viral).
   b) Severe reaction to smallpox vaccination (e.g., vaccinia gangrenosa, generalized vaccinia) or BCG.
   c) Severe reaction to varicella or rubeola or other virus infection.

3. *Physical examination*
   - Growth failure
   - Absence of tonsillar tissue; palpable lymph nodes
   - Evidence of successful smallpox or BCG vaccination
   - Evidence of recurrent infections (e.g., purulent otitis media, chronic gingivitis, scars of deep abscesses)
   - Persistent moniliasis.

Investigation

In all cases, initial examination of CBC including smear is essential: absolute no. of lymphocytes and granulocytes; cellular morphology.

Humoral Immunity

1. Serum protein electrophoresis.
2. Immunoelectrophoresis.
3. Quantitative immunoglobulins IgG, IgA, IgM.
4. Schick test.
5. Antibody titers; e.g., of isohemagglutinins, ASO, polio.
6. Secondary antibody response after booster injections; e.g., DPT.
7. Latex fixation test.
8. Bone-marrow or rectal biopsy, for plasma cells.
9. Immunofluorescence of peripheral blood, bone marrow, or lymph node, for immunoglobulin-bearing lymphocytes.

10. Detection of C_3 or F_C receptor on lymphocytes of peripheral blood, bone marrow, lymph node.
11. Lymph-node biopsy after antigenic stimulus.

Complement System

1. Total hemolytic complement.
2. $\beta_1 C$ globulin (C_3).
3. C_1 esterase inhibitor.
4. Complement-component titration; e.g., C_4 level.

Cellular Immunity

1. Absolute lymphocyte count.
2. Chest radiograph for thymic shadow.
3. Delayed hypersensitivity tests; e.g., monilia, strepto-kinase-streptodornase (SK-SD), PPD, mumps, phyto-hemagglutinin (PHA), dinitrochlorobenzene (DNCB).
4. Proliferation *in vitro*.
   a) nonspecific mitogens; e.g., PHA, concanavalin A, pokeweed.
   b) specific mitogens (e.g., *Candida,* SK-SD, PPD, tetanus toxoid).
   c) mixed leukocyte culture.
5. T-cell rosettes.
6. Lymphocytotoxic antibodies.
7. Lymphokine production; e.g., migration inhibition factor (MIF).
8. Lymph-node biopsy.
9. Skin-graft rejection.
10. Thymus biopsy.

Phagocytic System

1. Absolute neutrophil count.
2. Enzyme determinations, e.g., nitroblue tetrazolium (NBT), myeloperoxidase, glutathione peroxidase.
3. Phagocytosis and killing studies.
4. Chemotaxis; e.g., skin window (*in vivo*), Boyden chamber (*in vitro*).

Macrophage Function

1. Phagocytosis and killing studies.
2. F_c receptor.

Management

1. *Prevention*
   a) Patients with suspected cell-mediated immune (CMI) deficiency must be kept away from any source of infection, especially herpes, recent vaccination, chickenpox, measles, etc.
   b) Patients with CMI deficiency receive only irradiated blood or blood product (graft-vs-host reaction). Albumin may be given.

2. *For Hypogammaglobulinemia*
   a) Initial dose of gammaglobulins: 1.8 ml/kg, im.
   b) Maintenance: 0.6 ml/kg q4wk or more frequently, depending on symptomatic relief.

   Note. Administration of gammaglobulin is contraindicated in isolated IgA deficiency.

   c) An alternative method of therapy may be regular administration (q 3-4 wk) of plasma (10-20 ml/kg). *Plasma therapy carries the risk of transmission of hepatitis.*

TISSUE PATHOLOGY
Surgical Pathology

Routine Specimens
1. Place specimen (in 10% formalin) in refrigerator for pathology specimens (by directory, north of Elm St elevators, 3rd floor).
2. **Note.** If culture required for bacteria, fungus, or virus: send small portion of tissue, collected aseptically and unfixed, directly to Bacteriology and/or Virology.

Special Biopsies
Note. Schedule procedure as early in day as possible. Notify collection team (local 2268) in advance — they will pick up routine skin specimens and all special biopsy specimens except peroral intestinal and rectal.
1. *Peroral intestinal.* Place specimen in normal saline. Deliver to Pathology immediately (room 3102).
2. *Rectal.* Place in formalin; take to Pathology immediately (Histology, room 3102). After hours: place in formalin and treat as routine specimen.
3. *Skin.* If immunofluorescence or EM required, call ext 2268. Otherwise, treat as routine specimen.
4. *Brain.* Call Neuropathology (ext. 1661)

Quick Sections
1. *During day:* call 2268 (or 1661 for neuropathology).
2. *After hours:* consult staff pathologist on call (Locating, 2121).

Cytology
1. *Vaginal smear* for maturation index/tumor cells.
   a) Older child. Obtain specimen by vaginal or cervical scraping.
   b) Infant. Obtain by aspiration with eye-dropper. The specimen should be spread over an area no larger than a dime, to prevent drying before fixation.

   Note. Spray specimens immediately with Cytospray (to fix); the specimen must not dry.
   c) Put slide in appropriate envelope. Take with Histology form to Room 3102.

2. *Body fluids*
   a) Specimens should reach Pathology between 0830 and 1600 hr. (These fluids deteriorate rapidly and are unsatisfactory for diagnosis if not processed immediately)
   b) Place specimen in clear tube. Send immediately to cytotechnologist in Pathology.
   c) **Pleural tap.** If done after hours, dilute fluid with equal volume of 10% formalin (available in pathology specimen refrigerator, 3rd floor, Elm St wing). Leave specimen in this refrigerator.
   For EM: place small sample in glutaraldehyde (also in specimen refrigerator).

Special Investigations

1. Immunofluorescence
2. Electron microscopy
3. Biopsy of adrenals, pancreas, testes, kidney, liver

   } Consult pathologist; notify collection team. Call 2268 (1661 for Neuropathology)

4. Antinuclear factor and other autoantibodies: take 5 ml clotted blood to Pathology (specimen refrigerator, 3rd floor).
5. Chromosomes and tissue culture: see Genetics, p 86.

AUTOPSY SERVICE (p 18)

Consent

Requirement:

1. Consent signed by parent or legal guardian, and witnessed;
   or
2. Telegram stating: "I (name, relationship) consent to autopsy on (name of deceased)."; addressed to Medical Records, The Hospital for Sick Children.
3. A telephone or oral consent **is not acceptable.**

Restriction

1. If parents place any restriction in the consent, this must be strictly observed.
2. The present consent form does not permit removal of organs for transplant or for purposes other than diagnosis — informed special consent must be obtained for these.
3. If parents ask what to do after signing the consent, direct them to the undertaker of their choice to make the funeral arrangements.

Procedure

1. Make a brief summary of the history, for the patho-logist. State aspects requiring special attention.
2. All tubes, catheters, and drains must be left in place.
3. State name(s) of doctor(s) responsible for patient.
4. Call pathologist (staff or resident): discuss case and arrange a time that allows the resident responsible for patient's care during life to see at least part of autopsy.

Timing

1. a) Autopsies are begun 0830 and 1500 hr week-days and Saturdays, and between 0830 and 1200 hr Sundays and holidays.
   b) Immediate autopsy rarely justified (exception: cases of rare metabolic disorder). If autopsy wanted outside working hours, call staff patho-logist.
   c) If a pending autopsy is of special interest (e.g., renal or liver disease), both the clinical subspe-cialist and the pathologist subspecialist should be notified.
2. a) The gross autopsy takes 1½ to 2½ hr or more, depending on size of patient and complexity of dissection.
   b) The body can usually be released to undertaker about 3 hr after autopsy started. **Do not prom-ise** the family that the body will be released at a certain time.
3. a) Microscopic sections from general autopsy are usually available at the earliest on the third day after gross autopsy, but "overnight" or even in-stant diagnosis is available if necessary.
   b) Microscopic sections of brain take 17 to 21 days.
4. *Reports*
   a) Preliminary: available 24-48 hr after autopsy.
   b) Final (with detailed gross and microscopic de-scription of all viscera): available 1-2 mo after autopsy.

Sudden-infant-death Syndrome (SIDS; "Crib death")

1. Pathologists are available to explain SIDS to parents and can provide explanatory literature.
2. The pathologists can also refer newly-bereaved par-ents to a SIDS parents' group. See also p 95.

CHAPLAINCY SERVICE

Chaplains are available in the Hospital to provide emotional and spiritual support to patients and their families in times of stress or difficulty.

Office: (ext. 1498) Room 1403A, 1st floor Rotunda (Center wing). The chapel (interdenominational) is near the office in the Rotunda.

The Rev. Hugh Gemmell (home, 494-8414) is assisted by a Chaplain-Resident; in 1979-80 this is Chaplain John McKibbon (home, 690-6531). Denominational appointees are listed at the nursing stations.

A chaplain is usually on duty in the Emergency Dept from 7 to 11 p.m., 7 days a week. Also, chaplains engaged in training programs of clinical pastoral education are assigned to wards.

Family Counseling

Supportive care is provided for patients and/or their families when they are experiencing a crisis, such as awaiting the result of major surgery, in the ICU afterward, or after the diagnosis of a life-threatening disorder.

Terminally Ill Patient

Remember that the process of family bereavement usually starts some hours before the patient's death and is most acute at the time of death and during the next hour or so. It is most important that families are helped through this period. The chaplains are trained to function in a therapeutic manner throughout this time. They also provide support for staff who are closely involved in the patient's care.

"BEREAVED PARENTS OF ONTARIO"

This association, which is directed by Chaplain John McKibbon, is a self-help group, supported by a professional advisory committee, for persons who have experienced loss of a child within the family.

For further information, or for specific referrals of bereaved parents and families, call 928-0959 or contact the Director (ext. 1498; home, 690-6531).

SOCIAL WORK

Any staff member concerned that a patient's own or his family's life may be disrupted by the child's illness and hospitalization can make a referral to the Social Work Department. The social worker assigned will discuss the reasons for the referral with the doctor, and will assess the child's and family's strengths and help them use these in handling their problems. When necessary, the social worker contacts other services within the Hospital and in the community to help resolve these problems.

Individual social workers are available in:

Adolescent Clinic
Burns Service
Child Abuse Program
Child Development Center
Cystic Fibrosis Service
Diabetes Service
Emergency Dept
ENT & Hard-of-Hearing
    Service

Facial Treatment &
    Research Center
General Medical
    Outpatient Dept
Neonatology Service
Neurology Service
Neurosurgery Service
Dept of Psychiatry
Renal Dialysis &
    Transplant Unit

Referrals from other inpatient and outpatient areas: contact Social Work (ext 1471; off-hours, call Locating).

REHABILITATION MEDICINE

(PHYSIOTHERAPY & OCCUPATIONAL THERAPY)

Standing orders cover routine physiotherapy for thoracic surgery patients (see below).

Written medical referral is required for other services, which are provided for in- and outpatients: individual patient assessment, short-term treatment, and follow-up.

Family education can be provided, to facilitate home management and avoid complications. Recommendations can be made for follow-up in the community.

Hours of Service: Regular, 0830-1600 hr, Monday to Friday.

Physiotherapy for priority chest patients only:
1600-2100 hr, Mon. to Fri., and 0830-1600 hr, Sat. and Sun.

PHYSIOTHERAPY

Respiratory Care

1. *Surgical*
    a) Standing orders: routine exercises for thoracic surgery patients (inspiratory breathing, upper torso and arms, and posture).
    b) Pre- and postoperative assessment.
    c) Postoperative pulmonary complications.
2. *Medical*
    Complete services for patients with cystic fibrosis, pneumonia, bronchiectasis, asthma.
3. *Musculoskeletal*
    Complete services for patients with orthopedic conditions, burns, and specific hand problems.

OCCUPATIONAL THERAPY

1. *Developmental Program*
    For infants and children with developmental delay, failure-to-thrive, and CNS-related problems.

    Assessment, treatment, and follow-up, of gross and fine motor and adaptive skills, and activities of daily living (including oral motor feeding problems related to CNS damage).

2. *Physical Dysfunction*
   Specific retraining of upper extremity and functional activities, for patients with burns, musculoskeletal, and neurologic problems.

3. *Sensory Integration*
   For children with learning disabilities specific to gross and fine motor problems (*e.g.,* clumsiness). Includes liaison with school personnel, to help maximize learning potential in the classroom.

4. *Interpersonal Relationships*
   Individual and/or group involvement for psychosocially dysfunctioning patients and their parents.

COMBINED SERVICES

1. *Neurodevelopmental Therapy*
   For patients with sensorimotor dysfunction. Includes specific "handling" techniques to inhibit abnormal patterns of movement and facilitate more-normal ones.

2. *Splinting and Equipment*
   Consultation on design of resting/functional splints and adaptive equipment for patients with limb problems. Family education and follow-up included.

OPHTHALMOLOGY

Dilating the Pupil for Funduscopy
1. **Dilate rapidly** using:
   a) 0.5-1.0% tropicamide; **or**
   b) 0.5-1% cyclopentolate ophthalmic solution; **or**
   c) 2.5% Neo-Synephrine ophthalmic solution.
2. **Do not use** atropine (too long-lasting).

Antibiotics for Treating Eye Infections
1. *Conjunctivitis or blepharitis,* acute or chronic
   a) Gentamicin (p 412)
   b) Neosporin ophthalmic ointment or solution
   c) 10% sodium sulfacetamide ophthalmic ointment or solution.
2. *Intra-ocular infections*
   a) Give appropriate antibiotics in consultation with ophthalmologist.
   b) Do not patch infected eyes.
   c) Do not instill steroids into infected eyes.

Strabismus
1. As soon as suspected, refer child to ophthalmologist.
2. Treatment is by occlusion, glasses, or surgery, as early as 6 mo of age.
3. **Note.** A definite strabismus in infancy may indicate serious disease (e.g., retinoblastoma).
4. Patients who have strabismus appear to be at increased risk for malignant hyperthermia during anesthesia.

Emergency Eye Treatment

Burns (acid or lye)
1. Irrigate profusely with water immediately.
2. Evert upper lid; draw lower lid down, to irrigate conjunctival sac and foreign matter.
3. Notify Ophthalmology *stat.*

Foreign Bodies
1. In all cases: evert upper lid, and draw lower lid down.
2. FB not on cornea: remove with dampened gauze wick.

3. FB on cornea: apply topical anesthetic — use propara-caine HC1 (Ophthaine); remove FB with spud; then patch eye.
4. If FB struck eye with force, order radiograph of orbit *stat.*

Hyphema (blood in anterior chamber)
1. Complete bed rest.
2. Patch both eyes.
3. Look for lacerations of lids.
4. Rule out:
   a) perforation of globe
   b) intra-ocular FB(s)
   c) intra-ocular hemorrhage(s)
   d) fracture(s) of orbital walls.
5. Consult Ophthalmology.

Laceration of Lid, Cornea, or Globe
1. Do not manipulate eyelid excessively.
2. If laceration(s) of lid margin: suspect laceration(s) of globe or cornea.
3. Do not put any ointment or drops in eye.
4. Apply binocular bandages; (transfer child to hospital and) obtain Ophthalmology consult.

Abrasion of Cornea
1. Suspect if eye painful, red, tearful.
2. In many cases, sensation of FB.
3. Differentiation by fluorescein test: abrasion stains yellow-green.
4. Treatment: antibiotic drops, and patch over closed eye for 24 hr.
5. Obtain Ophthalmology consult if in doubt.

CAUTION: never patch an eye that has an insensitive cornea — danger of severe corneal abrasion and complications if lids open under patch.

Blocked Tear Duct
1. Massage the tear sac.
2. Instill antibacterial agents; e.g., 10% sulfacetamide sodium (Sodium Sulamyd) ointment.
3. If unimproved in 2-3 mo, consult Ophthalmology.
4. **Note.** Tearing is a common sign of congenital glaucoma.

Acute Glaucoma

Congenital. Eye is enlarged, and in many cases is tearful and photosensitive. Cornea may be hazy.
Refer to Ophthalmology.

Acquired. Eye acutely red and painful. Vision may be decreased.
Refer to Ophthalmology.

Absent Red Reflex by Ophthalmoscopy

Differential Diagnosis
1. Suspect tumor
2. Endophthalmitis } Refer to Ophthalmology
3. Congenital malformation

OTOLARYNGOLOGY

Adenotonsillectomy

1. Approx. 10% of children experience significant morbidity with upper respiratory tract infections and will benefit from adenoid and tonsil surgery.
2. Adenoid tissue is usually removed if tonsillectomy indicated.
3. Approx. 15% of children having surgery will need adenoidectomy only.

Indications for Adenotonsillectomy

Definite indications
1. Quinsy or peritonsillar abscess: 1 episode.
2. Tonsillitis (enlarged, inflamed, edematous tonsils, and cervical adenitis):
   a) With febrile convulsions.
   b) Recurrent tonsillitis:
      — under 7 yr of age: 5 episodes in 1 yr, or 3/yr for 2 yr
      — over 7 yr of age: 3 episodes/yr for 2 yr.

Possible indications
1. Strep tonsillitis with rheumatic fever in patients who comply poorly with prophylaxis.
2. Recurrent suppurative otitis media.
3. Possible malignancy (unilateral hypertrophy).
4. Dysphagia.
5. Bleeding, airway obstruction; diphtheria carrier; abnormal dental development with overbite; halitosis.

Indications for Adenoidectomy

1. Nasal obstruction
2. Secretory otitis media
3. Adenoiditis
4. Chronic sinusitis
5. **Rare, urgent:**
   a) Nasal obstruction by adenoids in the newborn.
   b) Cor pulmonale secondary to nasal obstruction.

Hemorrhage after Adenotonsillectomy

A. *Primary:* within 24 hr postop.
B. *Secondary:* between days 5 and 8 postop.
   a) Giving ASA in postop period significantly increases risk of secondary hemorrhage.
   b) Admit patient for at least 1 day for observation.

A or B: Clot usually in nasopharynx or tonsillar fossa.
- a) Make a paste of bismuth subgallate in epinephrine (1:1000) and apply it to pack.
- b) Remove clot, and insert pack in nasopharynx or tonsillar fossa for 10 min; also, post-nasal pack may be required.
- c) Check Hb immediately and again at 8 hr after control of hemorrhage (transfusion may be indicated).
- d) Start antibiotic therapy (p 406).

Foreign Bodies (FB)

Ear
Visualize with head mirror and attempt removal.
1. Soft material: use loop.
2. Hard, smooth object: use hook or loop.
3. Insect: kill it before removal, by instilling rubbing alcohol.
4. General syringing with warm water is helpful — but do not syringe if FB is vegetable matter (it may swell).

Nose
FB is the commonest cause of unilateral nasal discharge.
1. Visualize with head mirror or light.
2. Anesthetize nasal mucosa, and shrink it by inserting cotton packs soaked with 1:5 soln of epinephrine 1:1000 and cocaine 5%.
3. Suction off discharge surrounding FB.
4. Attempt removal.
   - a) Soft material (e.g., paper, cotton): use forceps.
   - b) Solid object: use a hook.

Larynx, Tracheobronchial Tree, and Esophagus
Note
1. Not all FB present as acute problems.
2. Keep possibility of FB in mind when assessing any child who has enigmatic chronic chest disease and dysphagia.

Diagnosis of FB aspiration established by:
1. History: choking cyanotic episode.
2. Examination: stridor or wheeze, unequal expansion of chest, decreased air entry unilaterally.

3. Radiology:
   a) Order inspiratory and expiratory chest films —
      - collapse suggests complete obstruction
      - look for FB shadow in trachea
      - hyperinflation suggests ball-valve obstruction.
   b) Fluoroscopy: unequal diaphragmatic movement.

Diagnosis of FB in esophagus
1. History: ingestion, dysphagia, regurgitation, vomiting, drooling.
2. Examination: usually nil abnormal; stridor if trachea compressed.
3. Radiology: AP and lateral views reveal position and number of FB only if radio-opaque.

Treatment
1. Remove FB endoscopically under general anesthesia in ENT OR.
2. FB in larynx may cause complete obstruction and require urgent bronchoscopy in Emergency Dept.
   - If bronchoscopist not immediately available, endotracheal intubation may be life-saving.
3. Stab tracheotomy = last resort. Use only for laryngeal/pharyngeal obstruction.

Acute Suppurative Otitis Media

Treatment
1. Systemic antibiotic therapy (p 406), po, x 10 days:
   a) Under 4 yr: amoxycillin: or, if allergy to penicillin: trimethoprim—sulfamethoxazole (TMP: SMX), or erythromycin.
   b) Over 4 yr, penicillin or amoxycillin; or, if allergy to penicillin, erythromycin, sulfamethoxazole, or trimethoprim.
2. Decongestants, local and systemic, x 5 days, if indicated.
3. Analgesics and antipyretics
4. *Myringotomy only if:*
   a) severe pain — **immediately**
   b) bulging drum and/or pain after 48-72 hr of therapy
   c) otitis media with complication (meningitis, facial paralysis)
   d) residual serous otitis 3-4 wk after acute otitis despite adequate medical therapy.
5. If discharge persists after 1 wk of adequate therapy: obtain specimens from deep in external canal (use toothpick culture sticks), for culture and sensitivity.

6. Mastoid radiographs not routine; usually obtained only if disease present for 3 wk or if acute mastoiditis present (surgery required if air-cell coalescence).
7. If symptoms or discharge persist beyond 1 wk: request ENT consult.

Mastoiditis

1. If subperiosteal abscess formation: surgical drainage usually required.
2. If erythema behind ear and no radiographic evidence of coalescence: give ampicillin iv, 400 mg/kg/day, divided q6h.

Serous Otitis Media

Commonest cause of hearing-loss in children.

In children, common accompaniment of adenoid hypertrophy, allergies, cleft palate, and cystic fibrosis.

Serous otitis media, inadequately treated, can delay onset of speech, cause major learning problems, and lead to chronic ear disease.

Treatment

Medical: first choice, unless —
    a) Symptoms present >6 mo at time of diagnosis.
    b) Bilateral hearing loss >30 db.
    c) Behavior or speech problem secondary to hearing loss.
1. Decongestants, systemic and local, for 3 wk.
2. Antibiotics po x 2 wk if regional infection.
3. Auto-insufflation — Valsalva maneuver.

Surgical: as above, and if medical management fails.

Assess each patient individually for requisite surgical procedure — e.g.:
1. Adenoidectomy or adenotonsillectomy with myringotomy
    — with or without insertion of middle-ear ventilation tubes.
2. Insertion of ventilation tube only.

Traumatic Perforation of Tympanic Membrane

Notify ENT resident immediately — emergency exploration and repair may be required.

External Otitis

Treatment

1. Debridement: gently, remove infective and epithelial debris from ear canal (by wet swabbing, gentle irrigation, or suctioning).
2. Topical antibiotic drops for up to 10 days only (longer may produce an allergic reaction).
   - Do not apply ointments (they prevent escape of moisture and heat, causing maceration of skin of ear canal).
3. If ear canal occluded by circumferential inflammatory edema: aluminum acetate 1% hygroscopic. Insert moist cotton wick into ear canal; keep it wet with this solution until canal has expanded sufficiently to permit debridement after 1-2 days. Then use topical antibiotic drops.
4. If periauricular swelling, regional adenopathy, signs of systemic infection: systemic antibiotic therapy.
5. Analgesics and sedatives.
6. If difficulty differentiating from furuncle of ear canal or mastoiditis with subperiosteal abscess formation: request ENT consult.

Facial Nerve Paralysis (VIIth Nerve)

Fairly common in children; due to Bell's palsy, trauma, acute otitis media, aural neoplasm, intracranial tumor.

Bell's palsy does not always resolve spontaneously in children.

Investigation may include:
- audiogram
- impedance studies
- nerve-conduction tests
- mastoid tomograms
- Schirmer's test
- salivary-secretion tests.

Therapy

1. Bell's palsy: refer child to ENT. (Steroid therapy is useful.)
2. Treat condition causing paralysis.
   - Transtemporal (mastoid) decompression of the facial nerve may be needed.

Epistaxis

Bleeding is usually from Little's area.

It is commoner during acute URI, allergy seasons, and in prodromal phases of exanthems.

Management

1. Facilitated by sedation prn (codeine 1 mg/kg/im), visualization (head mirror or light), and suction.
2. Control bleeding with pressure and cotton pledgets moistened with 1 part epinephrine (1:1000) in 5 parts cocaine (5%).
3. Then cauterize with silver nitrate stick behind bleeding point on vessel.
4. Pack nostrils (Oxycel, Gelfoam, Vaseline gauze) **only if cautery ineffective.**
5. If bleeding persistent, recurrent, or originating posteriorly: request ENT consult.
6. **Note.** Persistent bleeding may (rarely) represent clotting defect.
7. Children with blood dyscrasias should not have cautery with silver nitrate. Control bleeding with Oxycel gauze and pressure.

Fractured Nose

1. Examine nose for septal hematoma (causes major nasal obstruction and may result in late nasal deformity).
2. Radiograph may aid diagnosis.
3. Reduce deformity if no swelling, either early (within 2 to 3 hr of injury) or late (5 to 10 days after injury).
4. All cases from Emergency Dept with no ENT consultation: refer to ENT Clinic for 3-4 day follow-up to check for late septal hematoma, abscess formation, or deformity.

Corrosive Burns of Upper GI Tract

1. Observe for minimum of 6 hr.
2. Bear in mind:
   a) Esophagus may be damaged by the time the child arrives in Emergency.
   b) Degree of visible burns in mouth and pharynx may not be indicative of degree of esophageal involvement.

Management (see p 484)
1. Have an assistant notify ENT immediately.
2. Determine nature (acid/alkali/other) and form (solid or liquid) of ingested material.
3. **Do not** give emetic.
   Do not induce vomiting; **do not** attempt gastric lavage.
4. Promote ingestion of appropriate fluids:
   a) 1-5 yr: 1 to 2 cups. >5 yr, up to 1 qt.
   b) If alkali ingested: give milk, water, citrus fruit juices, dilute vinegar.
   c) If acid ingested: give milk, water, milk of magnesia (1 Tbsp to 1 cup of water), aluminum hydroxide gel.
   d) If bleach ingested: give water or milk.
5. Observe for respiratory distress secondary to laryngeal involvement (hoarseness, stridor, dyspnea).
6. Observe for shock: monitor vital signs.
   a) If shock developing, start iv infusion of fluids.
   b) Severe chest and abdominal pain are ominous signs — may be indicative of visceral perforation.

Note
1. Esophagoscopy is usually performed after oral burns improve (3-5 days), to assess extent of esophageal burn.
2. Esophageal stricture develops in approx. 15% of cases.

DENTISTRY

DENTAL TRAUMA

Principle

Displacement of deciduous teeth interferes with development and eruption of adjacent permanent teeth. Interference with blood supply results in pulpal necrosis (indicated by blue-black discoloration of crown) and infection. After age 20 mo, space-preservation is unnecessary in the anterior segment but imperative in the posterior segments of the deciduous dental arch.

Initial Assessment

1. Determine
    a) time of accident
    b) age of patient
    c) whether tooth/teeth deciduous or permanent
    d) whether tooth/teeth loose, out, or fractured, and whether dental pulp is visible.
2. In all cases, call dental resident.

Loosened/Displaced Anterior Teeth

A. Deciduous
Treatment: Remove the injured tooth.

B. Permanent
Treatment
1. Call dental resident immediately (who will immobilize tooth with acrylic splint, Risdon arch wires, or interdental ligation).
2. Every 4-6 wk, examine for signs of pulpal necrosis due to interference with neurovascular supply (less likely in younger children, in whom root-canal opening is relatively large).

    If necrosis develops: extirpation of the pulpal tissue, root-canal sterilization and obliteration are indicated.

Fractured Permanent Anterior Teeth

1. If temperature-sensitive, with/without pulp-exposure: should be treated by dentist on call.
2. Asymptomatic: should be referred to private dentist.

Avulsed Teeth

A. *Deciduous*

1. No treatment – unless:
2. If tooth is not found: radiograph for remnants in jaw, and chest film if indicated
3. Never re-implant.

B. *Permanent Teeth*

1. Ask patient to bring tooth – *kept moist.*
2. Call dentist, who will re-implant and immobilize.
3. Prognosis: varies with length of time tooth has been out – Eventually, tooth will be resorbed, but implantation will provide interim treatment until adult prosthetic replacement is possible.

Dental Pain

1. *Hyperemia:*
   Simple hyperemia due to trauma or large restorations.
   - Call dental resident
   - *Treatment:* Remove source of irritation.
2. *Pulpitis due to dental caries:*
   a) Serous pulpitis: tooth is sensitive to cold. Heat will relieve pain.
   b) Suppurative pulpitis: tooth sensitive to heat. Cold may relieve pain.
   - Call dental resident.
   - *Treatment:* Pulpectomy.
3. *Pulpal necrosis with abscess:*
   May occur without facial swelling or systemic signs.
   a) Call dental resident (who will decide which tooth is involved – by brief history, clinical examination, radiography).
   b) Give analgesics for pain (p 272).
   c) Give ASA for fever (p 418).
   d) Give systemic antibiotic (p 406).
   e) *Offending tooth should be removed stat,* to prevent continuing source of infection.
   - Re-examine within 24 hr.
4. *Periodontal abscess.*
   - Call dental resident
   - Treatment: Systemic antibiotic and surgical drainage, if necessary.

Dental Postoperative Hemorrhage

Bleeding longer than 4 hr or delayed recurrent bleeding.

1. Obtain consultation with dental resident on call.
2. Apply pressure: have the patient bite firmly on a folded 2" x 2" gauze pack positioned over the socket.
    — Check in 30 min for hemostasis.
3. Local infiltration of 2% Xylocaine with epinephrine 1:50,000
4. Try topical hemostatic agents (e.g., tannic acid) if necessary.
5. If necessary:
    a) Pack socket with Gelfoam gauze
    b) Suture closed under local anesthetic, then place a 2" x 2" gauze pack over this and apply pressure as in no. 2.

Temporo-mandibular Joint Pain

1. *Fractures*
    Treatment: Call Plastic Surgery.
2. *Dislocation of mandibular condyle*
    Treatment: Reduce dislocation.
3. *Trismus* — "locking" of mandible in open/closed position.
    Treatment: Eliminate muscle spasm, by massage and manipulation of mandible.
4. *Recurring episodes of pain, clicking, crepitis, trismus:*
    Treatment: Not an emergency. Refer to Dentistry for investigation.

INFECTIONS OF THE ORAL MUCOSA

Acute Herpetic Gingivo-stomatitis (Herpes Simplex)

Usually at age 1-3 yr. Rapid onset, dramatic pain, profuse salivation, halitosis, and fever. Red to grey-yellow membranous gingivitis with scattered ulcers on tongue and labial buccal mucous membrane.

Treatment (nonspecific):
1. Topical antiseptics (Dequadin)
2. Topical anesthetics (benzocaine)
3. ASA for fever (p 418).

4.   Idoxuridine 1% solution (Herpes Liquefilm) in water, applied every 2-3 waking hr for 5 days, may shorten duration of signs and symptoms.
5.   Systemic antibiotic therapy if necessary for secondary infection.

Acute Ulcerative Gingivitis
(Vincent's Angina)

Although associated with *Fusobact. fusiforme* and *Spirochaeta vincenti,* there is no positive evidence that it is contagious.

Rare under the age of 12.

Presents as gingival soreness and bleeding, and punched-out grey ulcers at tips of gingival papillae. Associated with poor oral hygiene.

Treatment
1.   *Acute phase:*
     a)   Irrigate with warm saline or dilute hydrogen peroxide.
     b)   Mouth wash: one capsule (250 mg) of chlortetracycline in 2 Tbsp of warm water qid for 3 days.
     c)   Systemic antibiotics for fever, malaise, and lymphadenopathy.
     d)   Metronidazole (Flagyl), 200 mg po tid for 7 days (p 415).
2.   *Residual phase:* institute optimal oral hygiene.
     —   Eliminate all dental and gingival sources of infection.

Thrush (Oral Moniliasis)

Due to *Candida albicans* infection and generally lowered tissue resistance, or antibiotic suppression of normal oral flora.

Superficial creamy-white crusted patches on mildly hyperemic mucous membranes of cheek, lips, tongue. The patches bleed when removed.

Diagnosis confirmed by smear or culture.

Treatment (local)
1.   Apply nystatin (p 415) in water or honey (100,000 U/ml), several times a day.

2. Also, amphotericin B lozenges (10 mg) sucked 4 times a day are effective.
3. 1% Gentian violet applications can be used.

PREVENTIVE DENTISTRY

Water Fluoridation
Natural or artifically fluoridated (1 ppm) drinking water for first 12 yr of life reduces caries by 60%. No proven contraindications exist for the ingestion of water containing fluorides at this level. Therefore, the fluoridation of all municipal water supplies where fluorides do not occur naturally is an essential public health objective.

Fluoride Supplements
Daily dietary supplements of sodium fluoride are beneficial for young children living in areas where community fluoridation programs are not feasible. However, as the supplement must be taken daily from infancy to 12 yr to be beneficial, strong parental motivation is essential. In addition, the dosage must be adjusted to complement the fluoride concentration occurring naturally in the drinking water.

Proprietary vitamin and sodium fluoride combinations are not recommended, because the dosage cannot be adjusted. Indiscriminate dosages could result in unesthetic dental fluorosis.

Adjusted Allowance of Water Fluoride for 3-year-old Child*

ppm	Sodium fluoride (mg/day)	Provides fluoride ion (mg/day)
0.0	2.2	1.0
0.2	1.8	0.8
0.4	1.3	0.6
0.6	0.9	0.4

*Halve the dose for child between 2 and 3 yr of age. Usefulness of fluorides for expectant mothers is questionable.

Topical Application of Fluorides
1. Semi-annual application of stannous fluoride solutions to dental surfaces inhibits caries.
2. Dentifrices containing stannous fluoride or sodium monofluorophosphate significantly prevent caries.

115

FLUID AND ELECTROLYTE THERAPY
GENERAL INFORMATION
Atomic Weights/Valence

Aluminum (Al)	26.9/3	Lead (Pb)	207.21/2,4
Barium (Ba)	137.4/2	Lithium (Li)	7/1
Calcium (Ca)	40.0/2	Magnesium (Mg)	24.3/2
Carbon (C)	12.0/2	Mercury (Hg)	200.6/1,2
Chlorine (Cl)	35.5/1	Nitrogen (N)	14.0/3
Copper (Cu)	63.6/1,2	Oxygen (O)	16.0/2
Fluorine (F)	19.0/1	Phosphorus (P)	31.0/3,5
Gold (Au)	197.0/1,3	Potassium (K)	39.1/1
Helium (He)	4.0/0	Silver (Ag)	107.9/1
Hydrogen (H)	1.0/1	Sodium (Na)	23.0/1
Iodine (I)	126.9/1	Sulphur (S)	32.1/2,4,6
Iron (Fe)	55.9/2,3	Zinc (Zn)	65.4/2

Definitions

1. Milliequivalent (mEq) = measurement of the electrical charge contributed by an ion

$$1 \text{ mEq of an ion} = \frac{\text{atomic wt (mg)}}{\text{valence}}$$

$$(\text{e.g., 1 mEq Ca} = \frac{40 \text{ mg}}{2} = 20 \text{ mg})$$

$$\text{mEq/liter} = \frac{\text{mg/dl x 10 x valence}}{\text{atomic weight}}$$

2. Millimole (mmol) = molecular weight of a substance (mg) (e.g., 1 mmol NaCl = 23 + 35.5 = 58.5 mg). For univalent ions 1 mmol = 1mEq; divalent ions 1 mmol = 2 mEq.

3. Milliosmole (mOsm) = mmol x number of particles produced by dissociation (e.g., 1 mOsm $CaCl_2$ = 1 mmol $CaCl_2$ x 3; 1 mOsm glucose = 1 mmol x 1)

4. Milliosmolarity (mOsm/kg) = no. of mOsm/kg solvent (e.g., plasma = 280-300 mOsm/kg)

Body Compartments

ECF = extracellular fluid
ICF = intracellular fluid
ISF = interstitial fluid

PV = plasma volume
TBW = total body water

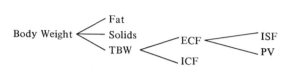

Average Normal Values for Various Compartments
(liters/kg)

	Newborn	Child	Adult Male	Adult Female
TBW	0.75	0.65	0.60	0.55
ICF	0.40	0.40	0.40	0.40
ECF	0.35	0.25	0.20	0.15
Blood volume	0.07-0.08	0.07-0.08	0.07-0.08	0.07-0.08

Caloric Expenditure

Body wt (kg)	*kcal/kg
3-10	110
>10-20	1000 + (50 for each kg > 10 kg)
>20	1500 + (20 for each kg > 20 kg)

*1 kcal (Cal) = 4.184 kjoules (kJ)

Components of Normal Water Requirements

Output	Water required (ml/100 kcal expended)
Insensible water loss (lungs 15 ml, skin 30 ml)	45
Sweat	0 to 25
Urine	50 to 75
Stool water	5 to 10
'Hidden' expenditure: water of oxidation	12
Normal activity (without sweating)	100

Note: Each C° of fever increases metabolic rate, and thus water output, by 12%.

Normal Maintenance Requirements

	per 100 kcal expended	per m^2
Water	100 – 125 ml	1500 ml
Na	2.5 mEq	60 mEq
K	2.5 mEq	50 mEq
Cl	5.0 mEq	100 mEq
Dextrose	5 g	150 g

Approximate Electrolyte Composition of Gastrointestinal Fluids (mEq/liter)

Fluid	H^+	Na^+	K^+	Cl^-	HCO_3^-
Gastric	80	40	20	150	0
Small-intestinal	0	130	20	120	30
Pancreatic	0	135	15	100	50
Diarrheal	0	40	40	40	40

ACUTE DEHYDRATION

A. History: determine duration and severity of the symptoms (vomiting, diarrhea, fever, polyuria).

B. Physical findings

Signs of Dehydration*

Approx. degree of isotonic dehydration	≤1 yr	>1 yr	Clinical signs
Minimal	<5%	<3%	thirst; mild·oliguria
Mild	5%	3%	dry mucous membranes, axilla, groin; tachycardia
Moderate	10%	6%	loss of skin turgor; soft, sunken eyeballs, sunken fontanels
Severe	15%	9%	CNS changes, poor peripheral circulation, low BP, fever

*adapted from Cockington, RA, et al.
Med J Aust 1:957-63, 1977.

C. General Management:

1. Determine acute weight loss from actual weights *and/or*
2. Clinically, assess percentage loss of total body wt.
3. Determine degree of dehydration:

	Amount of Water Loss (ml/kg body wt)	
	Infant	Adult
Mild (minimal signs)	50	30
Moderate (definite signs)	100	60
Severe (shock)	150	90

4. Define type of dehydration, by measuring serum Na or osmolality: estimated serum osmolality =

$$2\,[\text{Na}] + \frac{\text{glucose}}{18} + \frac{\text{BUN}}{3}$$

	Na^+ (mEq/liter)	Osmolality (mOsm/kg)
Isotonic	130 to 150	280 to 300
Hypertonic	>150	high
Hypotonic	<130	low

Water and Electrolyte Deficit in Moderate and Severe Dehydration

	Water (ml/kg)	each of Na^+ and K^+ (mEq/kg)
Isotonic	100 − 150	7 − 11
Hypertonic	120 − 170	2 − 5
Hypotonic	40 − 80	10 − 14

5. Measure serum K^+.
   Serum K^+ does not accurately reflect deficit in total body K^+; e.g., in metabolic acidosis, serum K^+ may be normal or high even when total body K^+ is low.

6. Determine acid−base status (p 124).

D. **General Principles of Treatment of Dehydration**

Phase	*Time*	
I	0 − 2 hr	Restore blood volume (i.e., treat shock).
II	2 − 24 hr	a) Partly correct water deficit. b) Correct remaining Na^+ deficit. (Subtract the Na^+ used in Phase I). c) Partly correct acid−base imbalance. d) Give maintenance requirement.
III	1 − 4 days	a) Replace remaining water deficit. b) Start K^+ repletion after child has voided. c) Give maintenance requirements.
IV	4 days to 1 − 3 wk	Restore body fat and protein.

E.   **Fluid Therapy**

Isotonic Dehydration

Phase I ("O" – 2 hr)
Give isotonic NaCl or lactated Ringer's solution, 20-30 ml/kg body wt. If dehydration severe, give plasma or blood (10-20 ml/kg).

Phase II (2-24 hr)
1.   Deficit fluid – give half to two-thirds of the deficit as "2/3:1/3" solution.
2.   Maintenance fluid – give 100 ml/kg/24 hr as "2/3:1/3" solution.
3.   Replace continuing losses (from stools, vomit, etc.) as required.
4.   If serum K^+ is low and renal function adequate, begin K^+ replacement (see Phase III).

Phase III (1-4 days)
1.   Fluid deficit – give remaining one-third to half of deficit fluid as "2/3:1/3" solution.
2.   Maintenance fluids – give 100 ml/kg as "2/3:1/3" solution.
3.   If renal function adequate, start K^+ replacement, 3-4 mEq/kg/day.

Note: "2/3:1/3" solution is used both for maintenance and to replace deficit fluid.

Hypotonic Dehydration
(Serum Na^+ <130 mEq/liter)

1.   Fluid therapy as for isotonic dehydration **plus**
2.   Correct hyponatremia
      a)   Calculate amount of Na^+ needed to bring serum Na^+ to normal:
            mEq of Na^+ required =
            normal serum Na^+ – observed serum Na^+
            x total body water (liters/kg: see p 117) x body wt (kg)
            (e.g., mEq Na^+ = (135 – 125) x 0.65 x body wt [kg]).
      b)   Give this additional Na^+ during first day (Phase II).
      c)   If patient symptomatic (e.g., convulsions) give N saline (or 3% NaCl).
      d)   Increase serum Na^+ by no more than 10 mEq/liter/hr.
      e)   Reassess frequently until serum is isotonic.

121

Hypertonic Dehydration
(Serum Na >150 mEq/liter)

Patient may have CNS disturbances: e.g., intracerebral and subdural hemorrhages.

1. Avoid rapid return of serum Na^+ to normal.
2. Decrease serum Na^+ ≤10 mEq/day by replacing fluid deficit over 2–3 days.
3. Calculate the water load (L_{H_2O}) necessary to produce a predictable fall in serum Na, using the formula:

$$L_{H_2O} = \frac{TBW_1 \, ([Na^+_1] - [Na^+_2])}{(Na^+_2)}$$

where TBW_1 = present total body water
(liters/kg; p 117)

(Na^+_1) = observed serum Na concentration
(mEq/liter)

(Na^+_2) = normal serum Na concentration
(mEq/liter)

e.g., $L_{H_2O} = \dfrac{0.65 \, (160 - 140)}{(140)}$

= 0.093 liter/kg body wt.

4. Maintenance: give 75 ml/kg/day (not 100 ml/kg/day)*
   - Less urine is excreted because of the hypertonic serum and increased ADH secretion.
5. Give only half the 'fluid deficit'.*
6. When metabolic acidosis is a problem, use 5% D/W with 30 mEq of $NaHCO_3$ per liter solution.
7. Complications:
   - Hyperglycemia and/or hypocalcemia, especially when hypokalemia present
     i) consider prophylaxis with Ca^{++} (10 ml of 10% Ca gluconate/500 ml iv solution)
     ii) do not mix Ca^{++} with a $NaHCO_3$ solution.
     iii) usually, insulin is not required.

*Note. Use solution containing 30-35 mEq/liter of Na^+ (e.g., 5% dextrose in 0.2% NaCl) for deficit and maintenance requirements; monitor rate of rehydration carefully.

122

F. **Electrolyte Imbalance**

Hyponatremia

Hyponatremia (Na^+ <130 mEq/liter) is usually secondary to loss of Na^+ (depletion) or gain of water (dilution).

Na^+ Depletion (Volume Contraction)

1. Features of dehydration (cool extremities, low BP, thirst, and CNS changes)
2. Causes: GI fluid loss, sweat (especially in patients who have cystic fibrosis; p 179), chronic renal disease (p 230), adrenal insufficiency (p 246), diuretics.
3. Treatment: correct Na^+ deficit (see hypotonic dehydration, p 121).

Acute Dilutional Hyponatremia
(Normal or Increased Volume)

1. Features of water intoxication (irritability, hyperactivity, somnolence, convulsions).
2. Causes
    a) Excessive iv administration of fluid without Na^+ (e.g., 5% dextrose/water).
    b) Failure to excrete water, due to various factors (drugs such as ADH, morphine), postoperative complications
    c) Compulsive water drinking.
3. Treatment: restrict fluid.
    a) If symptomatic, patient *may* require hypertonic saline.
    b) Increase serum Na^+ by no more than 10 mEq/liter/hr.
    c) Reassess until serum is isotonic.

Chronic Dilutional Hyponatremia;
Inappropriate ADH Syndrome (p 136)
(Normal or Increased Blood Volume)

1. Major features: hyponatremia, inappropriately concentrated urine, urine Na^+ loss; *no evidence* of dehydration, renal, or adrenal impairment.
2. Causes: CNS conditions (inflammation, trauma, neoplasm), lung disease, drugs, neonatal asphyxia, etc.

3. Treatment: fluid restriction sufficient to cause weight loss.
   a) If signs of water intoxication, give normal (or hypertonic) saline.
   b) Increase serum Na^+ by no more than 10 mEq/liter.
   c) Reassess frequently until serum is isotonic.

Hyponatremia with Edema
1. Causes: congestive heart failure, cirrhosis, nephrotic syndrome.
   Usually, total body Na^+ is increased and secondary hyperaldosteronism is present.
2. Treatment: Individualized Na^+ and fluid restriction, and diuretics.

"Artifactual" Hyponatremia
Seen in conditions in which solute accumulates in the extracellular fluid (e.g., hyperlipidemia, hyperglycemia).

Hypernatremia
(Na^+ >150 mEq/liter)

Causes
1. Limited intake of water (as in infant not given enough fluid)
2. Excessive water loss by evaporation (high temperature, tachypnea)
3. Excessive water loss by excretion (diarrhea, diabetes insipidus)
4. Salt loading (diet too high in Na or protein for the clinical condition)
5. Disorder of thirst center.

Treatment: as for hypertonic dehydration (p 122).

G. **Acid–Base Assessment.** pp 191, 243, 352 (ref values): Use the In Vivo Acid–Base Nomogram in single respiratory or metabolic acid–base disturbance for values derived from arterial, venous, or arterialized blood samples.

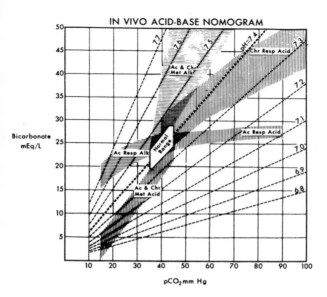

In vivo nomogram showing bands for defining a single respiratory or metabolic acid-base disturbance.

Arbus, G.S.: An in vivo acid-base nomogram for clinical use. Can Med Assoc J. 109:291, 1973. (With permission)

1. Each 'pathological' respiratory or metabolic acid–base disorder, and the appropriate range of "in vivo" (physiological) compensation, is represented as a shaded band.
   a) Usually, acid–base value falling within a shaded band indicates the single disturbance indicated on the shaded band.
   b) Occasionally, an acid–base value falling within a band indicates a mixed disturbance.
   c) Acid–base value falling outside the bands indicates there are at least two acid–base disturbances (i.e., mixed disturbance).

H. **Metabolic Acidosis** (see also Metabolic Tests p 55, Metabolic Disorders p 254)
1. Determine serum Na^+, K^+, Cl^-, pH, PCO_2, HCO_3^- values.
2. Confirm clinical impression using the In Vivo Acid—Base Nomogram.
3. Determine anion gap:

$$Na^+ - (Cl^- + HCO_3^-)$$

= 10 to 15 mEq/liter (normal).

4. Consult the metabolic acidosis flow chart to determine possible cause.

Treatment

1. Immediately, treat cause of acidosis (e.g., for diabetic ketoacidosis give insulin, p 243).
2. If serum HCO_3^- <8 mEq/liter **or** if patient is obviously in severe metabolic acidosis but serum bicarbonate levels not available (e.g., severe gastroenteritis, severe diabetes mellitus):
    administer $NaHCO_3$, 2 mEq/kg body wt over 10-120 min (depending on the severity of the acidosis).
3. Repeat the acid—base assessment after all the $NaHCO_3$ has been administered.
    a) If additional $NaHCO_3$ therapy is necessary, calculate:
        amount of $NaHCO_3$ needed = (desired serum HCO_3^- level — actual serum HCO_3^-) x body wt (kg) x 0.60.
    b) Give half the amount of HCO_3^- needed in the first 10—15 min and the remainder over the next 2 hr.
4. Reassess acid—base balance on completion of $NaHCO_3$ therapy.

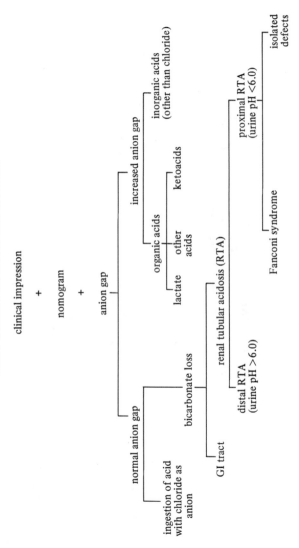

FLOW CHART FOR METABOLIC ACIDOSIS

clinical impression
+
nomogram
+
anion gap

normal anion gap
- ingestion of acid with chloride as anion
- bicarbonate loss
  - GI tract
  - renal tubular acidosis (RTA)
    - distal RTA (urine pH >6.0)
    - proximal RTA (urine pH <6.0)
      - Fanconi syndrome
      - isolated defects

increased anion gap
- organic acids
  - lactate
  - other acids
  - ketoacids
- inorganic acids (other than chloride)

127

COMPOSITION OF PARENTERAL SOLUTIONS (mEq/liter)

Solution	Na⁺	K⁺	Cl⁻	HCO₃⁻*	Others	Comments
Isotonic (0.9%) NaCl	154		154			a useful Na⁺ replacement fluid; also used for maintenance
Hypertonic (3%) NaCl	513		513			
3.33% Dextrose and 0.3% NaCl ("2/3:1/3" solution)	52		52		dextrose: 33.3 g	a useful Na⁺ maintenance fluid
5% Dextrose and 0.2% NaCl	34		34		dextrose: 50 g	
Darrow's solution, K lactate	123	35	105		lactate: 53	
7.5% NaHCO₃	893			893		
14.9% KCl		2000	2000			
1/6 M Na lactate	167			167	lactate: 167	
Lactated Ringer's solution	130	4	109	28	Ca⁺⁺: 3.0; lactate: 28	
NH₄Cl (2.14% in water)			400		NH₄⁺: 400	

*bicarbonate or potential bicarbonate

Other Frequently Used Parenteral Solutions
50% MgSO₄ (2 ml ampule: 4 mEq/ml) (p 447),
10% Ca gluconate (10 ml ampule: 0.47 mEq/ml) (p 425),
10% CaCl₂ (10 ml ampule: 1.8 mEq/ml).

128

COMPOSITION OF ORAL SOLUTIONS (mEq/liter or as noted, see p 322)

Solution	Na$^+$	K$^+$	Cl$^-$	HCO$_3^-$*	Others
human milk	7	14			
cows' milk	25	35	28	30	
ginger ale	3.5	0.1		3.6	
Coca Cola	0.4	13		13.4	
orange juice	0.2	49		50	
apple juice	0.5	25			
tomato juice	100	59	150	10	
Pedialyte	30	20	30	28	Sucrose 60 g
Cooke mixture†	30	20	30	20	Sucrose 50 g

*bicarbonate or potential bicarbonate
†Order from Pharmacy (Sucrose 50 g, NaCl 1.7 g in 1 liter soln + KHCO$_3$ 2.0 g)

Other Frequently Used Oral Solutions
MgCl$_2$: Mg citrate solution (HSC preparation): 0.8 mEq/ml
Ca Sandoz syrup (110 mg elemental Ca/5 ml): see p 426
K-lyte/Cl: see p 455
Slow-K (K$^+$ and Cl$^-$: 8 mEq each per tablet): see p 455
Citrate solutions A, B: see p 431

129

INFECTIOUS DISEASES
PURULENT MENINGITIS

A medical emergency — a good result depends upon:
1. Early diagnosis
2. Immediate optimal specific therapy
3. Intensive supportive therapy

It is convenient to separate patients by age: childhood meningitis (> 1 mo of age; see below) and neonatal meningitis (birth to 1 mo; pp 139, 168).

CHILDHOOD PURULENT MENINGITIS
(over 1 mo of age)

1. About 95% of cases caused by *Haemophilus influenzae* type b, meningococcus, pneumococcus; streptococcus (group A) infrequently; other bacteria rarely.
2. Peak incidence between 6 and 12 mo of age.
3. Transmission by direct contact or infected droplets; nasopharyngeal infection commonly precedes the meningitis. Communicability of the nasopharyngeal reservoir ceases within 24 hr of the start of effective antibiotic therapy.

Diagnosis

A. *Signs and Symptoms*
   Depend primarily on age of child; the younger the child, the less specific the clinical picture.
1. Fever with altered state of consciousness is the hallmark of CNS infection.
2. Preceding URI; headache (older child) or irritability; convulsions; vomiting; oculomotor palsies (very late sign).
3. Meningismus may be revealed by neck stiffness going on to opisthotonos, and positive Kernig's and Brudzinski's signs (many of these infants cry when their hips are flexed while their legs are straight during diaper change). Meningismus commonly absent under 1 yr of age.
4. Petechial rash or purpuric eruption favors diagnosis of meningococcal infection, but may develop with pneumococcal and certain viral infections.

B. *Diagnostic Tests*

Lumbar puncture should be performed as soon as the possibility of meningitis is considered, especially in patients presenting with convulsion and fever. **If papilledema is present,** consult neurologist before performing LP.

1. Spinal fluid: cell count and differential; Gram stain on centrifuged specimen; chemistry (protein and sugar); bacterial and viral cultures.

2. Blood culture.

3. Culture swabs of nasopharynx and any other focus of infection.

4. Hb, WBC total and differential, smear.

5. Blood sugar and serum electrolytes.

6. If indicated by shock: platelet count, PT, PTT, and fibrin split products.

   The following, also, may be indicated:
7. Gram stain of petechial smear.

8. Chest film and tuberculin test (5 TU).

9. Skull film — if history of recent head injury, or possibility of infection in mastoids, sinuses.

10. Urine electrolytes, urine and serum osmolality (to check for inappropriate ADH syndrome).

11. Counterimmune electrophoresis (CIE) on CSF, serum, urine.

12. CSF lactic acid.

13. Continuing diagnostic studies, see p 133.

C. *Differential Diagnosis* see p 132

C. Differential Diagnosis

1. Viral meningoencephalitis and tuberculous meningitis (see table).

	Purulent	Viral	Tuberculous
Spinal Fluid			
Cells/mm³	Increased (30- to 50,000); 95% polys.	Increased (<2000); initially polys ±; later lymphs.	Low cell count (20 to 500); mostly lymphs.
Sugar	Greatly decreased.	Normal	Decreased
Protein	Increased.	Normal or slightly increased.	Greatly increased. Pellicle formation.
Gram stain	Usually positive.	Negative.	± (Ziehl-Neelsen +)
Culture	Positive.	Negative.	Only isolation of tubercle bacilli provides absolute diagnosis.
Lactic acid	>2.5 mM	<2.0 mM	Probably >2.5 mM
Peripheral WBC			
	Increased.	Normal.	Slightly increased.

2. Brain abscess or extradural focus: suspect if congenital heart disease, chronic ear or sinus infection, dermal sinus, recent staph infection, recent head injury — all suggested if CSF purulent but sterile in absence of antibiotics.

3. Papilledema on admission: suggests brain abscess, tuberculous meningitis, or brain tumor.

4. Diffuse meningeal tumor: pleocytosis, decreased CSF sugar, increased ICP, mental deterioration, meningismus, multiple cranial nerve signs and **absence of infection.**

5. Fungal infection: very rare, usually cryptococcal; CSF sugar decreased, cell count variable. Diagnosis is made by demonstrating the organism, which in a wet preparation is often mistaken for lymphocytes.

D. Continuing Diagnostic Studies

Day 2: 1. Repeat CSF studies (if indicated by unsatisfactory clinical course or conflicting lab. results).
2. WBC total and differential; ESR.
3. Acute viral serology ⎱ if viral meningitis possible.
4. Viral auger suction ⎰

Day 7: 1. Repeat CSF studies.
2. Hb, WBC total and differential, smear; ESR.

Other: Skull films, EEG, CT scan, or subdural and ventricular taps (by neurosurgeon), at any time, as indicated by clinical course.

Treatment

A. Antibiotic Therapy

Each iv dose of antibiotic should be administered in less than 30 min. This is conveniently done with a Pedatrol.

Asterisk* indicates that it is rarely necessary to treat beyond the 7 days.

a) *Unknown Purulent** (i.e., specific etiology not established by bacteriology)

1. Ampicillin (dose as for *H. influenzae)* for 7 days minimum.
   and
2. Chloramphenicol (dose as for *H. influenzae*).
   If patient is allergic to penicillin, give chloramphenicol as sole antibiotic.

b) *H. influenzae Type b**
Always start with combined therapy:

1. Ampicillin, 400 mg/kg/day, iv, divided q4h:
   and
2. Chloramphenicol, 100 mg/kg/day, iv, divided q6h.
   – If organism sensitive to ampicillin, discontinue chloramphenicol.
   – If patient allergic to penicillin, give chloramphenicol as sole antibiotic.
3. *Continue therapy with appropriate antibiotic for 7 days minimum.*

c) *Meningococcus**

1. Aqueous penicillin G, 250,000 units/kg/day, iv, divided q4h, for 7 days minimum.
   or
2. If patient is allergic to penicillin, give chloramphenicol (dose as for *H. influenzae*).

133

d) *Pneumococcus or Streptococcus**
   1. Aqueous penicillin G (dose as for meningococcus) if etiology is established. Continue for 7 days minimum.
      or
   2. If patient is allergic to penicillin, give chloramphenicol (dose as for *H. influenzae*).

e) *Staphylococcus aureus*
   1. Cloxacillin, 300 mg/kg/day, divided q4h, iv, and 5 mg daily as indicated.
   2. Aqueous penicillin G (dose as for meningococcus).

B. Supportive Therapy

SPEED is important — irreversible shock may develop in minutes.

PROPHYLAXIS: Because many complications progress to serious sequelae, supportive therapy is directed particularly at their prevention.

a) *Nursing Care*
   1. *Constant nursing care essential for:*
      All patients under 2 yr of age; and
      Those who are semi-comatose, convulsing, or in shock — **regardless of age.**
   2. *Other patients over 2 yr:* may have shared nursing care at discretion of attending staff. Fully conscious, oriented patients do not require special nursing unless deterioration occurs.

The nurse has 3 main responsibilities:
   1. Monitor vital signs.
   2. Temperature control.
   3. In the event of vomiting, maintain a clear airway and prevent aspiration.

b) *Normothermia*
   Hyperthermia increases the rate of brain metabolism and, therefore, O_2 requirement, and may result in febrile convulsions.

   Monitor temperature continually — try to achieve normothermia:
   1. Lower room temperature
   2. Antipyretics when practicable
   3. Patient unclothed
   4. Tepid sponge-baths (only for hyperpyrexia, $T > 40.5°C$)
   5. **Do not** direct fan at child.

134

CONVULSIONS

Treatment

**An acute episode is an emergency — START TREAT-
MENT IMMEDIATELY**

1. Guard against cerebral hypoxia, vomiting, and aspiration.
2. Give *stat:* diazepam 0.30 mg/kg (maximum, 10 mg),
   iv over 2 min.

   or

   paraldehyde, 0.30 ml/kg (maximum, 10 ml), im.

   then:

3. After 10 min, if still convulsing:
   a) Consult Anaesthesia re respiratory function.
   b) Notify Neurology.
   c) Repeat diazepam.
4. After 15 min, if still convulsing:
   a) infuse 5% paraldehyde soln iv, rapidly, until
      seizure ceases (12.5 ml paraldehyde in 250 ml
      hypotonic infusion fluid — *make up fresh for
      each infusion*).
5. **Watch for respiratory depression** — Pay attention to
   the following at all times:
   a) Semi-prone positioning and adequate airway
   b) Need for assisted ventilation (for respiratory
      acidosis)
   c) Whether cooling is needed
   d) Need for O_2 by mask.

Prophylaxis

1. *Diphenylhydantoin* (Dilantin): not recommended as
   routine in meningitis, but can be given after initial
   convulsion has been controlled with diazepam, etc.

   Give 6 mg/kg iv *stat;* repeat in 6 hr; then 3 mg/kg
   q6h, iv, at $\leqslant$ 50 mg/min, until patient can take it
   orally (pp 174, 436).

CEREBRAL EDEMA

1. Anticipate if convulsions repetitive or prolonged, if
   hypoxia or hyperpyrexia, and if therapy delayed >24
   hr after onset of meningitis.
2. Consider cerebral edema present if an unconscious
   patient has abnormal pupillary reflexes, respiratory
   irregularity, hypertension, or signs of cerebral/cerebel-
   lar herniation.

Treatment

1. *Mannitol* (20% solution: Osmitrol). Patient must be catheterized (because of diuresis).
    a) *Test dose:* 1 mg/kg – infuse over 5 min: give only if urinary function is in doubt. Should result in urine output exceeding 40 ml/hr.
    b) *Therapeutic dose:* 1.0-1.5 g/kg – infuse at 1 g/min. Repeat q4-6h as needed.
2. *Dexamethasone* (Decadron): 1.25 mg/kg *stat;* then 0.5 mg/kg/day, divided q6h. (If steroid therapy does not exceed 72 hr, gradual withdrawal is unnecessary.)
3. *Supportive measures:*
    a) Temperature control.
    b) Extreme care to avoid overloading with fluids given iv.
    c) Correct respiratory acidosis: assisted ventilation and/or oxygen.

Prophylaxis

When edema is suspected but no life-threatening situation exists, mannitol is usually unnecessary.

SEPTIC SHOCK

Outline of Management (detailed protocol on p 472).

1. Hydrocortisol (Solu-Cortef), 50 mg/kg, iv. *stat.* May repeat hourly x 4; then give maintenance dose of 15 mg/kg, iv. q3h for 24 hr, and re-assess.
2. Insert a central venous pressure catheter (normal CVP = 6-12 cm H_2O)
    a) If CVP <6 cm:
        – Expand blood volume with Rheomacrodex until whole blood or plasma is available.
    b) If CVP >12 cm:
        – Digitalize (p 201); and
        – Give dopamine iv: 2-10 μg/kg/min by pump infusion, or give isoproterenol (Isuprel) iv: 1 mg in 250 ml of 5% dextrose in water, at 0.5-1.0 ml/min.
        – Use ECG monitor.
3. If cardiac failure present, digitalize (p 201).
4. Correct metabolic acidosis with sodium bicarbonate.
5. Do not give vasopressors.

INAPPROPRIATE ADH SECRETION (p 123)

Incidence: 80-90% of cases of bacterial meningitis.

1. Obtain serum electrolytes on admission.
2. Restrict fluid intake to 1/2 to 2/3 maintenance requirement **after** cautious correction of prior losses.
3. **Note.** When calculating fluid orders, include fluid given iv with antibiotics.
4. If serum Na <130 mEq/liter, obtain urine and serum electrolytes and osmolality.

SUSPECTED FULMINATING MENINGOCOCCAL SEPSIS

Management
(see also p 472)

A.	Status	1.	*Stat* lab studies
B.	Sepsis	2.	Ampicillin and chloramphenicol
C.	Shock and disseminated intravenous coagulation	3. 4. 5. 6. 7.	Central venous line Intravenous fluids Steroids Dopamine (or Isoproterenol) Digoxin
D.	Acidosis	8.	Bicarbonate
E.	Monitor status	9.	Helpful indices

1. Stat Lab Studies
 a) Blood culture (2-5 ml blood).
 b) Type and cross-match (1-3 ml).
 c) CBC, smear, platelet count (1 ml).
 d) Electrolytes, blood gases, sugar, BUN, Ca (2 ml).
 e) PT & PTT (2 ml) & fibrin split products (2 ml clotted).
 f) *Defer CSF studies until shock is controlled.*

2. Antibiotics
 a) *Immediately,* start a temporary iv line (not a cutdown)
 b) *Stat,* give *first ampicillin dose* iv (about 70 mg/kg over 20 min).
 c) After 20 min, give *first chloramphenicol dose* iv (25 mg/kg over 20-30 min).
 d) Continue ampicillin iv: 400 mg/kg/day, divided q4h, for 7 days minimum.
 e) Continue chloramphenicol iv: 100 mg/kg/day, divided q6h, until meningococcus proven.

3. **Central Venous Line**
   a) Use central venous line as permanent iv line (*not* an ankle cutdown).
   b) Measure central venous pressure every 5-30 min — depending upon status and infusions.
   c) Normal CVP = about 6-12 cm water.

4. **Intravenous Fluid Therapy**
   Expand blood volume (to increase peripheral perfusion and cardiac output): administer expanding fluids until patient out of shock *or* CVP exceeds 12 cm water.
   a) *Plasma* or fresh frozen plasma — 20 ml/kg.
              or
   b) *Saline* or Ringer's lactate soln (20 ml/kg within 1 hr) until plasma available.
              or
   c) *Whole blood* (20 ml/kg), if Hb <10 g/dl — it takes about 90 min to cross-match.

5. **Steroids** (are vasodilators and positive inotropic agents when given in large dose).
   a) Hydrocortisol (Solu-Cortef), 50 mg/kg *stat*, into iv drip-tubing.
   b) *Repeat* this dose q1h, for 4 doses — if needed.
   c) *Then* reduce dose to *15 mg/kg* q3h, up to 48 hr.

6. **A:** **Dopamine** (a sympathomimetic drug) — **give only if intensive care available.**
   In shock, with CVP > 12 cm water, dopamine dilates renal and mesenteric vessels and increases cardiac contractility. Results = CVP falls and cardiac output rises.

   Give 2-10 μg/kg/min by continuous iv pump infusion with *constant* ECG oscilloscope, CVP, and BP monitoring.

   OR, if bradycardia present give

6. **B:** **Isoproterenol** (Isuprel) — constant medical and nursing care essential. In shock with elevated CVP, isoproterenol dilates peripheral vessels (CVP falls and cardiac output rises).
   a) **Do not give** if heart rate >200 beats/min (*see* digoxin, below).
   b) Give by continuous pump infusion, 0.01-1.0 μg/kg/min starting at lowest dose and adjusting upward, while monitoring ECG, BP, CVP. If possible, use ECG oscilloscope.
   c) **If constant medical and nursing care not available** GET HELP IMMEDIATELY (e.g., consult anesthetist).

7. **Digoxin**

When CVP elevated (>12 cm water) and tachycardia present (>200 beats/min), digoxin increases cardiac output and decreases heart rate.

a) Digitalize rapidly, iv (p 201).

b) As heart rate falls (<200/min), give dopamine (or isoproterenol) as needed (above).

8. **Bicarbonate** (7.5% sodium bicarbonate)

a) Can give *stat* dose before results of blood studies known — 2 mEq/kg (2 ml/kg) in iv drip.

b) Further needs according to blood-gas analyses.

9. **It is helpful to follow:**

a) Temperature/color of extremities.

b) Peripheral pulse strength, heart rate, BP.

c) CVP

d) Urine output

e) Bodyweight

f) Laboratory studies.

NEONATAL MENINGITIS

(Bacterial meningitis within 30 days of birth)

1. Most cases caused by *E. coli* K_1 and streptococcus group B.

2. Infection contracted from maternal birth canal, other sick infants, nursery personnel, or contaminated equipment.

a) Within 2 wk of birth: Gram-negative bacteria, streptococcus group B, and *Listeria* infections.

b) During wk 3 or 4: staphylococcal and pneumococcal infections.

3. Consider possibility of meningitis if:

a) prolonged rupture of membranes, or

b) maternal infection, or

c) premature or traumatic delivery.

Diagnosis

A. **Signs and Symptoms**

1. Initially, usually signs of sepsis, poor feeding, poor activity, apneic episodes, respiratory distress, jaundice.

2. Later, convulsions may occur.

3. **Note.** Neck stiffness, fever, and bulging of anterior fontanelle *may be absent.* Therefore, *strong suspicion* in any neonate not doing well *justifies lumbar puncture.*

B. *Diagnostic Tests*

As for Childhood Meningitis (p 130).
— Perform LP *stat.*

C. *Differential Diagnosis*

Septicemia, CMV infection, toxoplasmosis, systemic herpes, hepatitis, and myocarditis of the newborn.

General Management

1. Patient may be admitted to Neonatal Intensive Care or Infectious Disease Ward. If the latter, deterioration in patient's condition will necessitate transfer to a ward providing intensive care.
2. Notify ward chief of admission.
3. Initiate *stat* or continue treatment (p 139).
4. Repeat LP daily until CSF is sterile.
5. 48 hr after start of therapy: if CSF still unsterile, suspect ventriculitis. Arrange CT scan with enhancement (contact Neuroradiology resident on call; also, p 83).

Treatment

A. *Antibiotic Therapy*

---

*Gentamicin:
1. Give dose slowly, over 1 hr.
2. Monitor peak and trough blood levels, and adjust dosage as necessary (therapeutic range of peak values = 4-10 μg/ml).

†Ampicillin: whenever practicable, give dose in <30 min.

Initially (maximum, 48 hr):
1. *Postnatal age 0-7 days*
   Gentamicin* 7.5 mg/kg/day, divided q12h, iv
   plus
   Ampicillin† 100 mg/kg/day, divided q12h, iv.
2. *Postnatal age >8 days*
   Gentamicin* 7.5 mg/kg/day divided q8h iv — and up to 10 mg/kg/day, if indicated by blood level.
   plus
   Ampicillin† 200 mg/kg/day, divided q6h, iv.

140

Continuing antibiotic therapy (after 48 hr):

1. In each individual case, this is determined in consultation with Infectious Disease Division. Continue appropriate antibiotic regimen for *minimum of 3 wk.*

2. If organism sensitive to ampicillin and gentamicin, continue these as in initial therapy.

3. If streptococcus group B is causal organism:
   a) Switch to aqueous penicillin G
      <1 wk of age, 100,000 units/kg/day iv q8h
      >1 wk of age, 200,000 units/kg/day iv, q6h.
      Treat for 3 wk.
   b) Gentamicin can be continued for 1 wk, as synergy with penicillin has been demonstrated *in vitro*.

4. If *H. influenzae* type b: ampicillin can be continued as *sole* antibiotic (if organism sensitive; otherwise, use chloramphenicol).

5. If pneumococcus or meningococcus, switch to penicillin G.

6. *If organism resistant to ampicillin:*
   a) *for Pseudomonas:* continue gentamicin as above
      plus
      Ticarcillin, given iv:
      – Infant <2000 g: initial dose, 50 mg/kg; then, until 7 days of age, 110 mg/kg/day, q8h;
        after 7 days, 200 mg/kg/day q6h
      – Infant >2000 g: initial dose, 50 mg/kg; then, until 3 days of age, 150 mg/kg/day q6h
        after 3 days, 200 mg/kg/day q6h.

   b) *for Klebsiella:* continue gentamicin as above

      plus

      Additional antibiotic(s) as indicated by sensitivities. If ventriculitis develops, instillation of antibiotics directly into ventricles will be necessary (1-5 mg of gentamicin, *or* 25 mg of cephaloridine, in 1 dose/day).

B. Supportive Therapy

As for Childhood Meningitis (p 130).

141

RABIES

Every exposure to possible rabies infection must be carefully and individually evaluated by the attending physician.

Factors to be Considered in Relation to Rationale of Treatment

1. *Species of biting animal*
   Most likely to be infective are carnivores, especially skunks, foxes, coyotes, raccoons, dogs, cats and bats. Bites of rodents such as rats, hamsters, etc., are unlikely to be infective.

2. *Biting incident*
   An unprovoked attack is more likely to indicate the animal is rabid.

3. *Extent and location of bite*
   a)   Severe: multiple or deep puncture wounds, any bite on head, neck, face or hands.
   b)   Mild: scratches, lacerations, or *single bite on areas other than listed under 'severe',* or abrasions contaminated with saliva.

4. *Vaccination status of biting animal.* If the animal has been immunized, the risk of its transmitting the disease is minimal.

5. *Whether rabies known or suspected in the geographic area.*

Local Treatment of Wounds

1. *First Aid*
   Flush and cleanse wound with copious amounts of soap and water or any solution with high alcohol content.

2. *Treatment under Direction of Physician*
   a)   Flush and cleanse wound thoroughly with soap and water, then irrigate with aqueous benzalkonium chloride solution 1:1000 or other quaternary ammonia compounds.
   b)   Tetanus prophylaxis (p 146)
   c)   Measures to combat bacterial infection as indicated.
   d)   Prevent primary closure of wound.
   e)   Rabies vaccine, if indicated.

Post-exposure Prophylaxis with Rabies Vaccine

1. Duck-embryo vaccine (DEV)
2. Nervous-tissue vaccine (NTV)
3. Human diploid-cell vaccine (HDCV)

Efficacy of Vaccine

1. DEV is the least immunogenic, but is associated with significantly fewer CNS reactions than NTV. (Severe CNS reactions are NTV's major drawback.) Efficacy of DEV and NTV in preventing rabies after proven exposure has never been demonstrated in controlled trial.

2. HDCV is most immunogenic of the 3 vaccines and has fewest side-effects. It is not yet licensed, but limited amounts are available for persons who have been bitten by a rabid animal and who have severe reactions to DEV or NTV.

GUIDE* TO TREATMENT AFTER ESTABLISHED OR POSSIBLE EXPOSURE TO RABIES

(**NOTE.** RIG and DEV — use substitute human-derived vaccine and sera if at all possible)

Species of Animal	Condition of Animal at Time of Attack	Treatment of Exposed Human
Wild Skunk Raccoon Fox Bat Coyote	Regard as rabid	RIG + DEV[†]
Domestic Dog or cat:	Healthy Unknown (escaped) Rabid or suspected rabid	None — but[#] RIG + DEV RIG + DEV[†]
Other	Consider individually	

*See text for details and dosages. (MMWR, 25:405, 3 Dec., 1976; *and* Proc. Int. Symp. on Rabies, Lyon, 1972, ed. by R. H. Regamey *et al.* Basle, Karger, Symp. Series on Immunobiol. Standardization, v.21, 1974).

†Discontinue vaccine if fluorescent antibody tests of the animal — *if killed at/after time of attack* — are negative.

#Begin treatment immediately if evidence of rabies develops in the biting dog or cat during holding period (10 days).

Administration of Vaccine
1. *DEV and NTV:*
    a) Give as 1 sc injection daily x 14 days, in abdomen, lower back, or lateral thigh; rotate sites;

    or

    b) If exposure is severe or antiserum is used: give 14 doses during first 7 days, and 7 doses during days 8-14.
    c) Give booster 10 and 20 days after primary course completed.
    d) Antihistamines, epinephrine may be needed to control hypersensitivity reactions.
2. *HDCV:* give on days 0,3,7,14,30 & 90.
3. Give *steroids* only if life-threatening reaction develops (in animal models, they increase risk of rabies).

Hyperimmune Serum
1. Hyperimmune serum + vaccine is the best post-exposure prophylaxis.
2. Equine antirabies serum causes serum sickness in up to 40% of recipients − careful history and tests for hypersensitivity must be performed before use.
3. Human rabies immune globulin (RIG) is preferred over equine serum, because of freedom from hypersensitivity reactions. Dose is 20 U of human RIG or 40 U of equine antirabies serum, per kg bodyweight.
4. If antirabies serum is given, at least 5 ml of total dose should be thoroughly infiltrated around the wound.

TETANUS (LOCKJAW)

Caused by *Clostridium tetani,* a spore-forming anaerobe. Source may be soil, dust, animal or human feces, plaster, unsterile sutures. Transmitted by direct or indirect contamination of an obvious or unrecognized wound.

Differential Diagnosis

1. Reaction to phenothiazine or anti-emetic drugs
2. Meningitis; encephalitis
3. Rabies

4. Hypocalcemic tetany
5. Hysteria
6. Poisoning (strychnine).

Treatment

Specific
1. (Human) tetanus immune globulin (TIG), 250 U/vial: 3,000 – 6,000 U im.
   – Infiltrate part of dose locally around wound.
2. If TIG unavailable, give tetanus antitoxin (TAT), equine or bovine: 50,000 – 100,000 U.
   First, give part of dose (20,000 U) iv (test for immediate sensitivity – skin and eye signs).
3. Antimicrobials: give penicillin G (p 406) or a tetracycline parenterally for 10-14 days.

Nonspecific
1. Constant nursing care in quiet, semi-darkened room, with minimal auditory and visual stimuli.
2. *Mild Cases*
   a) Sedation and muscle relaxation.
   b) Diazepam, 0.2 mg/kg im or iv, repeated in 3-4 hr as necessary. Larger doses may be required more frequently.
   c) Chlorpromazine, 25-50 mg (or 0.5 mg/kg) x q4-6h, po. Drug can be diluted and given iv. Maintenance dosage can be given po or pr.
   d) Mephenesin, po or iv, in conjunction with sedatives, provides muscle relaxation.
      – 30 to 150 ml 2% solution iv, infused at 6-7 ml/min, provides 2-3 g daily for adults; for infants and small children, give proportionately smaller dose based on age and weight.
3. *Severe Cases*
   a) Treatment of choice (when facilities available) is *d*-tubocurarine to produce paralysis, with tracheotomy and artificial ventilation. Concomitant sedation with diazepam is essential.
   b) Hypotensive drugs to control hypertension and cardiac arrhythmias.
   c) Maintain clear pharyngotracheal airway and adequate ventilation. Avoid respiratory depression, and treat quickly if it occurs.

4.   *Debridement of Wound* (surgical consultation is necessary)
     Indicated if foreign material or necrotic tissue present. Debride only after sedation, antimicrobial therapy, and tetanus immune globulin.

5.   *Other Adjuncts to Therapy*
     a)   Maintain adequate fluid, electrolyte, and caloric intake;
          – po if possible; otherwise, iv, or by NG tube, or by gastrostomy.
     b)   Tracheotomy recommended if patient has respiratory problems associated with difficulty in swallowing, laryngospasm, accumulation of secretions, and severely altered level of consciousness.

6.   *Booster Injections of Tetanus Toxoid at Time of Injury*
     a)   After 4 doses of tetanus toxoid, antitoxin persists at protective levels for at least 5 yr. In wound management, booster injections are not needed more often than every 5 yr – but if tetanus immunization is incomplete at time of injury, complete the recommended series.
     b)   Passive protection with TIG or antitoxin: give only if the patient has had 0 or only 1 injection of tetanus toxoid or if the wound has been unattended longer than 24 hr.
          – TIG dosage: 250-500 U im.
          – TAT (if TIG unavailable): 3,000-5,000 U im after testing for sensitivity.

GUIDE TO TETANUS PROPHYLAXIS IN WOUND MANAGEMENT

(USPHS Advisory Committee on Immunization Practices)

History of tetanus immunization (doses)	*Clean, minor wounds* Tetanus toxoid	TIG	*All other wounds* Tetanus toxoid	TIG
Uncertain	Yes	No	Yes	Yes
0 or 1	Yes	No	Yes	Yes
2	Yes	No	Yes	No*
3 or more	No[†]	No	No[‡]	No

*Unless wound more than 24 hr old.

[†]Unless more than 10 yr since last dose.

[‡]Unless more than 5 yr since last dose.

WHOOPING COUGH (PERTUSSIS)

A relatively common and potentially serious infectious disease, particularly in infants under 2 yr.

Agent: Bordetella pertussis

Source: discharge from respiratory tract of infected person.

Transmission: direct contact with infected person or indirectly by contact with freshly contaminated articles.

Incubation period: 5-21 days, usually <10 days.

Communicability is greatest during initial 2 wk of the disease (catarrhal stage). The incidence of *B. pertussis* isolation decreases rapidly during the paroxysmal stage, and thus is rarely recovered after the 4th wk of illness. Duration of communicability is shortened in patients receiving specific antimicrobial agents.

Diagnosis

1. Any child with a paroxysmal cough or whoop must be considered to have pertussis until this is bacteriologically disproven or the definitive diagnosis established.
2. Conditions simulating pertussis include viral and mycoplasma respiratory-tract infections, allergic disorders, cystic fibrosis, and inhaled foreign body.
3. Bacteriologic confirmation is essential for diagnosis:
   a) By demonstrating the organism by immunofluorescence in mucus obtained by nasopharyngeal aspiration (auger suction).
   b) By culture.
4. Increased WBC count and absolute lymphocytosis are of diagnostic significance (but not present in all confirmed cases).
5. A rise in agglutinating antibody to the organism is of diagnostic help in some cases.

Treatment

1. Isolate patient.
2. If paroxysms severe, constant nursing care is essential to provide suction and removal of secretions from the oropharynx. O_2 may be necessary during paroxysms.
3. Cool moist air (as in a croup tent) is usually helpful. Benefit of sedation, cough syrups, atropine and steroids not proven.
4. Hydration, nutrition, and electrolyte balance require careful observation and attention.

5. Erythromycin, 50 mg/kg/24 hr for 10 days, abbreviates communicability. Bacteriological complications (e.g., staph pneumonia) may require additional antimicrobial therapy.
6. Pertussis immune-globulin (human).
   Despite anecdotal support, effectiveness unproved in controlled trials.

Isolation of Patient

Patients with diagnosis of pertussis should be isolated for a minimum of 3 wk from onset of illness or until 10-day course of erythromycin completed.

Quarantine and Care of Contacts

1. Regulations vary, but advisable to quarantine non-immunized contacts for 2 wk after intimate exposure.
2. Contacts under 6 yr of age previously immunized against pertussis should receive a booster dose of vaccine and a course of erythromycin.
3. Contacts not previously immunized should be given erythromycin for 10 days; **or, if contact maintained,** as long as the patient has the cough.

HEPATITIS A

(INFECTIOUS HEPATITIS)

Incubation period: 15-45 days (average, 25-30 days).

Clinical picture: Characteristically, abrupt onset with fever, malaise, anorexia, nausea, abdominal pain, vomiting, and jaundice. Morbidity is age-related, with asymptomatic and anicteric infection predominating in childhood. Mortality in clinically recognized cases is <1%.

Transmission: primarily by fecal–oral route; occasionally via contaminated food and water.

Communicability: Hepatitis A virus (HAV) in stool during late incubation period and early prodromal phase. Viral excretion and communicability decreases rapidly a few days after onset of jaundice. Maximal infectivity period is 2 wk before onset of jaundice to (maximum) 1 wk after onset.

Diagnosis
1. Bilirubin in urine.
2. Total and direct bilirubin elevated.
3. Serum ALT and AST elevated early (pp 353, 358).
4. WBC count normal or low; ESR normal.
5. Antibody assay for anti-HAV will soon be available.

Prophylaxis
1. Immune serum globulin (ISG) given before or 1-2 wk after exposure prevents illness in 80-90% of cases.
2. ISG >2 wk after exposure is useless.
3. ISG (0.02 ml/kg) recommended for all household contacts, *especially adults — in whom the disease may be more severe.*
4. ISG not routinely recommended for school contacts or hospital personnel.

HEPATITIS B (HBV)
(SERUM HEPATITIS)

Incubation: 60-180 days (average, 90 days).

Clinical picture: Onset usually insidious, with anorexia, malaise, nausea, vomiting, abdominal pain, jaundice, arthralgia or arthritis, rash. More severe and prolonged than hepatitis A. Mortality increases with age.

Transmission by:
1. Direct percutaneous inoculation by needle of contaminated serum or transfusion of infected blood/blood products.
2. Percutaneous transfer of infected serum or plasma through even minute cuts and abrasions.
3. Introduction of blood or serum into ocular or buccal mucosa.
4. Sexual contact.
5. Indirect transfer of serum or plasma via vectors or environmental surfaces.
6. Airborne transmission rare, if ever; transmission via intestinal tract never.
7. *Blood of infected person is extremely infectious:* there may be 10^6-10^8 infective virus particles per ml.

Diagnosis

1. Hepatitis B surface-antigen (HB_SAg; formerly Australia antigen) demonstrated in serum; or
2. Rising titer of variety of antibodies to HBV.
3. Follow-up for persistence of antigenemia and development of chronic hepatitis is important.

Prophylaxis

Lots of ISG currently manufactured in Canada and USA contain detectable antibody to HBV. Hepatitis B-immune globulin (HBIG) with anti-HB titer of 1:100,000 or more is available.

1. *Acute exposure* (accidental needle-stick or mucosal exposure to blood known to contain HB_SAg)
   a) HBIG, 0.05-0.07 ml/kg, as soon as possible within 7 days; give 2nd dose 25-30 days later.
   b) If HBIG is unavailable, give ISG in same dosage.
2. *Fetal exposure:* infant born to mother who contracted acute HBV hepatitis in 3rd trimester or is chronic carrier.
   a) Give HBIG 0.13 ml/kg within 7 days of birth.
   b) If HBIG is unavailable, give ISG 0.5 ml/kg.
   c) Can repeat at 1 mo of age.

GONORRHEA

Agent: Neisseria gonorrheae

Source: exudate of infected mucosal surfaces.

Transmission: intimate contact, including parturition, nonsexual intimate physical contact, and sexual contact.

Diagnosis

Ideally, swabs should be plated directly on to Thayer–Martin agar plates, or Trans-Gro CO_2 vials, or placed in transport medium.

1. Gram stain of exudate from conjunctivae, prepubertal child's vagina, or male urethra.

2. Gram stain of endocervix of pubertal/adult women unreliable (because of other *Neisseria* species).

3. Urethral swab in male; vaginal and urethral swabs in female.

4. Pharyngeal and rectal swabs, especially on homosexuals.

Uncomplicated Gonorrhea

(Urethral, Cervical, Pharyngeal, Rectal)

1. *Treatment of choice*
   a) Probenicid po, in the age-related dose outlined in table, preferably 30 min before penicillin injection.
   b) Aqueous procaine penicillin im, in the age-related dose outlined, injected at different sites if necessary, at one visit.
   c) Long-acting forms of penicillin have no place in the treatment of gonorrhea.

2. *Alternative therapy*
   a) Ampicillin as a single dose po, in the age-related dosage as outlined, preferably before a meal.
   b) Probenicid, in the age-related dose, simultaneously.

3. When penicillin and ampicillin are contraindicated: give spectinomycin or tetracycline HCl (see schedule for dosage, p 152).

4. Adolescent or child with resistant organisms or with complications of gonorrhea (e.g., salpingitis – PID): Large doses of aqueous crystalline penicillin G (20-30 million U daily for 5-7 days), iv.

Recommended Guide for the Antimicrobial Treatment of ACUTE GONORRHEA in Children, Adolescents, and Adults

Age	Aq Procaine Penicillin	Ampicillin	Spectinomycin	Tetracycline
<6 yr*	100,000 U/kg	50 mg/kg	not recommended	not recommended
6 yr	1.2 million U	1000 mg	not recommended	not recommended
9 yr	2.4 million U	1500 mg	not recommended	not recommended
12 yr	2.4 million U	2000 mg	not recommended	not recommended
15 yr	4.8 million U	3000 mg	male: 2000 mg (2 g) female: 4000 mg (4 g)	1500 mg initially & 500 mg qid x 4 days
Adult: 4.8 million U† a) single dose (± divided injection) b) im c) with probenecid#		3500 mg a) single dose b) po c) with probenecid# d) preferably ac	as for 15 yr a) single dose b) im	as for 15 yr a) one 4-day course (9 1/2 g) b) po

152

NOTE:
*Children under 6 yr of age with gonorrhea will achieve a higher cure-rate if treated in hospital for 4 days with penicillin daily im in the above dosage.

†Increasing number of treatment failures with this regimen, due to emergence of gonococcus strains resistant to even these high doses of penicillin. For this reason some centers initiate therapy with other antimicrobial regimens (e.g., tetracycline).

#Probenecid: We recommend giving with both ampicillin and penicillin routinely (higher antibiotic levels, longer duration). Suggested probenecid dosage schedule:

Age (yr)	<6	6	9	12	15	Adult
Dose (mg)	10/kg	250	250	500	750	1000

Give probenecid as single dose po 30 min before penicillin/ampicillin.

Gonorrheal Ophthalmia Neonatorum

Prophylaxis
1. Infected mother: prenatal treatment with penicillin or erythromycin.
2. Infant: instill 1% silver nitrate soln into each eye immediately after birth.

Treatment
1. Aqueous penicillin G, 50,000 units/kg/day im q12h for 5-7 days.
2. Topical antibiotic — may be unnecessary (because of rapid response to systemic penicillin).
3. If recovery slow:
   a) Apply 0.5% tetracycline or gentamicin opthalmic ointment every 4-6 hr.
   b) Cleanse discharge from eyes; use cotton pledgets moistened with sterile saline soln of 1:1000 benzalkonium chloride.
   c) If cornea appears threatened, dilate pupils with atropine sulfate and request ophthalmologic consultation.

Gonorrheal Vulvovaginitis

Occurs in prepubertal female (in contrast to urethritis and cervicitis in adolescent or adult female; p 263)

Treatment
1. Isolation.
2. Prevent child from infecting eyes.
3. Systemic antibiotic therapy as outlined.
4. Local — perineal and vulvar cleanliness.
5. Topical antibiotic (gentamicin cream) to vulvar area.
6. Intravaginal medication not necessary.

Follow-up of Patients with Gonorrhea

Males: Obtain anterior urethral swabs 7 days after completion of therapy.
Females: Obtain cervical and rectal swabs 7 and 14 days after therapy, and a third specimen after a menstrual period.

Treatment of Contacts of
Patients with Gonorrhea

Those with known exposure to gonorrhea should receive the same treatment as those who have gonorrhea.

Possibility of Syphilis

1. All gonorrhea patients should have a serologic test for syphilis at the time of diagnosis.
2. Patients receiving treatment other than the recommended parenteral penicillin schedule should have a follow-up serologic test for syphilis each month for 4 mo (the treatment may be masking syphilis).

SYPHILIS

Diagnosis

Although dark-field examination of smears from ulcerative lesions on genitals or perianal, rectal, or oropharyngeal areas may yield positive results, syphilis is usually diagnosed serologically.

1. If the screening test (e.g., VDRL) is positive, seek confirmation with the *Treponema pallidum*-immobilization (TPI) test, or (better) the more accurate and sensitive FTA-ABS test (fluorescent treponemal antibody-absorbed).
2. If serology is negative in suspected patient, do serologic follow-up weekly x 4 wk, then monthly x 3 mo.

Recommended Specific Therapy

1. *Congenital syphilis.* **Treat:**
    a) Infants and children who have established diagnosis of congenital syphilis.
    b) Infants of mothers with untreated syphilis, who have reactive serology at birth or any clinical or radiographic evidence of syphilis.
2. *Early, asymptomatic syphilis without CNS involvement*
    Benzathine penicillin G, 50,000 U/kg single dose im; **or** procaine penicillin G, 10,000 U/kg, single dose im daily x 10 days (but see below also).

3. *Syphilis with possible/definite CNS involvement*
   a) Early stage: Procaine penicillin G, 50,000 U/kg, single dose im daily x 10-14 days.

   As spirochetes have been isolated from 'normal' CSF of infants who have congenital syphilis without evidence of CNS involvement, some authorities recommend the higher dose (see above) for all infants.
   b) Late stage: Over 30 kg (12 yr and older), same therapy as for adult:
      - If CSF is reactive: treat as for neurosyphilis.
      - If CSF is nonreactive: treat as for late latent syphilis.
4. *Acquired syphilis, primary or secondary*
   a) Benzathine penicillin G, 2.4 million U im (1.2 million U into each buttock); **or**
   b) Aqueous procaine penicillin G, 600,000 to 1 million U im daily x 10 days.
5. *Latent syphilis* (This stage is now being reported in adolescents.)
   a) Nonreactive CSF: treat as for primary syphilis.
   b) Reactive (or unknown) CSF (i.e., neurosyphilis): treat with either
      - Benzathine penicillin G, 9.6 million U (2.4 million U/wk x 4 wk); **or**
      - Aqueous procaine penicillin G, 9 million U (600,000 U/day x 15 days)

Allergy to Penicillin

Tetracycline or erythromycin 30 to 40 mg/kg/day (in equally divided doses, qid) x 10-15 days. **Note.** If possible, avoid giving tetracycline to patients under 7 yr of age.

Note

1. As treponemes cannot enter the fetal circulation before the 16th to 18th wk, treatment of the mother before the 5th mo of pregnancy almost invariably protects the child from infection.
2. Giving therapy before the 3rd or 4th mo of intrauterine life avoids development of the periodontal/periosteal stigmata of congenital syphilis.
3. Florid signs and symptoms at birth predict a poor prognosis despite therapy.

4. The later the signs/symptoms of active disease after birth, the better the outlook. Treatment in older children will result in cure, but prognosis depends on extent of prior damage — adequate therapy may not prevent interstitial keratitis, nerve deafness, or Clutton's joints.

OTHER VENEREAL DISEASES

Specific Therapy

Adolescent and Adult Patients

1. *Lymphogranuloma venereum*
Tetracycline, 1 g daily x 30 days

2. *Chancroid*
Tetracycline, 1 g daily x 15-20 days

3. *Herpes simplex genitalis*
A common disease, but no treatment at present.
   - Pregnant virus-positive females: consider cesarean section at onset of labor.

4. *Hepatitis B (serum hepatitis)* and *Cytomegalovirus (CMV) infection*
Indirect evidence that these viral infections can be transmitted by sexual intercourse. No treatment at present.

5. *Nonspecific urethritis*
Whether postgonococcal or caused by the TRIC (chlamydial) organisms or mycoplasma: responds well to tetracycline (if symptoms warrant therapy).

PARASITIC DISEASES

Disease	Parasite	Diagnosis	Treatment	Special Instructions
Ascariasis	*Ascaris lumbricoides*	Intact worms or ova in feces	1. Pyrantel pamoate 11 mg/kg (max, 1 g) po, in 1 dose **or** 2. Mebendazole 100 mg bid po for 3 days **or** 3. Piperazine 75 mg/kg/day (max, 3.5 g) x 2 days.	
Giardiasis	*Giardia lamblia*	Ova in stool, or trophozoites in duodenal aspirate	1. Quinacrine dihydrochloride (Atabrine) 6-8 mg/kg/day x 5 days (max, 300 mg/day) **or** 2. Metronidazole (Flagyl) 10 mg/kg/day x 10 days.	Treat only if infestation heavy/symptomatic
Hydatid disease	*Echinococcus granulosus* (larval stage)	Eosinophilia; complement-fixation Casoni (intradermal) test	Surgery where indicated. *No chemotherapy.*	

158

Hookworm	*Necator americanus*	Ova in stool; iron-deficiency anemia	1. Mebendazole 100 mg bid po x 3 days **or** 2. Pyrantel pamoate 11 mg/kg x 2 doses **or** 3. Thiabendazole 25 mg/kg bid x 2 to 4 days **or** 4. Bephenium hydroxynaphthoate (Alcopar) 100 mg/kg/day x 2 days	Treatment not necessary for light infections in nonendemic areas. 4. Give on empty stomach; rest for 1 hr afterward
Pneumocystis pneumonia	*Pneumocystis carinii*	Sputum smear Bronchial or tracheal aspirate Lung biopsy, plain film, blood gases	Trimethoprimsulfamethoxazole (TMX) 20 mg TMX/kg/day x 10 days	
Pinworns (oxyuriasis)	*Enterobius vermicularis*	Live worms around anus or vulva. Ova obtained by application of Scotch tape to anus	1. Mebendazole 100 mg po in 1 dose. Repeat in 10-14 days. **or** 2. Pyrvinium pamoate 5 mg/kg (max, 250 mg) in 1 dose **or** 3. Pyrantel pamoate 11 mg/kg po (max, 1 g) in 1 dose **or** 4. Piperazine (Antepar, Vermisol, Entacyl)	Maintain good hygiene.

cont'd on p. 160

159

Disease	Parasite	Diagnosis	Treatment	Special Instructions
			50-75 mg/kg/day, in 1 dose (before breakfast) x 5-7 days. May need to repeat.	Saline purge and anti-emetic before medication. Saline purge 2 hr after medication. Light diet for 48 hr after medication.
Tapeworm (taeniasis)	*Taenia solium; Taenia saginata*	Proglottids or ova in stool	Quinacrine (Atabrine) 15 mg/kg, divided into 2 doses. Give the doses 1 hr apart, on empty stomach, with equal amount of Na bicarbonate	
Toxoplasmosis	*Toxoplasma gondii*	Serum Sabin–Feldman dye test; complement-fixation test; skin test – not reliable	*Congenital:* no treatment. *Acquired* – 1. Sulfadiazine 150-200 mg/kg/day, in 4 divided doses, x 1 mo. 2. Pyrimethamine (Daraprim) 1 mg/kg/day x 4 days, then 0.5 mg/kg/day x 1 mo. 3. Supplement with folinic acid, 1-2 mg/day.	Watch for leukopenia: treatment according to individual case.

Trichinosis	*Trichinella spiralis*	1. Complement-fixation test 2. Skin test: read in 20 min and 24 hr 3. Biopsy of muscle	Thiabendazole 25 mg/kg bid for 3-7 days	Steroids: value controversial
Visceral larva migrans	*Toxocara canis; Toxocara cati*	1. Eosinophilia 2. Isohemagglutinins increased 3. Low serum albumin 4. Skin biopsy (for cutaneous larval migrans)	Thiabendazole 25 mg/kg bid until symptoms abate. Prednisone 20-40 mg/day for symptomatic relief	No specific treatment demonstrated of value
Whipworm	*Trichuris trichiura*	Ova or parasites in stool	Mebendazole 100 mg po bid x 3 days. Same dosage for all ages. Repeat in 3 wk if eggs still present	

SKIN PARASITES: see Dermatology, p 267

NEONATOLOGY

NEONATES OF NORMAL AND LBW
(LOW BIRTH WEIGHT)

Resuscitation

1. Avoid cooling. Dry, and immediately place the ill neonate under radiant warmer.
2. Clear upper airway with gentle suction
    a) if not pink and crying well, administer O_2 by funnel or mask
    b) if no improvement within 1 min, resuscitate with bag and mask.
3. If pale and toneless, with bradycardia (<100/min): intubate; suction; resuscitate with bag, giving sufficient O_2 to keep baby pink.
4. If heart rate <60/min or umbilical artery not pulsating:
    a) Apply external cardiac massage, with 2 fingers over midsternum, at 100/min (4 pressures to each respiration).
    b) Intracardiac epinephrine 0.5 ml (1:10,000 solution) may be necessary.
5. If liquor and/or baby is meconium stained, suspect meconium aspiration:
    –   intubate and suction trachea before resuscitation.
6. All other instances: assess and record Apgar score at 1, 5, and 10 min.

Factor	Apgar Score		
	0	1	2
Heart rate	Absent	<100/min	>100/min
Respirations	Absent	Weak cry	Crying lustily
Muscle tone	Flaccid	Some flexion	Well flexed
Irritability	No response	Some motion	Cry
Color	Blue, pale	Blue hands & feet	Entirely pink

Apgar at 1 min

7: Baby normal, but rough technique could cause vagal inhibition. Observe.

3-6: a) If apneic: suction, and ventilate with bag on a mask.
     b) If breathing: search for causes of airway obstruction.

0-3: Intubate, IPPV. Apply external cardiac massage (p 468) as necessary.

7. Bicarbonate may be necessary to correct metabolic acidosis.
    a) If continued hypotonia, pallor, poor respiratory effort: give via umbilical vein, at 1 ml/kg/min, 7.5% Na bicarbonate 1-2 ml/kg diluted with equal quantity 5% dextrose soln. (Maximal safe dose of bicarbonate = 8 mEq/kg/24 hr.)
8. All infants: give 0.5 mg vitamin K_1 im.
9   *Analeptics have no place in management.* – Give naloxone (Narcan), $5\mu g$/kg body weight, for narcotic depression.

Transportation

1. Notify referral center by prior physician/physician contact.
2. Obtain all necessary details of pregnancies, labor, delivery, drugs, Apgar score and subsequent progress.
3. Accompanying nurse must have neonatal experience and have been instructed in respiratory emergencies.
4. Essential apparatus includes stethoscope, bag & mask, NG tube, iv pump, suction facility, low-reading thermometer, laryngoscope, appropriate nasotracheal tubes.
5. Check O_2 reserves, including ambulance reserve tank.
    a) Monitor O_2 where possible.
    b) Be generous with O_2 unless journey unduly long.
6. Avoid cooling: optimal temperature = at least 36°C for all but fit large neonates (35°C).
7. Stabilization before transfer is critically important.
    a) Severe RDS, recurrent apnea, diaphragmatic hernia: ensure adequate airway – prophylactic NT intubation.
    b) Correct metabolic acidosis, hypotension, severe anemia, hypoglycemia.
8. Air transport: ascertain cabin pressure; adjust F_1O_2 appropriately.

Important Aspects of Examination

1. *At birth:* Apgar score at 1, 5, 10 min (see p 162).
2. *Admission to nursery:*
    a) Note general appearance, whether true premature or small for GA (SGA), skin color, tone, posture, respiratory rate and pattern, and BP (see Fig).
    b) Do full physical examination.

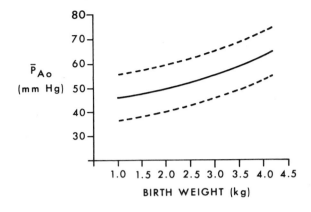

Parabolic regression (middle line) and 95% confidence limits (broken lines) of mean aortic BP plotted against birth weight in normal neonates during hours 2–12 of life.

3. *Discharge from nursery*
   a) Check weight gain, activity, feeding pattern; and if male, urinary stream.
   b) Exclude: persistent jaundice, residual infection, moist umbilicus, edema, heart murmur, unstable hips, hepatosplenomegaly, renal enlargement, undue increase in head circumference, increase in fontanel tension.

NEONATES OF LOW BIRTH WEIGHT (LBW)

Management
1. Use aseptic technique, clean gown, and wash hands with antibacterial soln, for handling each baby.
2. Assess whether appropriate or SGA, using Dubowitz's scoring system (Pediatrics 77:1, 1970).
3. Maintain rectal temp at 37°C, using incubator or infants' servo-controlled system with plastic heat-shield if necessary.

4. Start feeding within 2 hr (by NG radio-opaque tube, if necessary).
   a) First feed 1-5 ml water, depending on birth weight.
   b) If tolerated, continue with breast milk or artificial formula:

80 ml/kg in first 24 hr	Frequency of feeds
120 ml/kg to day 4	depends upon birth
150 ml/kg to day 10	weight — hourly if
Increase to 200 ml/kg	necessary in smallest
by day 14	infants

5. If these total volumes are not tolerated enterally, supplement to daily requirement with iv dextrose (5% or 10%, guided by blood glucose and absence of glycosuria).
6. Monitor respirations and/or heart rate for apnea.
7. Monitor O_2 indices:
   a) Monitor environmental O_2 concn hourly.
   b) Measure PaO_2 frequently in all infants given O_2 supplement.
   c) Umbilical artery PaO_2 should be kept below 90 mm Hg, and radial artery PaO_2 below 100 mm Hg. PaO_2 should be above 40 mm Hg.
   d) Arterialized heel-prick samples are unreliable in prevention of hyperoxia.
8. Monitor blood biochemistry:
   a) Blood glucose at least twice daily for first 3 days.
   b) Bilirubin at least daily while clinical jaundice lasts.
   c) Serum Ca daily for first 3-4 days.

Prophylaxis

1. Vit K_1 0.5 mg im, single dose (p 464).
2. Antibacterial ophthalmic ointment (Na sulfacetamide 10%) on admission and day 5.
3. Vit A, B, C, D, E daily trom 2 wk of age.
4. Oral Fe preparation: start at 1 mo (e.g., Fer-in-Sol 0.3 ml po tid).

NEONATES SMALL FOR GESTATIONAL AGE (SGA)

Weight >2 SD below the mean for GA (Usher chart).

Special Problems
High incidence of hypoxia, meconium aspiration, temp. instability (hypothermia/fever), hypoglycemia, hypocalcemia, other electrolyte disturbances, intrauterine infections, pulmonary hemorrhage, hyperviscosity syndrome, etc.

Management
1. Assess blood glucose with Dextrostix q6h for first 48 hr. Maintain blood glucose over 40 g/dl.
2. Early feeding if necessary, supplemented with dextrose 5-6 mg/kg/min iv.

RESPIRATORY DISTRESS SYNDROME (RDS)

Diagnosis
1. *Exclude other causes* of respiratory distress: pneumonia (strep B sepsis), transient tachypnea, massive aspiration, pneumothorax, pneumomediastinum, diaphragmatic hernia, cardiac disease, choanal atresia, micrognathia, cerebral asphyxia.
2. *Investigations*
    a) PaO_2, note concentration of inspired O_2 — fractional inspired O_2 (F_IO_2), $PaCO_2$, pH, HCO_3^-, glucose and BUN, Ca^{++}, Na^+, K^+, Cl^-, Hct.
    b) Chest film. RDS characterized by diffuse ground-glass appearance or reticulogranular pattern with air bronchogram.

Management
1. Catheterize umbilical artery (tip at L_{5-4}); check radiographically.
2. Nurse the baby in an Isolette.
3. Place in head-box: monitor carefully — warmed humidified mixture of 50% O_2 in air.
4. Increase F_IO_2 every 2 min by 10% steps until central cyanosis is relieved. Maintain PaO_2 between 50 and 80 mm Hg.

5. Assess severity of RDS by noting response to F_IO_2 0.9 for 15 min. If possible, monitor PaO_2 with umbilical artery or transcutaneous electrode.
6. Monitor BP. Correct hypotension with fresh frozen plasma or whole-blood transfusion.
7. a) **Note.** Correction of metabolic acidosis is rarely necessary and should not be attempted until the above are managed. Use only half correction. *(See also* use of bicarbonate, p 163).
    b) Monitor acid–base PaO_2, $PaCO_2$: every 4 hr and after any therapeutic manipulation (e.g., bicarbonate administration).
8. Maintain NG feeds if possible; supplement prn with 5% or 10% dextrose.
    a) Total (NG and iv) fluids should not exceed 80-100 ml/kg/24 hr while in severe respiratory distress.
    b) Monitor blood glucose regularly for hypo- and hyperglycemia.
9. Antibiotics are indicated only for suspected or proven infection.

ASSISTED VENTILATION

Indication: failure to maintain $PaO_2 > 50$ mm Hg in F_IO_2 of 50% by other means. Methods include:

1. Continuous distending pressure (CDP, CPAP).
    a) Maintain with nasopharyngeal tube (NPT), endotracheal tube (ETT), or continuous negative-pressure breathing (CNPB).
    b) Start with 5 cm water pressure; increase by 2-3 cm every 10-15 min to maximum of 12 cm (as indicated by PaO_2 response).
2. IPPV with positive expiratory pressure (IPPV with PEP):
    a) If CPAP or CNPB fails (PaO_2 <40 mm Hg in 0.8 O_2 with CPAP 10 cm water)
    b) if baby moribund
    c) if hypercarbic respiratory acidosis, or
    d) if continuous bagging needed for apnea.
3. Suction airways as frequently as indicated by stethoscopic evidence of secretions, poor color, excessive indrawing, poor chest-wall movement.
    a) **Note. Excessive suctioning may be harmful.**
    b) Avoid sudden changes in F_IO_2 and hypoxia.
    c) Antibiotics not routinely indicated with NT intubation.
    d) Too high CPAP may interfere with cardiac return and hence cardiac output. Lowering CPAP may improve oxygenation in some cases.

INFECTION

1. *High risk* of infection —
   a) if infant LBW
   b) if labor difficult or complicated
   c) if rupture of membranes >24 hr (especially if amnionitis or asphyxia)
   d) if infant requires resuscitation, intubation, catheterization, or surgical procedures.
2. *Symptoms and signs* (often minimal) include unexplained jaundice, respiratory distress, apnea, lethargy, feed-refusal, abdominal distention, vomiting, weight loss, thermal instability, metabolic acidosis.

Investigations

1. Chest film.
2. Culture and sensitivities — umbilical swab, blood, CSF, and urine (preferably obtained by suprapubic aspiration, p 78).
3. WBC total and differential. Note especially the percentage of band forms.
4. If infant <24 hr, aspirate stomach and external auditory canal (for smear and culture).
5. *Gastric-aspirate "shake test"*, to differentiate RDS from group B strep. infection:
   a) Add 0.5 ml gastric aspirate to 0.5 ml 0.9% saline with 1.0 ml 95% ethanol.
   b) Shake for exactly 15 sec.
   c) Read in 15 min. Negative in RDS (less than one-third of surface covered with foam).

Treatment

1. *Minor infections* (e.g. isolated pustules, conjunctivitis) may require local treatment only, but:
   a) Obtain cultures in all instances before treatment.
   b) Re-institute bathing with antibacterial soln if sepsis staphylococcal.
2. *Major infections;* see also p 139.
   Use antibiotic combinations to avoid emergence of resistant strains.
   a) Ampicillin and gentamicin (p 412) provide the best coverage. (Ampicillin should be given iv to be fully effective.)
   b) Modify according to organism sensitivities.
   c) Proven septicemia requires therapy for minimum of 2 wk; proven meningitis, 3 wk.

3. Provided infant (or mother) has not received antibiotics recently: if cultures negative, antibiotics used in prophylaxis for suspected infection can be discontinued after 48 hr.
4. Supportive therapy includes fluid and electrolytes iv, incubator isolation, use of strict sterile technique whenever spread of organism likely (e.g., abscess, fecal or urinary excretion of pathogenic organisms).

SEPTIC SHOCK

See under Meningitis, p 136.

APNEA

1. May be due to primary immaturity of respiratory control *or* symptomatic of a biochemical disturbance, sepsis, pneumonia, hypoventilation/hypoxia, severe anemia, late metabolic acidosis (severe), congestive cardiac failure, or convulsions.
2. *Clear airway* by suction.
3. *Stimulate:* flick sole of foot, stroke epigastrium.
4. *Ventilate* manually with bag, using environmental O_2 concn.
   a) Consider aminophylline:
      - Loading dose = 6 mg/kg; maintenance = 1.3 mg/kg q6h.
      - Monitor blood levels of drug.
      - Side-effects: tachycardia, gross GI hemorrhage.
   b) CPAP (at 3-5 cm) or IPPV may be necessary.

NEONATAL CONVULSIONS

See under Neurology, p 177.

ANEMIA

Measure Hb weekly in hospital and monthly thereafter.
a) *Early anemia:* Hct <35 within 3 days of birth.
   - In small prematures, may result from blood sampling.
b) *Anemia of prematurity*
   - Hb usually lowest $2 - 3$ mo after birth.
   - Transfuse only if recurrent apneic attacks result.
   - Often due to vitamin E deficiency $-$ give vit E 25 U po, daily, up to $1 - 2$ mo age.
c) *Late anemia*
   Iron deficiency will occur at age $6 - 12$ mo, particularly in prematures and twins, unless Fe prophylaxis.

HEMOLYTIC DISEASE

Rh-neg mother with Rh antibodies, *or* group 0 mother with group A or B infant.

1. Suspect ABO incompatibility if hemolytic hyperbilirubinemia with negative or weakly positive direct Coombs' test and positive indirect Coombs' test.
2. Clamp cord early.
    a) Cord specimen for Hb, bilirubin, Coombs' tests.
    b) Sample of maternal serum.
3. Pallid, edematous infant:
    a) Give immediate small exchange with packed cells to correct anemia.
    b) Paracentesis may be necessary if abdominal distention severe.

Exchange Transfusion

Indications

1. Cord blood Hb <12 g/dl, bilirubin >5 mg/dl, strongly positive Coombs' test.
2. Affected sib and positive Coombs' test.
3. Unconjugated bilirubin >20 mg/dl.
4. Prematurity: if bilirubin >1 mg/dl/100 g body wt, especially with acidosis, hypoxia, or hypoglycemia.

Procedure

1. Check for incompatibility of donor/baby's blood (p 26) and maternal serum.
2. **Before starting exchange:**
    a) **Check availability of suction and resuscitation equipment.**
    b) Draw blood for serum Ca and platelets.
    c) **Note.** Albumin priming (1.5 to 2.0 g/kg) 2 hr before will increase efficacy of exchange transfusion for hyperbilirubinemia.
3. Warm donor blood to 37°C, and adjust pH to 7.2 with THAM.
4. During exchange, monitor temp, ECG, color, respiratory rate, CVP (normal, 3 – 10 cm), and acid–base status.
5. Exchange 160 ml/kg, at a rate not exceeding 1.6 ml/kg/min, in aliquots of 5 – 20 ml according to size and state of infant.

6. With ACD blood, add 5 ml of 2% Ca gluconate per 100 ml exchange (to prevent hypocalcemia).
   a) Monitor cardiac rate carefully.
   b) Halfway thru exchange, draw blood for serum Ca.
7. If jaundice is severe, repeat microbilirubin every 3 – 4 hr after exchange.
8. Antibiotic prophylaxis (ampicillin and gentamicin, p 407) may be considered for potential septic complications.

HEMORRHAGE; SHOCK

1. Immediately after birth:
   a) May be due to fetal, twin-to-twin, placental, feto-maternal hemorrhage.
   b) Hct normal in acute stage.
   c) If hemorrhage suspected, check BP and monitor arterial pressure closely.
   d) If BP falling, transfuse with whole blood.
      – Otherwise, transfuse with packed RBC.
2. Postnatal hemorrhage – mainly due to vit K deficiency.
      – Correct with fresh frozen plasma 10 ml/kg and vit K.

DISSEMINATED INTRAVASCULAR COAGULATION (DIC)

1. Usually associated with asphyxia, severe RDS, or severe infection.
2. Platelets reduced; PT and PTT prolonged; factors V, VIII and fibrinogen decreased.
3. Notify Hematology.
4. Treat with exchange transfusion of fresh heparinized blood.

NECROTIZING ENTEROCOLITIS (p 280)

Causes

Multifactorial – acidosis, asphyxia, hypotension, umbilical-vessel catheterization, extreme prematurity, etc.

Diagnosis

1. Unstable temperature, increased apneic episodes, abdominal distention, bloody stools, delayed gastric emptying.
2. Plain film of abdomen typically shows gas in gut wall; later, gas in hepatic portal venous system, and pneumoperitoneum.

Management

1. If radiological findings definite, laparotomy indicated in most neonates **weighing more than 1500 g — but infants <1500 g withstand surgery poorly.**
2. Conservative treatment includes Gomco suction, iv alimentation, antibiotics as for neonatal sepsis (p 168). Surgery for abscess or stricture can be performed later.

CLINICAL APPROACH TO METABOLIC DISORDERS

Presentation	Metabolic Disorders
Neurological	Maple-syrup-urine disease (MSUD)
	Hyperammonemia
	Non-ketotic hyperglycinemia
Metabolic Acidosis	Congenital lactic acidosis
	Organic aciduria
	Defects of cytosolic gluconeogenesis
Hepatic Dysfunction	Galactosemia
	Hereditary fructose-intolerance
	Tyrosinemia

Investigations appropriate to each disorder are discussed in Tests of Metabolic Function (p 55) and/or Metabolic Disorders (p 254).

NEUROLOGY
(Drug Therapy, see p 174)

CONVULSIVE DISORDERS

Centrencephalic or Idiopathic

Represent nonprogressive CNS abnormality. All have EEG spike-and-wave phenomenon, though not always present in routine tracing.

A. *Grand mal seizures*

B. *Petit mal seizures*

1. Short staring spell or "absence"; may have rhythmic blinking or rolling up of eyes. Onset after 3 yr and usually cease about 15 yr. Grand mal seizures develop in 5%.

2. Akinetic or drop attacks

3. Myoclonic spasms.

C. *Status epilepticus*

Recurrent grand mal seizures, with no intervening recovery of consciousness, progressing to deepening coma and hyperthermia.

Focal seizures

Represent local and, in some cases, progressive CNS disease. Seizure activity usually only focal but may spread to adjacent areas, or to opposite side, or become generalized.

A. *Jacksonian motor seizures*

1. Usually begin in finger, face, or toe, and "march" to adjacent motor areas.

2. May leave transient focal weakness.

B. *Temporal-lobe or psychomotor epilepsy*

1. Aura: altered perception, unpleasant smell or taste, *déjà vu,* "dreamy state", fear, or complex hallucination.

2. Patient confused, out of contact, and cannot respond, but carries out habitual or repetitive acts.

3. Convulsive component: chewing; lip-smacking; swallowing; grimacing; perhaps rubbing, patting, or picking at something.

4. Postictal: confusion, drowsiness.

C. *Other types*

Adversive or postural movements, focal seizures affecting sensory, visual, auditory or speech areas.

COMMON ANTICONVULSANTS

Drug	Use	Dosage	Therapeutic serum level	Side-effects
phenobarbital	Grand mal, focal seizures	3 – 6 mg/kg/day	15 – 50* μg/ml	Drowsiness, irritability, hyperactivity
diphenylhydantoin sodium (Dilantin)	Grand mal, focal seizures	4 – 6 mg/kg/day	10 – 20 μg/ml	Ataxia, gingival hypertrophy, rash, hirsutism
primidone (Mysoline)	Grand mal, focal seizures	5 – 20 mg/kg/day	5 – 15* μg/ml	Drowsiness, vertigo, ataxia, rash, anorexia
acetazolamide (Diamox)	Petit mal	12 – 25 mg/kg/day	NA†	Lassitude, anorexia, headache, paresthesia
ethosuximide (Zarontin)	Petit mal	20 – 30 mg/kg/day	20 – 80 μg/ml	Nausea, rash, drowsiness, disturbed vision
trimethadione (Tridione)	Petit mal	20 – 40 mg/kg/day	NA†	Rash, bone-marrow depression, nephrosis, photophobia
diazepam (Valium)	Auxiliary drug in many disorders	0.1 – 1.0 mg/kg/day	NA†	Drowsiness, ataxia

carbamazepine (Tegretol)	Temporal lobe, grand mal seizures	20 mg/kg/day. Start with 5 mg/kg and increase over 4 wk.	4 – 10 μg/ml	Fatigue, malaise, dizziness, lethargy
clonazepam (Rivotril)	Infantile spasms, myoclonic seizures, absence attacks, grand mal seizures	0.5 mg tid x 3 days (average dose for 10-yr-old). Increase daily dose by 0.25 mg (total dose based on 0.5 mg/kg/day tid), q3-5 days; to build up slowly to 0.5 mg/kg/day tid if needed.	—	Ataxia, drowsiness, wt gain, dysarthria, irritability
nitrazepam (Mogadon)	Minor motor seizures	0.6 – 1.2 mg/kg/day	—	Hepatotoxicity
valproic acid (Depakine)	Minor motor, temporal lobe, grand mal seizures	1st wk: 25–50 mg/kg/day [handwritten: 20 30] 2nd wk: 75–100 mg/kg/day [handwritten: 30 3rd wk 40mg/kg/day] Slowly, increase to total 2-6 g/day prn	50 – 100 μg/ml	Nausea, vomiting, drowsiness, wt gain, tremor, hepatotoxicity

*Not fully established

†NA – test not readily available

175

Minor Motor Seizures

A. *Myoclonic seizures:* brief jerks (usually flexor) of extremities.

B. *Akinetic seizures:* caused by sudden loss of tone. There may be a head-nod or sudden collapse on to the floor.

A,B: *Myoclonic–akinetic seizures:* most relate to a fixed lesion; others, associated with degenerative disease.

In many cases, deterioration in intellect, resulting in mental retardation (Lennox–Gastaut syndrome).

Treatment is difficult, often requiring combination of anticonvulsants (p 174): clonazepam (Rivotril), valproic acid (Depakine), and nitrazepam (Mogadon) may be useful.

A ketogenic diet may be prescribed.

C. *Infantile spasms (salaam attacks):* probably the commonest etiology is perinatal anoxia, but many other causes (e.g., tuberous sclerosis, inherited metabolic disease).

1. Usually start between 3 and 9 mo.
2. May be flexor or extensor.
3. May be multiple daily, often in flurries.
4. EEG usually very abnormal; may be classical hypsarrhythmia.
5. Treatment: includes ACTH, prednisone; more recently, clonazepam, valproic acid, and nitrazepam.
6. Prognosis poor: progression to mental retardation in >90%, and spasms may become generalized after age 2 yr.

FEBRILE CONVULSIONS

Type & Characteristics

A. **Typical or Benign**
1. Patient is neurologically normal before convulsion.
2. Age range: 6 mo-4 yr
3. Generalized convulsion during fever
4. Convulsion brief (<10 min)
5. May have
   - positive family history
   - no CNS signs afterward
   - normal EEG and lab studies.

B. **Atypical or Malignant**
   1. Age <6 mo or >4 yr
   2. Seizure local or asymmetrical
   3. Seizure prolonged (>10 min)
   4. May have residual Todd's paralysis or other abnormal CNS signs
   5. Persistent EEG abnormality is common.

Management
1. *Investigations* – **all first febrile convulsions:**
   a) LP (to rule out meningitis)
   b) Blood sugar, calcium, BUN, phosphorus (p 376)
   c) EEG
   d) Skull radiographs.
2. *Treatment*
   A. **Typical**
      a) Reassure parents,
      b) Treat fever and/or infection
      c) Give phenobarbital, 5 mg/kg/day, for present illness.
         Note. Intermittent anticonvulsant therapy during subsequent febrile illness is of no value.
      d) If patient has 4 or more seizures: start continuous anticonvulsant regime.
   B. **Atypical**
      a) Start continuous anticonvulsant therapy.
      b) Arrange follow-up.

Prognosis
A. **Typical:** normal CNS development; but, commonly, recurrent febrile seizures.
B. **Atypical:** epilepsy develops in 40%, other CNS sequelae common.

CONVULSIONS IN THE NEONATE

Type & Characteristics
A. *Subtle* – easily overlooked
   1. Very common, especially in premature infants
   2. Signs may include: apnea, tonic posturing, tonic eye deviation, fluttering of eyelids, drooling or lip movements.
B. *Multifocal*
   1. Common, but only in first month of life

2. Succession of clonic jerks migrating from limb to limb
   3. EEG: multiple foci migrating bilaterally.
C. *Focal* **Note:** may represent generalized or metabolic disease
   1. Well localized to one part
   2. Patient may not lose consciousness
   3. Prognosis is good.
D. *Tonic*
   1. Focal or generalized stiffening, or decerebrate posturing
   2. EEG grossly abnormal
   3. Prognosis is poor.
E. *Jitteriness* – **not a seizure disorder**
   1. Confined to neonatal period
   2. Patient is exquisitely stimulus-sensitive
   3. "Tremors" – rhythmic alternating movements of equal rate (clonic jerks have rapid flexion and slow return)
   4. No tonic deviations or jerks.

Etiology includes:

   −   ischemic injury
   −   cerebral contusion
   −   periventricular hemorrhage
   −   hypoglycemia, hypocalcemia, hypomagnesemia, other metabolic disorders
   −   infection
   −   congenital malformation
   −   drug-withdrawal.

Treatment

1. Correct sugar and Ca levels
2. Give phenobarbital:
    a) Loading dose: 10 ml/kg; repeat once if necessary.
    b) Maintenance dose: 5 mg/kg/day.
3. If convulsion persists, give either:
    a) 3% soln magnesium, iv, **or**
    b) pyridoxine, 25 mg iv.

Prognosis – varies with etiology

1. Normal CNS development in (approx.) 50%
2. CNS damage in 25%
3. Death in 25% of cases.

RESPIROLOGY
CYSTIC FIBROSIS

Genetics
Autosomal recessive. In Caucasians, carrier rate = 1:20, and incidence 1:1600 live births.

Both parents heterozygous: with each conception, 25% chance of having a CF child, 50% chance of heterozygote child, and 25% chance of child with no abnormal genes for CF.

Diagnosis
1. Birth weight: commonly, low at term compared with normal sibs.
2. Meconium ileus and/or volvulus: 5%.
3. Failure to thrive despite good appetite.
4. Stools large, foul, and contain increased quantities of fat, protein, and starch.
5. Rectal prolapse not otherwise explained.
6. Frequent respiratory infections; mucus plugging and secondary infection result in patchy atelectasis and hyperinflation.
7. Usually, clubbing of fingers and toes.
8. Initial infecting organism in lungs usually *Staph aureus*.
9. Sinusitis in almost 100% of cases.
10. Nasal polyps in children <14 yr old are indicative of CF.
11. Cirrhosis of liver may be a presenting feature.

Investigation
1. Sweat chloride high (p 404); >60 mEq/liter significant.
    a) A high level before 3 mo old important, but a low level in same age group does *not* rule out CF.
    b) False positive sweat chloride tests: Addison's disease, nephrotic syndrome, glycogen-storage disease, etc.
2. Stool analysis (5-day fecal fat collection), plus calculation of dietary fat content, to determine % fat excreted and stool chymotrypsin content.
3. Pancreatic secretion analysis for trypsin, chymotrypsin, and bicarbonate. Arranged by Gastroenterology.

Nutritional Management

1. Normal diet for age.
2. Vitamins
    a) Double dose of A, D, C and B.
    b) Vitamin E: infant, 50 U tid; children, 100 U tid.
3. Enzyme replacement (Cotazyme; p 453)
    a) Infants: 1 capsule/4 oz of formula
    b) Young children: 1 capsule/kg body wt, to maximum of 27 capsules daily.
    c) Older children, adults: 27-30 capsules daily (6 with each meal and 3 with snacks).
4. If improved absorption needed, on nutritional grounds or because of persisting diarrhea, a trial of sodium bicarbonate or cimetidine supplementation should be considered.
5. Add salt to diet, particularly during hot weather and fever (excessive salt loss in sweat).

Treatment of Respiratory System

1. Frequent *sputum cultures* to determine organisms and their sensitivity.
2. *Inhalation therapy* may be bland, bronchodilator, mucolytic antibiotic, or combination therapy. It is given by mask and nebulizer tid.
    a) Bland therapy: 2-3 ml normal saline or 2-3 ml buffered nebulizing vehicle (BNV = 10% propylene glycol; 90% of 1/8% phenylephrine).
    b) Bronchodilator therapy: salbutamol 0.01 - 0.03 ml/kg, up to 1 ml maximum, added to 2 ml normal saline or BNV in nebulizing mask.
    c) Mucolytic therapy: 2-3 ml of 20% N-acetyl-cysteine solution.
    d) Antibiotic therapy: cephaloridine 500 mg or lincomycin 300 mg added to 2-3 ml of vehicle solution in nebulizing mask.
    e) Combination therapy: antibiotic and bronchodilator can be combined with bland nebulizing solution or mucolytic agent.
3. *Postural drainage:* tid after mask inhalation therapy.

    All lobes drained; particular attention paid to those most involved.
4. *Systemic antibiotics:* type depends on culture and sensitivity reports.
    a) Antistaphylococcal- drugs such as cloxacillin; anti-pseudomonas drugs such as tobramycin iv with carbenicillin or ticarcillin; in special cases, trimethoprim—sulfa might be indicated.

b) Give antibiotics continuously or intermittently, depending on particular case and severity of involvement.
c) Recommended doses: consult Infectious Disease Service.
d) Peak and trough serum levels of parenteral antibiotics, especially aminoglycosides: monitor twice weekly.

EPIGLOTTITIS

Characterized by abrupt onset of fever, respiratory obstruction, and difficulty swallowing.

Do NOT examine throat (risk of inducing gagging and obstruction) unless ENT personnel and equipment are present.

The swollen epiglottis may be readily visible: looks like a large strawberry.

Do NOT order any radiographs until maintenance of adequate airway is ensured.

Treatment
1. Ensure maintenance of adequate airway:
   a) Endotracheal tube preferred, but tracheotomy may be necessary.
   b) Send ETT secretions for culture and sensitivity.
2. Admit patient to ICU, where airway will be secured.
3. Blood culture, CBC.
4. Give antibiotics iv. *H. influenzae* is common infecting agent; when culture results are available, antibiotics can be adjusted accordingly:
   a) ampicillin 100 mg/kg/day q4h **PLUS**
   b) chloramphenicol 100 mg/kg/day q6h.

ACUTE LARYNGOTRACHEOBRONCHITIS (CROUP)

Admitting Department
1. **Immediately,** notify pediatric admitting resident.
2. **If case severe,** also notify ICU medical resident and ENT resident.
3. *If indicated,* film of chest and neck to rule out foreign body and lung collapse.
4. Examine throat: hazardous – do once only. Remember possibility of diphtheria.

5. Start treatment:
   a) Croupette – with O_2 in all but very mild cases.
   b) Antibiotic not routinely necessary. If indicated, ampicillin (p 407).
   c) Sedation (not routinely, but may be helpful if child frightened or agitated):
      Secobarbital, 50 mg pr, in child 1-3 yr.

Ward

1. Take pulse and respiratory rate q 15 min for 4 hr or until settled.
2. **Watch for** restlessness, rising pulse, and increased in-drawing: these indicate critical compromise of air-way and need for assistance by:
   a) 2% Racemic epinephrine (0.5 ml in 2-3 ml N sa-line) by nebulized aerosol or IPPB.
      - Notify senior medical resident, who will notify Anesthesia and arrange transfer to PAR. (This treatment is not being given on the ward at present.)
      - This treatment necessitates constant-care nursing and frequent monitoring of vital signs.
      - Racemic epinephrine gives only temporary relief and may need repeating.
      - Assess patient frequently and carefully:
        If apparently tiring, or considerable respi-ratory distress continuing, another means of airway maintenance is needed; such as:
   b) Endotracheal intubation
      - Notify ICU and ENT (intubation may be done by ICU staff)
      - Patient will be monitored in ICU.
   c) Or, if endotracheal intubation not possible, tra-cheotomy:
      - ENT will perform surgery and follow pa-tient.
3. Encourage clear fluids po. Give iv if not taking fluids well.
4. Order chest film if temperature elevated after 24 hr or if rales present.
5. If patient moderately to severely ill: Monitor arterial-ized pH, pO_2, and pCO_2.

BRONCHIOLITIS

Severe respiratory infection in infants <2 yr, involving terminal bronchioles and surrounding alveoli.

Produces signs of lower respiratory obstruction – expiratory grunt and/or wheeze, tachypnea, dyspnea and fine crepitant rales.

Etiology: usually viral, rarely complicated by bacterial superinfection.

Differentiate from:
1. Asthma
2. Foreign body:
   a) high obstruction = inspiratory distress
   b) low obstruction = unilateral signs
3. Cardiac failure (p 200)
4. Severe acidosis
5. Salicylate intoxication (p 485).

Management
1. Croupette, high humidity; and O_2 in all but very mild cases
2. Constant-care nursing if necessary
3. Suction nasopharynx **gently** prn, and turn patient frequently
4. Start iv to correct dehydration; do not overload (p 119)
5. Salbutamol by nebulized aerosol may be tried (p 186)
6. Bronchoscope suction rarely necessary
7. If child seems moderately ill: monitor arterialized pCO_2, O_2, and pH.

TUBERCULOSIS

Pulmonary

Uncomplicated
1. Conservative therapy:
   a) Isonicotinic acid hydrazide (INH: Isoniazid) 10 mg/kg/day in 1 or 2 doses, not to exceed 300 mg daily.
   b) Close follow-up mandatory (Chest Clinic).
2. Continue therapy for at least 1 yr.

Progressive

1. If involvement beyond hilar nodes: give INH plus rifampicin (10-15 mg/kg/day, not to exceed 600 mg/day, in 2 doses).
2. Streptomycin sulfate may be added: 15-30 mg/kg/day im (maximum daily dose = 1 g):
   a) in 2 daily doses for 1 wk
   b) then total dose once daily for 1-2 wk
   c) then 3 times weekly for 1-2 mo.
3. Chemoprophylaxis: All children who have a positive 5 TU >10 mm induration (even if child had BCG as infant) after 48 hr should receive INH according to above regimen.

Tuberculous Adenitis

1. Whether due to TB bacilli or atypical mycobacteria, give INH (same dose as above) plus rifampicin for 1 yr.
2. If gland suppurative: apply 10% PAS ointment locally.

Tuberculous Meningitis

(Purulent Meningitis, *see* p 130)

1. Early diagnosis mandatory.
2. During acute illness: 5 TU test may be falsely negative, due to allergy. 250 TU intradermally may be necessary to demonstrate tuberculin hypersensitivity.
3. CSF cell count, differential, and sugar content essential.

   Note. TB meningitis is characterized by lymphocytic response with sugar <50 mg/dl. CSF from suspected cases should be hung for pellicle formation, and pellicle should be sent for Ziehl–Neelsen staining.
4. Serum electrolytes may reveal inappropriate ADH secretion (p 136). Low serum electrolytes are correctable by fluid restriction.
5. Drug therapy (triple therapy):
   a) INH, rifampicin, and streptomycin (dosages as above).
   b) Steroids: prednisone 1-2 mg/kg/day qid X 6-12 wk, or longer if indicated.
      (CSF block: hydrocortisone may be given intrathecally.)

184

ASTHMA

Asthma is characterized by increased reactivity of the airways to various stimuli and is manifested by slowing of forced expiration. The degree of severity may alter spontaneously or as a result of therapy.

Acute Asthma

Assessment
1. Restlessness
2. Fatigue
3. Cyanosis
4. Respiratory rate
5. Use of accessory muscles of respiratiom
6. Pulsus paradoxus (>10 mm Hg signifies severe airway obstruction)
7. Peak expiratory flow rate before and after bronchodilator (in children old enough to co-operate)
8. Arterial blood gases: serial measurement mandatory
9. Chest films.

Management
1. *Oxygen – humidified*
   Inspired O_2 concn:
   a) initially, Ventimask 35%
   b) subsequently, as dictated by serial arterial O_2 tension measurement.
2. *Intravenous fluids*
   a) Establish an iv line early, using a conventional hypotonic replacement solution, to administer drugs and to correct dehydration and electrolyte imbalance.
   b) Metabolic acidosis should be corrected as soon as possible, with sodium bicarbonate 0.3 mEq x body weight (kg) x base deficit.
   c) **Do not fluid-overload.**
3. *Drugs*
   a) β-Adrenergic bronchodilators (Table I)
      i) salbutamol (Ventolin) by nebulizer; **or**
      ii) metaproterenol (Alupent) by nebulizer; **or**
      iii) epinephrine (1:1000) subcutaneously.

      Note. Do not use salbutamol and epinephrine within 1 hr of each other (possibility of cardiac arrhythmia).

TABLE I. β-ADRENERGIC BRONCHODILATORS

Drug	Formulation & Dosage		
	Metered aerosol*	Nebulizer†	Oral preparation
salbutamol (Ventolin)	100 μg/puff. for age 6 - 14 yr: 1 puff up to qid >14 yr: 2 puffs qid	0.5% solution; 0.01 – 0.03 ml/kg, up to max. of 1.0 ml, prn to q4h.	0.05 – 0.1 mg/kg/dose up to tid
metaproterenol (Alupent)	750 μg/puff. for age 6 - 14 yr: 1 puff up to qid >14 yr: 2 puffs qid	5% solution; 0.01 ml/kg up to max. of 1.0 ml, prn to q4h.	0.5 mg/kg/dose up to tid
Epinephrine (1:1000)	Subcutaneously: 0.125 – 0.20 ml *stat*; and prn q 10 min x 2		

*Metered aerosols have a potential for abuse and psychological dependence. Their use should be carefully explained.
† All solutions made up to 2 ml with distilled water.
Note. Intravenous preparations of salbutamol and isoproterenol are available for use in very severe attacks and where constant monitoring is possible.

186

b) Theophylline — see Precautions (below)
   - iv loading dose 6 mg/kg over 20 min;
   - thereafter, **either**
     i) intermittent bolus q4-6h, to maximum 24 mg/kg/24 hr; **or**
     ii) 3 hr after initial loading dose, start continuous infusion (1.0 mg/kg/hr) and monitor serum theophylline level.

Note. iv drug is aminophylline: 100 mg of this is equivalent to 80 mg theophylline.

Precautions
   i) Contraindicated if patient has known theophylline idiosyncrasy.
   ii) Reduce loading dose to 3.5 mg/kg if patient has used theophylline products in previous 12 hr.
   iii) Heart failure, liver disease, viral disease, and erythromycin *decrease* theophylline metabolism and may produce toxic serum levels with conventional doses.
   iv) Smoking and phenobarbital *increase* theophylline metabolism and may result in inadequate serum levels with usual doses of theophylline.
   v) In obese patients, use a lean-weight estimate.

c) Steroids: give either
   i) hydrocortisone, 4 mg/kg iv q4-6h; **or**
   ii) methyl prednisolone, 1 mg/kg iv q4-6h.

d) Antibiotics:
   Bacterial infections are an unusual cause or complication of acute asthma. Therefore, antibiotics are rarely indicated.

4. *Failure of management*
   is manifested by worsening clinical signs, progressive hypoxemia, and a rising arterial CO_2 tension.

   This may indicate:
   a) need for β-agonists iv and/or assisted ventilation
   b) complication(s) such as pneumothorax, emphysema.

CHRONIC ASTHMA

Patients with mild, infrequent (once or twice a yr) episodes of asthma can be treated with bronchodilators intermittently. However, once treatment has been instituted, it should be continued at full dosage for a minimum of 2 wk.

TABLE II. THEOPHYLLINE PREPARATIONS

Brand name	Strength	Effective "free" theophylline (%)
Liquids		
Elixophyllin	5.3 mg/ml	100
Elixophyllin – paediatric suspension		
Slo-phyllin GG	20 mg/ml	100
Quibron	10 mg/ml	100
*Somophyllin	10 mg/ml	100
Choledyl paediatric syrup	18 mg/ml	85
Choledyl elixir	10 mg/ml	64
Theophyl-225	20 mg/ml	64
	7.5 mg/ml	100
Tablets		
Theolair	125 mg/tablet	100
Theolair	250 mg/tablet	100
Slo-phyllin	100 mg/tablet	100
Slo-phyllin	200 mg/tablet	100
Theophyl	225 mg/tablet	100

*Aminophylline	100 mg/tablet	80
*Aminophylline	200 mg/tablet	80
Choledyl	100 mg/tablet	64
Choledyl	200 mg/tablet	64
Rectal Solution		
Somophyllin	60 mg/ml	80
SUSTAINED-RELEASE PRODUCTS		
Gyrocaps		
Slo-phyllin	60 mg	100
Slo-phyllin	125 mg	100
Slo-phyllin	200 mg	100
Tablets		
Theo-Dur	100 mg	100
Theo-Dur	300 mg	100

*Theophylline products available in HSC Pharmacy.

The asthmatic patient who has more frequent attacks should be managed with long-term continuous therapy.

1.   *Theophylline* (see Table below)

THEOPHYLLINE DOSAGE

Age (yr)	*Dose (mg/kg/dose), given q6h	
1-9	6	*If serum theophylline levels are not obtained within 4 days of starting this drug, it is suggested that the dose be 25% lower.
9-12	5	
13-16	4.5	
>16	3.25	

a)   Aim for therapeutic serum levels of theophylline (between 10 and 20 mg/liter).
b)   *Rectal suppositories are contraindicated* (unreliable absorption and rectal irritation).
c)   *Rectal solutions are reliable and useful* but are not yet available in Canada.

2.   *β-Adrenergic bronchodilators* – salbutamol and metaproterenol can be administered as oral preparations, nebulized solutions, or by metered aerosol (see Table I).
3.   *Disodium cromoglycate* (Intal). Dose: 1 Spincap (20 mg) qid
      a)   This drug is a prophylactic agent: it will not reverse bronchoconstriction once this has occurred.
      b)   Intal is inhaled as a powder from a Spinhaler.
      c)   Patients who experience exercise-induced asthma attacks can often prevent them by inhaling the drug 10 min before exercise.
4.   *Corticosteroids*
      a)   Inhalations: Beclomethasone by metered aerosol is a prophylactic agent and should never be used for acute attacks.
           Dose is 2 puffs (100 μg) qid.
      b)   Systemic: few patients require this form of therapy. Prednisone, 0.5 mg/kg daily on alternate days, is the preferred method of treatment. This may not provide satisfactory control, necessitating daily doses of steroids.

190

RESPIRATORY FAILURE

Definition
Inability of the pulmonary system to meet the body's metabolic demands. Approx. 1/3 of all episodes of resp. failure occur in the neonatal period, and another 1/3 during the 1st yr of life.

Assessment
Difficult and often unreliable, except when patient is *in extremis*.

Aids to diagnosis
1. Knowledge of diseases in which resp. failure is a likely complication.
2. Clinical alertness to the possibility.
3. Arterial blood-gas measurements.

Causes
1. Obstruction of upper resp. tract (e.g., croup)
2. Obstruction of lower airways (e.g., bronchiolitis)
3. Pulmonary parenchymal disease (e.g., pneumonia)
4. Extrinsic pressure on lung (e.g., pneumothorax)
5. Neurologic disease (e.g., Guillain–Barré syndrome)
6. Systemic disease (e.g., sepsis)
7. Postoperative state (e.g., after cardiac, thoracic, or abdominal surgery).

Signs
1. *Clinical*
   a) general: fatigue, sweating
   b) respiratory: wheezing, expiratory grunting, decreased breath-sounds, nasal flaring, chest-wall retractions, tachypnea/bradypnea/apnea, cyanosis.
   c) cardiac: brady- or excessive tachycardia, hypo-/hypertension, pulsus paradoxus >12 mm Hg, cardiac arrest.
   d) cerebral: restlessness, irritability, headache, mental confusion, convulsions, coma.

2. *Laboratory*
   a) hypoxemia, acute or chronic
   b) hypercapnia, acute or chronic
   c) acidosis, respiratory and/or metabolic
   d) vital capacity <30% predicted *or* <3 x tidal volume
   e) maximal inspiratory pressure above −20 cm H_2O.

3.   *Arterial blood-gas measurements (ABG)*
     Indicate 2 types of resp. failure — **always,** must be
     interpreted with known inspired O_2 concn (F_IO_2).
     a)   Type I failure = low arterial pO_2 with normal
          or low pCO_2.
          Caused by ventilation–perfusion mismatch, in-
          trapulmonary shunting, and/or impaired diffu-
          sion — these are clinically indistinguishable.
     b)   Type II = low arterial pO_2 with high pCO_2.
          Caused by hypoventilation.
     c)   Without intracardiac shunt, *if* arterial pO_2
          <50 Torr, *and/or* arterial pCO_2 >50 Torr, =
          resp. failure.

          Exception: decreased pO_2 is normal when F_IO_2
          is low (at high altitude).

4.   *Hyperoxic test:* to exclude R-to-L intracardiac shunt-
     ing as cause of hypoxemia.
     a)   give 100% O_2 for 15-20 min; repeat ABG.
     b)   Hypoxemia of pulmonary origin will be partly
          corrected, whereas hypoxemia of intracardiac
          shunt will not change.

5.   The alveolar–artificial O_2 difference is a measure of
     resp. failure; it can be determined from nomogram
     on p 193.

Management

1.   When patient's condition is stable, transfer him to
     area where skilled nursing, ABG, radiography and an-
     cillary facilities are constantly available.

2.   Prevent deterioration during transport. Provide:
     a)   protection of airway
     b)   assisted ventilation prn
     c)   continuous supply of O_2
     d)   suction pump (for removal of pharyngeal secre-
          tions)
     e)   reliable iv line for drugs, fluids.

3.   Ventilation (see also 12, Assisted Ventilation)
     a)   Arterial pCO_2 is the measurement of alveolar
          ventilation: ↑pCO_2 = hypoventilation; ↓pCO_2
          = hyperventilation.
     b)   Supplemental O_2 must be humidified; and its
          concn is dictated by serial ABG.
     c)   Required O_2 concn varies for different diseases;
          but, in general:
          —   extrathoracic disease rarely necessitates
               >30% unless intubation or other assistance
               is required
          —   most intrathoracic diseases require more.

192

Alveolar Air Equation Nomogram

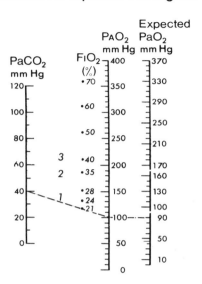

Solution of alveolar air equation, assuming sea level and R=0.8. To determine alveolar oxygen tension, locate $PaCO_2$ to the left, and F_IO_2 in the middle. Join the points with a ruler, and read PAO_2 at the right. At the far right are approximate values of PaO_2, assuming normal values for the (A-a) O_2 gradient. If the observed PaO_2 is lower than the PaO_2 on the far right scale, the (A-a) O_2 gradient is increased.

The dash and dot lines illustrate sample calculations:

Example	$PaCO_2$	F_IO_2	PAO_2	Expected PaO_2
I	40	21%	102	92
II	80	21%	54	44
III	60	40%	216	186

Prepared by Dudley F. Rochester, M.D. (Reproduced with permission of American Thoracic Society — Medical Section of the American Lung Association).

4. **Special notes re use of O_2**
   a) Premature neonates — retrolental fibroplasia may occur if arterial pO_2 >150 Torr for ≥4 hr.
   b) Pulmonary O_2 toxicity — F_IO_2 ≥60% for >60 hr with high ventilatory inflation pressures (>30 cm H_2O) may cause this.
      - But pulmonary toxicity is relatively uncommon, develops slowly, and often is reversible. Fear of causing this must *never* prevent treatment of hypoxia.
   c) Chronic obstructive pulmonary disease (e.g., cystic fibrosis). In patients with chronic CO_2 retention, high inspired O_2 may remove hypoxic drive, causing further hypoventilation. Low-flow O_2 (24-28% by mask, or 2-3 liters/min by nasal cannuli) can increase such patients' O_2 saturation to safe levels without cutting off their hypoxic drive.

5. Humidify all inspired gases — helps loosen viscid secretions, particularly if systemic dehydration is present.

6. Aerosol therapy
   a) Bronchodilating agents for asthma (p 186).
   b) Racemic epinephrine for croup (p 181).
   c) No proven indication for giving antimicrobial or mucolytic agents as aerosol.

7. Pharyngeal suction
   a) Perform gently, frequently, to remove secretions that tend to pool in pharynx in the very ill.
   b) Stimulates coughing and expulsion of tracheobronchial secretions.
   c) Contraindicated in epiglottitis, croup, or laryngeal spasm.
   d) Occasionally, patients with retained secretions need periodic endotracheal suction without prolonged intubation.

8. Physiotherapy
   a) Include chest-clapping and -vibrating, hyperinflation, and positioning for postural drainage.
   b) Useful in any situation where:
      i) acute mucus plugging of major bronchi is potential problem; *or*
      ii) copious bronchial secretions are part of disease process that led to resp. failure.

9. Fluids
   a) When dyspnea present, stop ingestion po and substitute feeding via NG tube. **But:**
   b) If dyspnea severe of palato-pharyngeal incoordination present, stop tube-feeding (risk of aspiration);

c) In which case, iv usually preferred route. But remember (especially if patient is small infant):
   i) humidification of inspired gases prevents resp. fluid losses;
   ii) with mechanical ventilation, full maintenance fluid needs = approx. 50% of requirement during spontaneous breathing.

10. Treatment of specific etiology: as indicated clinically.

11. General care, observation, and monitoring
   a) Nurses must be available for constant supervision.
   b) Handle child gently, and position as clinically appropriate (e.g., slight head-up tilt if cerebral edema present; sitting if gastro-esophageal reflux suspected).

12. Assisted ventilation
   a) Indications according to natural history of the disease and clinical assessment of the child.
   b) Mechanical assistance increases the complexity of management and introduces its own complications, which must be weighed against its advantages.
   c) Mechanical ventilation: usually reserved for patients unlikely to survive without it but who have a disease process that is reversible within a few days/weeks.
   d) Methods: select the one that is clinically appropriate (and dependably available)
      i) artificial airway: intubation, tracheotomy, or (neonate) nasal cannula.
      ii) IPPB by ventilator
      iii) CPAP: continuous constant pressure to the airway during spontaneous breathing
      iv) intermittent or continuous negative-pressure respiration — using a body-enclosing box
      v) CPPB: IPPB combined with PEEP.

13. General rules for intubation
   The formula for correct endotracheal tube size (apart from the exception below) is:

   $$\text{mm inner diam. (ID)} = \frac{\text{age (yr)}}{4} + 4$$

   a) **Exception:** in upper-airway obstruction, use very small tube:

Age (yr)	Tube size (mm ID)
<2	3.5
2-5	4.0
>5	4.5

b) The smallest endotracheal tube through which suctioning is possible = 3.0 mm ID (suitable for all but the most premature neonates).

c) In emergency, quick orotracheal intubation is preferred; the tube can be changed later to the NT route.

d) When endotracheal tube (ETT) inserted, do not secure until you have checked:
   i) tube positioned correctly — listen for equal air entry into both lung fields during inflation.
   ii) presence of air-leak around tube.

d) As soon as feasible, confirm position of ETT radiographically.

CARDIOLOGY

Interpretation of Electrocardiogram

Overloading (Hypertrophy/Dilation)

    Right atrial
Either:

1. Peaked P waves 3 mm or more in any lead; or
2. qR pattern in right chest leads (see RV hypertrophy also).

    Left atrial

1. Bifid P in any lead;
or 2. P duration more than 0.09 sec;
or 3. Late inversion of P in right chest leads (1 mm or more).

    Right ventricular

1. qR pattern in right chest leads,
or 2. R in V_1 20 mm or more at all ages;
or 3. S in V_6

0-7 days	14 mm	
8-30 days	10 mm	or more
1-3 mo	7 mm	
3 mo-16 yr	5 mm	

or 4. R/S ratio in V_1

0-3 mo	6.5	
3-6 mo	4.0	
6 mo-3 yr	2.4	or more
3-5 yr	1.6	
6-15 yr	0.8	

or 5. T positive in V_1 after 3rd day of life, if R/S > 1.0.

    Left ventricular

1. S in V_1 more than 20 mm at all ages.
or 2. R in V_6

0-6 mo	16 mm	
6-12 mo	19 mm	or more
1-16 yr	21 mm	

or 3. R/S ratio in V_1

under 1 yr	0.8	
1-5 yr	0.2	or less
6-13 yr	0.1	

or 4. Secondary T inversion in V_5 or V_6.
or 5. q more than 3 mm in V_5 or V_6.

Combined ventricular
Either:

1. Direct signs of right and left ventricular overload

or 2. Direct signs of right ventricular overload, **plus**
   a) q = 2 mm or more in V_5 or V_6; **or**
   b) inverted T in V_6 (after positive T in right chest leads).

CARDIAC AXIS

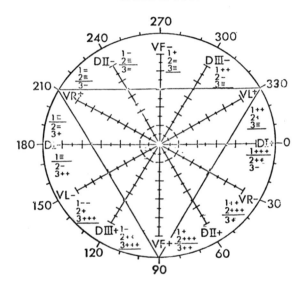

Orientation of ECG leads. It should be used to calculate the mean frontal axis of the QRS and the T-wave.

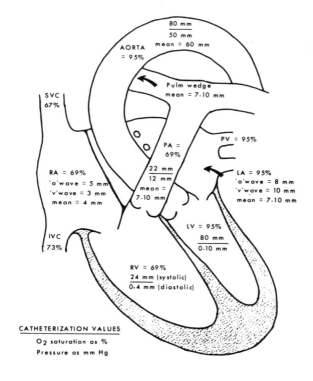

AORTA
= 95%

80 mm
50 mm
mean = 60 mm

SVC
67%

Pulm wedge
mean = 7-10 mm

PA =
69%

PV = 95%

22 mm
12 mm
mean =
7-10 mm

RA = 69%
'a'wave = 5 mm
'v'wave = 3 mm
mean = 4 mm

LA = 95%
'a'wave = 8 mm
'v'wave = 10 mm
mean = 7-10 mm

IVC
73%

LV = 95%
80 mm
0-10 mm

RV = 69%
24 mm (systolic)
0-4 mm (diastolic)

CATHETERIZATION VALUES
O₂ saturation as %
Pressure as mm Hg

Electrolyte Changes Affecting the ECG
Hypokalemia (pp 243, 351)
1. T waves low, flat, or inverted.
2. ST segment depressed.
3. QT interval increased.
4. U waves prominent.

Hyperkalemia
1. Tall peaked T waves.
2. Widening QRS: signs of intraventricular block.
3. Lengthening PR interval.
4. Diminishing size of P & R waves.
5. Depression of ST segment.
6. Gradual prolongation of QT interval.

Hypocalcemia (p 248)
1. Enhances effect of any K depletion that is present.
2. QT prolonged but RST segment unchanged.

Hypercalcemia
1. QT shortened.
2. Cardiac arrhythmias.
3. Enhances digitalis effect.

Digitalis toxicity – if severe, treat with KCl (p 204)
1. Scooping ST segment.
2. Inversion of first portion of T waves.
3. Various degrees of heart block.
4. Arrhythmias.

Congestive Heart Failure

Treatment
1. Bed rest.
2. Oxygen as required.
3. *Diuretics:*
   a) Furosemide (Lasix): give either iv, 1-2 mg/kg, slowly in 5-10 min; **or** im or po, up to 2 mg/kg/day in 2 doses.
   b) Aldactone: 2 mg/kg/24 hr, together with Diuril 20 mg/kg/24 hr.

c) Furosemide or aldactone: watch serum K level. If this is low:
   i) give 1-2 mEq/kg/day as 'slow K' tabs or 'K-lyte/Cl' solution (p 455), **or**
   ii) give spironolactone with other diuretics.
4. *Digoxin* (p 436)
   a) Total digitalizing dose =
      prem infant, 0.03 mg/kg.
      term neonate to 2 yr, 0.05 mg/kg.
      > 2 yr, 0.04 mg/kg, up to 1.5 mg.
   b) Initial digitalizing dosage: give 1/3 *stat,* 1/3 at 6 hr later, 1/3 at a further 8-12 hr later, depending on clinical state.
      — First dose can be given im.
   c) Total daily maintenance dose = 1/5 of total digitalizing dose. Can be increased to 1/4 if necessary.
   d) Availability: as elixir, tablets, and ampules (p 436).
   e) Chronic renal disease: reduce dose according to serum creatinine or BUN levels. Monitor dose by serum digoxin levels (therapeutic levels = 0.8 − 1.8 ng/ml).

Acute Pulmonary Edema Due to Left Ventricular Failure

Treatment
1. Sit patient upright.
2. Morphine:
   a) give 0.2 mg/kg sc. Can be repeated q4h prn.
   b) maximal dose in child = 10 mg.
3. Oxygen.
4. Furosemide (Lasix); give iv (p 441)
5. Digoxin (p 436)
6. Consider positive airway pressure.

Congenital Heart Disease

Investigation
1. *Special points in history*
   a) Mother, during this pregnancy: rubella, other virus infections, vaginal bleeding, medications or radiation during 1st trimester.

b) Cyanosis: age at onset, relation to exertion.
c) Dyspnea – respiratory rate.
d) Anoxic spells.
e) Exercise tolerance – be specific.
f) Murmur – age first detected.
g) Growth and development – weight gain.
h) Squatting.

2. *Routine*
a) Film of chest at 2 m FFD
b) ECG

3. *Other as indicated:*
    – echocardiography
    – cardiac catheterization
    – angiocardiography

For these procedures:
a) Discontinue feeding 4 hr before study.
b) Sedation
    – none under mo
    – half dose if child cyanosed
    – give CM3 sedative mixture (p 273) – but **not if patient has tetralogy of Fallot,** in which case give morphine, 0.1 mg/kg sc (maximum, 2 mg/dose).

'Blue Spells' in Cyanotic Infants with Congenital Heart Disease

Remember that paroxysmal anoxic attacks in cyanotic heart disease are not due to heart failure – they are due to infundibular spasm.

Treatment

1. Place child in knee–chest position.
2. Propranolol: 0.05 mg to 0.1 mg/kg, iv over 10 min – to relieve infundibular spasm.
3. Morphine: 0.2 mg/kg, sc, to maximum 10 mg. Can be repeated q4-6h as needed.
4. Oxygen.
5. **NO digitalis.**
6. Draw 2 ml arterial blood for pH, pCO_2, pO_2 (p 71).
7. Treat metabolic acidosis with soda bicarbonate (p 126).

Rheumatic Fever

Diagnosis is based on arbitrary criteria in child with proven recent streptococcal infection.

Major manifestations
1. Carditis
   a) development of significant murmur
   b) heart size increased
   c) pericarditis
   d) congestive heart failure.
2. Polyarthritis — 2 joints or more
3. Chorea
4. Nodules
5. Erythema marginatum.

Minor manifestations
1. Fever
2. ESR elevated
3. Recent strep infection:
   a) positive culture of nose and throat swabs
   b) history of sore throat with fever
   c) ASO titer 250 or more
   d) scarlet fever.
4. PR interval prolonged in relation to age and rate (see Table, p 206).
5. Definite history of rheumatic fever.

Diagnosis
1. One major plus 2 minor, or 2 major manifestations, usually are required (diagnosis can be made if Sydenham's chorea and no accompanying manifestations).
2. If *only* polyarthritis, fever, and elevated ESR, other causes must be considered (lupus, anaphylactic purpura, periarteritis, leukemia, viral infection).

Routine Investigations
1. ESR
2. ECG
3. Film of chest at 2 m FFD
4. Throat swab for hemolytic strep.
5. Sleeping pulse daily
6. ASO titer immediately and in 7-10 days.

Treatment

1. *Bed rest*
   a) may feed himself unless extremely ill or restless
   b) minimum of 2-4 weeks.

2. *Penicillin*
   a) therapeutic doses for 10-14 days
   b) then, 1,200,000 U of benzathine penicillin G, im, every 2nd week while in hospital.

3. *Acetylsalicylic acid (ASA),* 60 mg/kg daily, for 3 mo or until ESR normal.

4. *Prednisone* – if carditis severe, with heart failure or pericarditis.
   a) Consult cardiology about dose.
   b) Add ASA after heart failure is controlled (dose as in 3. above); continue for 1 mo after prednisone discontinued.
   c) Treat heart failure with digoxin and diuretics **in low doses** (myocardium is particularly sensitive to toxic effects of digitalis).

5. **Continue therapy until:**
   a) ESR (weekly) normal.
   b) Weight gain satisfactory.
   c) Patient looks well.
   d) No tachycardia.
   e) No heart failure.
   f) Murmurs constant for 3-4 wk.
   g) No progression in cardiac enlargement.

6. **Continuous prophylaxis.** After the initial penicillin treatment, continue with:
   a) sulfadiazine – if child under 30 kg, 0.5 g po each morning; **or**
   b) benzathine penicillin G, 1,200,000 U im, once monthly; **or**
   c) penicillin G, 250,000 U bid po; **or**
   d) if penicillin sensitivity, erythromycin (p 411)

Routine Treatment of Digitalis Poisoning (p 496)

Note. Symptoms occur 30 min to 6 hr after ingestion (usually nausea and vomiting initially).

General management

1. Determine amount and kind of digitalis received, and time it was taken.

2. Inquire about history of vomiting or gastric lavage. Empty stomach with syrup of ipecac or by immediate gastric lavage. Give activated charcoal.

3. Establish during first 2 hr after digitalis received whether patient can take fluid po and retain it, and whether patient voids.

    Specific therapy
1. If amount of digitalis ingested was large, or if fluids po are not retained, or if patient has been vomiting or is clinically dehydrated: start iv fluids.
2. Draw blood for serum electrolytes and digitalis level (>2 ng/ml can be toxic).
    a) If serum K low and child voiding: give KCl iv, 0.5 mEq/kg in 1st hr. The total should not exceed 2 mEq/kg/day. (Solution: 40 mEq KCl in 500 ml of 5% glucose in water.)
    b) **NOTE:** Do not give KCl if heart rate <55/min or ECG evidences AV block.
3. If heart rate significantly slowed, or if ECG abnormal (p 197), or if large amount of digitalis ingested: keep patient in recovery room, connected to an ECG monitor and have an external pacemaker available.
4. If ECG and heart rate normal on admission and dose ingested small: observe child closely, and repeat ECG q4h or as indicated.
5. If tachycardia:
    a) give iv
        i)   propranolol (p 202) **or**
        ii) by slow push, **either**
             – diphenylhydantoin (Dilantin), 1-5 mg/kg/dose, to maximum 500 mg in 4 hr; **or**
             – lidscaine (Xylocaine), 0.5-1.0 mg/kg/dose; repeat q5-10 min prn.
    b) if tachycardia severe, a pacemaker, artificial ventilation, or chelation with EDTA, may be needed.
6. Hypothermia may be necessary in certain cases.

Maximal PR Intervals (in sec)
in Relation to Heart Rate and Age

Age		70	71 – 90	91 – 110	111 – 130	131 – 150	151
	Heart Rate/min						
1 mo				0.11	0.11	0.11	0.11
1 – 9 mo				0.14	0.13	0.12	0.11
10 – 24 mo				0.15	0.14	0.14	0.10
3 – 5 yr		0.18	0.16	0.16	0.16	0.13	
6 – 13 yr			0.18	0.16	0.16		

HEMATOLOGY

Glucose-6-PO$_4$ Dehydrogenase Deficiency (G-6-PD)

G-6-PD is a hereditary X-linked abnormality in which the stability and activity of this enzyme in the tissues is diminished. The red blood cells are severely affected, causing episodic hemolytic anemia, especially after exposure to certain drugs or fava beans, with infections, and in newborns.

Drugs/chemicals known to cause hemolysis
Antimalarial drugs: primaquine, etc.
Analgesics: ASA, phenacetin, antipyrine
Sulfonamides and sulfones
Other: nitrofurantoin, PAS, naphthalene, methylene blue, nalidixic acid.

Sickle-cell States

The red blood cells 'sickle' when de-oxygenated, causing clinical manifestations.
1. Sickle-cell anemia is the homozygous state for the sickle-cell gene (HbSS): it is the more common form and usually more severe, and manifests as chronic hemolytic anemia with symptomatic episodes.
2. Sickle-cell trait is the heterozygous state (HbSA) and usually is asymptomatic.

Sickle-cell anemia
1. Painful or thrombotic crisis due to vaso-occlusion.
2. Aplastic crisis.
3. Sequestration crisis: hypovolemia caused by sudden pooling of blood in the liver or spleen.
4. Hemolytic crisis.

Testing
   "Sickle-cell preparation"
1. Sulfite method.
   a) On a slide, mix 1-2 drops Na metabisulfite or Na hyposulfite with 1 drop of patient's blood.
   b) Apply coverslip.
   c) Read at 15, 30, 60 and 180 min and 12 hr.
2. "Sickledex": a solubility test using dithionate reduction of HbS.

Note.   Positive result indicates that some or all of patient's blood is HbS.
           If result positive, determine amount of HbS, using Hb electrophoresis.

General Therapy

1.   Prevention of crises
     a)   Order folic acid supplement.
     b)   Treat infection promptly.
     c)   Ensure adequate hydration.
2.   Maintain Hb>10 g/dl by transfusion.

Disseminated Intravascular Coagulation (DIC)

Treatment of DIC (controversial)

1.   Heparin
     a)   Give 100 U/kg *stat* into iv.
          This will heparinize the patient for about 2 hr.
     b)   Consult Hematology if coagulation studies are abnormal or additional heparin is required.
2.   Monitor
     a)   vital signs
     b)   fluid balance
     c)   body wt
     d)   CVP
     e)   **lab** results.

Hemophilia and Related Disorders

Replacement Therapy

Factor VIII-rich cryoprecipitate ("Cryo")

For treatment of classical hemophilia (AHG factor-VIII deficiency, von Willebrand's disease, and some hypofibrinogenemic disorders (e.g., congenital afibrinogenemia).

1.   One unit of Cryo is produced from 1 unit of whole blood.
2.   Blood Bank reconstitutes 2-3 ml Cryo with a small vol of N saline.
     –   Several units may be pooled in a single pack.
3.   When giving cryoprecipitate
     a)   Using a plastic syringe, withdraw the material from the pack and inject it immediately iv. (A glass syringe would jam.)

b) Administer cryoprecipitate as soon as received (avoid loss of potency and bacterial contamination).

4. Dosage varies according to severity of bleeding, potency of units, and individual response.
   a) Common hemorrhages into joints and muscles
      - treat child as outpatient
      - give single injection of 1.0-1.5 units/10 kg body wt (3-4 units/m²)
      - child to return for second injection the next day if not improved.
   b) Bleeding from mucous membranes (e.g., dental extraction): give 1 dose of Cryo daily (1.0-1.5 units/10 kg) until lesion has healed (3-7 days).
   c) Persistent bleeding: give larger doses more frequently (e.g., q8-12 hr).

5. Management depends on replacement according to the factor's half-life and the amount necessary for hemostasis.

Factor VIII concentrate (hemophil)

A dried, concentrated preparation of antihemophilic factor, used for replacement therapy in classical hemophilia.

1. Used more for routine bleeding problems, especially severe hemorrhage or intracranial hemorrhage; also convenient to carry while traveling.

2. Each vial contains approximately 300 clinical units of factor VIII
   a) reconstitute with diluent immediately before iv injection
   b) dosage and administration vary according to treatment indicated.

   Read instructions in package before using.

Single-donor fresh frozen plasma

Used mostly for replacement therapy in Christmas disease (factor IX deficiency) and factor XI deficiency

Factor IX concentrate

For treating deficiency of one or more factors of the prothrombin complex (II, VII, IX, and X), whether congenital or acquired.

1. Used mainly for replacement therapy in Christmas disease when there is uncontrollable hemorrhage or intracranial bleeding.

2. Also used during surgery if fresh frozen plasma may not suffice or volume load is a consideration.

3. Each bottle contains about 500 clinical units
    a) reconstitute with sterile water immediately
        before iv injection
    b) dosage/administration vary according to treat-
        ment indicated. Before giving this therapy, read
        instructions in package.

Management of Replacement Therapy
Blood Groups
1. Although cross-match procedures are not necessary
    for routine replacement therapy, use ABO and Rh
    specific products whenever possible.
2. As the blood group of each hemophiliac is recorded
    in the Blood Bank, you do not require a specimen
    from the patient.

Side-effects
1. Febrile reactions:
    —   treat with antipyretics. Do not give ASA —
        acetaminophen (Tylenol, Tempra) is a safe, ef-
        fective substitute (p 417).
2. Allergic manifestations (urticarial, angio-edema, or
    anaphylactoid):
    a) first, try antihistamines such as diphenhydra-
        mine (Benadryl; p 437) po or iv. (Avoid the im
        route in 'bleeders').
    b) if response to Benadryl inadequate, inject epine-
        phrine 1:1000 sc (p 440).
3. Discontinue infusion if reaction is severe (unusual).
4. When patient is receiving plasma, watch for fluid
    overload
    a) if it develops, stop therapy and administer diuret-
        ics
    b) digitalization may be helpful.

Laboratory control
To assess the efficacy of replacement therapy, measure
the increase in the deficient factor after a course of treatment.
1. Take specimen just before and about 15 min after
    giving therapy
2. Also, obtain screening tests (p 20).

Neoplastic Disorders

Leukemia and other types of neoplasia are treated with specific therapy (chemo- and/or radiotherapy), supportive medical therapy, and supportive psychological therapy.

Supportive Medical Therapy

A. **Bleeding secondary to thrombocytopenia**
1. Platelet transfusions (p 27)
    a) give 1 unit platelets/5 kg body wt
    b) order must be authorized by Hematology.
2. Dose and duration of response to transfusion depend on whether child has fever, active bleeding, and/or platelet antibodies.
3. Do not give injections im.
4. Replace blood loss.

B. **Neutropenia**
1. Definition: an absolute neutrophil count <1000-1500/mm^3 is abnormally low and may predispose patient to infection.
2. Fever (38.5°C)
    a) consider due to bacterial infection until disproved
    b) obtain cultures of blood, urine, and any suspicious-looking lesions.
3. Start antibiotic therapy if Gram-positive or -negative organisms — especially pseudomonas and staphylococcus.
4. If organism identified, adjust therapy according to sensitivities.
5. If no organism identified, decision to stop antibiotics depends on patient's clinical status.
6. If patient's condition deteriorates despite antibiotics, consider possibility of unusual (nonbacterial) infections.

C. **Hyperuricemia: uric-acid nephropathy may result**
1. It is important to consider and prevent this before and during antineoplasia chemotherapy.
2. Suspect if WBC count high and organomegaly present.
3. Avoid uric-acid precipitation in kidney, by hydrating patient well:
    a) fluids iv: 3000 ml/m^2 body surface area/24 hr
    b) fluids po as tolerated.

(cont'd on p. 215)

DRUGS FOR TREATMENT OF ACUTE LEUKEMIA

DRUG	MAIN USE	USUAL DOSAGE	TOXIC EFFECTS (order of frequency)
prednisone	1. To induce remission 2. Additive treatment	40 to 60 mg/m^2 po daily	1. Diabetes mellitus 2. Hypertension 3. Peptic ulceration
vincristine sulfate	1. To induce remission	1.5 to 2 mg/m^2 iv weekly (maximal dose not to exceed 2 mg)	1. Alopecia 2. Obstipation 3. Ileus 4. Paresis 5. Irritation with extravasation
methotrexate	1. To induce remission 2. To maintain remission	1. 6.0 mg/m^2 po daily 2. 20 mg/m^2 po q4 days 3. 12 mg/m^2 intrathecally, q3-4 days.	1. Bone-marrow suppression 2. Mouth ulcers 3. Hepatitis 4. Pulmonary infiltration
mercaptopurine	1. To induce remission 2. To maintain remission	75 mg/m^2 po daily	1. Bone-marrow suppression 2. Hepatitis 3. Mouth ulcers

212

Drug	Purpose	Dose	Side effects
cyclo-phosphamide	1. To induce and maintain remission 2. Rapid reduction of blast count	1. 1 g/m^2 iv once only; **or** 2. 100 mg/m^2 po daily	1. Bone-marrow suppression 2. Nausea and vomiting 3. Alopecia 4. Cystitis
cytosine arabinoside	1. To induce remission; and 2. in combination with cyclo-phosphamide in myelo-genous leukemia	1. $100\text{-}150 \text{ mg/m}^2$ iv 2. 25 mg/m^2 iv q8h x 12, repeated q14 days	1. Bone-marrow suppression 2. Nausea and vomiting 3. Mouth ulcers 4. Esophagitis
daunomycin	1. To induce remission 2. Additive treatment	1. 30 mg/m^2 iv daily, x 3-5 days 2. 40 mg/m^2 iv, once a mo.	1. Bone-marrow suppression 2. Cardiomyopathy
L-asparaginase*	1. To induce remission	6000 units/m^2 iv, 3 times a wk	1. **Acute allergic reactions, including anaphylactic shock (treatment, see p 469)** 2. Liver malfunction 3. Coagulation defects 4. Pancreatitis

*Allergic reactions common. Nurse must be with patient, and dr must be on ward, throughout infusion and for 30 min afterward.

OTHER DRUGS TO TREAT NEOPLASIA

DRUG	DISEASE	USUAL DOSAGE	TOXIC EFFECTS (order of frequency)
vinblastine sulfate	Hodgkin's disease Histiocytosis X	0.15 mg/kg/wk iv Can be increased by 0.05 mg/kg weekly iv if tolerated, but do not exceed 0.5 mg/kg.	1. Bone-marrow suppression 2. Irritation with extravasation
actinomycin D	Wilms' tumor	15 μg/kg/day iv, for 5 days	1. Nausea and vomiting 2. Bone-marrow suppression 3. Irritation with extravasation
bulsulfan (Myleran)	Chronic myelogenous leukemia	0.1-0.2 mg/kg/day po	1. Bone-marrow suppression
nitrogen mustard	Hodgkin's disease	0.4 mg/kg total dose; iv, via tubing of running saline drip	1. Nausea and vomiting 2. Bone-marrow suppression 3. Irritation with extravasation
procarbazine	Hodgkin's disease	3 mg/kg po daily for 14 days	1. Bone-marrow suppression
adriamycin	Osteogenic sarcoma	(Under study)	1. Bone-marrow suppression 2. Cardiomyopathy

4. Decrease uric-acid formation, by giving allopurinol (hypoxanthine oxidase inhibitor), 50-100 mg po tid; **or,** if po not possible, 100-200 mg pr tid.
5. Alkalinization of urine acts as an uricosuric:
   a) give $NaHCO_3$ 50 ml/500 ml of iv solution, with po supplement if necessary and/or
   b) Diamox (acetazolamide), po or im, 5 mg/kg q4h x 3 (be alert for acidosis).
   c) Test urine pH q1-2h and adjust alkalinizing agents accordingly.
6. Monitor urine output, BUN, serum creatinine, uric acid, and electrolytes.

D. Meningeal leukemia

1. Can cause headache, vomiting, cranial-nerve palsy, and hyperphagia.
2. The most useful therapy is intrathecal administration of methotrexate, 0.4 mg/kg (12 mg/m^2); maximal dose = 10 mg (in special cases, 15 mg):
   a) dissolve methotrexate 10 mg in 10 ml N saline
   b) perform LP; measure opening pressure, and remove CSF equal to volume of methotrexate to be given; send CSF for usual studies (p 74) plus cytology
   c) instil methotrexate (as a precaution, ensure that CSF flow is good and nontraumatic before giving the drug)
   d) repeat q3-4 days until cell count, pressure, and/ or clinical status improved.
   e) other systemic chemotherapy may have to be stopped for 24 hr after each methotrexate instillation.
3. Radiotherapy to the cranium is an adjunct to treatment.
4. Seizures due to CNS leukemia:
   a) give diazepam (Valium) 0.3 mg/kg/dose iv (see Neurology, pp 173, 471)
   b) if CSF pressure very greatly increased, give 25% mannitol iv, 1 g/kg/dose, in 15 min (p 136) **and/ or**
   c) dexamethasone iv, 2-4 mg/dose.

E. Focal leukemia

Local radiotherapy may relieve gonadal and bone pain secondary to infiltration.

Supportive Psychological Therapy

1. Keep the initial interview with the parents brief; be frank and sympathetic
   a) help them to allay guilt feelings
   b) stress the positive side, such as effective drugs, continuing research, and the ever-increasing median duration of survival.

2. Counselors, such as the social worker, chaplain, nurse specialist, are important members of the therapeutic team (see Support Services, pp 95, 96).

3. Try to reinstate the child into a normal environment while his condition is in remission; encourage him to play and to return to school.

4. Be prepared to help the child and his family deal with the emotional aspects of fatal illness.

5. Take care that discussions with patients and their parents, by nurses, residents, and staff physicians, are consistent — do not give conflicting facts or statements.

GASTROENTEROLOGY

ACUTE DIARRHEA

Definition: excessive loss of fluid and electrolytes in the stool.

A. *Etiology* (usually infectious)
   1. Bacterial
      a) invasive: *Salmonella, Shigella, E. coli*
      b) toxigenic: *Vibrio cholerae, E. coli, Clostridium perfringens, Cl. botulinis, Klebsiella*
      c) pathogenic: *Yersinia, Campylobacter, E. coli*
   2. Viral: rotavirus, parvovirus, mini-reo virus, adenovirus, calicivirus, astrovirus, etc. (p 64)
   3. Protozoan: *Giardia,* amebae, etc.

B. *Pathophysiology*
   Note. Primarily the small intestine is affected; in some infections, also the colon.
   1. Water moves passively from the lumen across the intestinal epithelium in response to transport of solutes.
   2. Enterocytes lining the villi have transport pathways for Na and glucose.
   3. Mature villous cells have highly developed transport capacity; when damaged (viral or bacterial invasion, radiation, etc.) they are replaced by less-effective immature cells from the villous crypts.
   4. Bacterial toxins stimulate intestinal epithelial-cell secretion (through cAMP activation or other mediators).
   5. Because of the transport delay and the increased osmolar load in the lumen, there is a net flow of water into the lumen.

C. *Management*
   Note. Appropriate management requires careful history and clinical examination, and an understanding of the pathophysiology.

History

1. Record duration of symptoms, no. and character of stools, oral intake, vomiting, oliguria, etc.

2. Accept and record mother's story even if clinical picture doesn't seem to fit.

Assessment

1. Patients with mild to moderate diarrhea (most cases) need not be hospitalized.

2. Moderate to severe diarrhea is cause for hospitalization
    a) assess degree of hydration (see Fluid and Electrolytes, p 116); weigh stat and daily
    b) physical examination may reveal weight loss, sunken eyeballs and fontanel, rapid shallow respirations, greyish cyanosis, loss of tissue elasticity, dry tongue and mucous membranes, lack of tears, drowsiness, eyes rolling up, and/or oliguria.

3. In patients who have severe diarrhea there may have been rapid onset of multiple watery stools, but patient's hydration may not seem poor (tissue may feel doughy rather than dehydrated).
    a) patient may be unduly thirsty and take fluids well, but soon vomits or pools fluids in his gut, or
    b) patient may refuse all fluids po;
    c) patient usually has disproportionate water loss and condition may progress rapidly to coma, convulsions, hyperpyrexia, and death (hypertonic dehydration with hypernatremia, see p 122).

Rehydration

1. In mild to moderate diarrhea, rehydrate orally; give oral solution with low osmolar load (reduces luminal osmolar load and, thus, obligatory small intestine water loss)

2. In moderate to severe diarrhea, rehydrate with iv fluids (see Fluid and Electrolytes, p 116)
    a) If shock-like state present: start with Ringer's lactate; as soon as it is available, give fresh frozen plasma (10-20 mg/kg).
    b) **If hypernatremia present:** rehydrate carefully as outlined in Fluid and Electrolytes (p 124).
    c) All other cases: start hydration with 2/3–1/3 soln or equivalent; if volume depletion moderate or severe, the amount of fluid given iv over 24 hr must compensate for:
        i) *deficit:* usually 100 ml/kg in 1st 24 hr
        ii) *maintenance* (p 118)
        iii) *continuing losses* (vomiting or diarrhea).

d) After patient voids, start KCl, 5 mEq/250 ml iv solution.

Note. If diarrhea is bloody, suspect dysentery organisms, but always consider possibility of intussusception (rectal examination mandatory).

Investigations (necessary if illness moderate or severe)
1. Blood:
   a) serum Na^+, K^+, Cl^-, venous blood gases, and BUN, *stat* and serially, depending on clinical situation; and serum protein, Ca^{++}, and Mg^{++} may be necessary.
   b) Hb, Hct, CBC, and blood smear.
      i) Serum electrolytes and HCO_3^- are needed to check for hypo-/hypernatremia and for calculating anion gap [Anion gap = Na^+ − (Cl^- + HCO_3^-). Normal gap = 5-15 mEq/liter. >15 mEq/liter indicates additional anions (usually H) and occurs with retention of a strong acid, as in ketosis. <5 mEq/liter may indicate hypoproteinemia or lab error.]
      ii) Blood gases may indicate acidosis/alkalosis (p 124). Correction of acidosis with $NaHCO_3$ is necessary if serum HCO_3^- <15 mEq/liter (0.3 x kg body wt x base excess = mEq $NaHCO_3$ needed for half correction).
      iii) Increased Hb, Hct suggest hemoconcentration and, as volume depletion is corrected, will fall to more accurate values. Therefore, repeat these indices when dehydration corrected.
      iv) Decreased Hb and abnormal blood film might indicate bleeding or hemolytic process.
      v) Elevated BUN indicates volume depletion: if renal dysfunction is suspected, check serum creatinine and urinalysis (including microscopy).
2. Stool: smear (p 80), culture for bacteriology; electron microscopy (Virology) of fresh specimen may show virus particles and is useful for virus identification. Check stool for pH and reducing substances (p 32), on admission and daily if diarrhea persists.
3. Additional studies, according to individual case.

Oral Feedings
1. Start oral feedings when vomiting/ileus ceases, or after 12-24 hr.

2. Traditional dietary advancement: 5-10% sugar solution or flat gingerale; then, dilute milk solutions, such as 1/2-strength formula, as stooling or other GI symptoms decrease over the 24-72 hr after admission.

3. Then, fairly rapid advancement (over the next 24-48 hr) to semi-solid and solid foods is of nutritional benefit to the ill child. Monitor for disaccharidase deficiency if stooling persists and dietary advancement unsuccessful (p 32); adjust diet accordingly.

Potential Problems in Management

1. Impaired kidney function: expansion of intravascular compartment with correction of the volume depletion may not lead to normal kidney function if underlying pathology exists.

2. Shock (p 472)

3. Twitching or convulsions may occur if too rapid correction of volume depletion, especially in hypernatremic dehydration. See management of convulsions (p 470) and check for hypocalcemia and hypoglycemia, as well as for electrolyte problems.

CHRONIC DIARRHEA

Definition: loose stools which persist >3 weeks.

Careful History (essential)

1. Clinical history: enquire about night pain or diarrhea, abdominal symptoms, appetite, frequency and consistency of stools (? bulky, pale, foul, frothy, floating), presence of blood, mucus.

2. Dietary history: precise information regarding total calorie intake, relationship of symptoms to ingestion of food and of particular foods.

Clinical Assessment (very important)

1. Some important signs are easily overlooked: undernutrition, mouth sores, smooth tongue, finger clubbing, skin changes, edema.

2. Rectal examination: inspect perianal region and test fresh stool.

Usual Etiology *

1. Infection: bacterial, viral, fungal, parasitic.
2. Postinfectious: carbohydrate intolerance.
3. Dietary: allergy (*e.g.*, milk, soy protein), celiac disease.
4. Carbohydrate malabsorption: lactose, sucrose, isomaltose, galactose, glucose.
5. Malnutrition: starvation, maternal nutritional deprivation.
6. Endocrine: hyperthyroidism, adrenal insufficiency.
7. Pancreatic insufficiency: cystic fibrosis, Schwachman's disease.
8. Metabolic: endocrine tumors, galactosemia, neuroblastoma, ganglioneuroma, abetalipoproteinemia.
9. Hepatic disease in which bile salts are absent.
10. Antibiotic-related
11. Inflammatory: regional enteritis, ulcerative colitis.
12. Anatomical lesions: short-gut syndrome, blind loop, malrotation.
13. Toxicity due to radiation or chemotherapy.
14. Immune deficiency: hypo- or agammaglobulinemia, combined immune deficiency, defective cellular immunity.
15. Other: lymphangiectasia; associated with otitis or urinary tract infection; protein-losing enteropathy.

---

*adapted from Gryboski, J. J., Chronic Diarrhea *In* Current Problems in Pediatrics, Vol. 9, No. 5, March 1979.

Investigations

1. Stool
    a) do gross and microscopic examinations; also, test for occult blood and reducing substances (p 32).
    b) send bacterial and viral cultures; electron microscopy gives rapid viral identification.
    c) obtain fresh specimen for ova and parasites (e.g., amebae, *Giardia*).
2. Blood. Order
    a) CBC, smear, ESR
    b) serum electrolytes (Na, K, Cl, Ca, Mg, PO_4)
    c) serum iron (p 372), B_{12}, and/or folate studies
    d) quantification of blood loss (^{51}Cr tagging — p 85)

3. Urine. Order
   a) routine urinalysis: check for reducing substances
   b) special tests: VMA, catecholamines, 5-hydroxy-indolacetic acid, inclusion bodies, amino acids.
4. Absorptive function.
   Note. Patient must receive adequate calorie intake for at least 3 days before testing.
   a) Fat: microscopic exam; 5-day fecal-fat collection (p 45).
   b) Carbohydrate: D-xylose absorption (p 44), oral glucose tolerance (p 53), oral disaccharide tolerance (p 44).
   c) Protein: consult Gastroenterology for special tests to measure protein absorption. Also, order serum protein electrophoresis, quantitative immunoglobulins.
5. Plot growth curves.
6. Order sweat chloride testing (p 45).
7. Order radiography
   a) chest: to check for cystic fibrosis, tumor
   b) abdominal: plain A-P and lateral films to check for obstruction, calcification (lateral shows pancreatic calcification)
   c) Ba studies (cineradiography, air-contrast enema): to find inflammatory disease, anomalies
   d) bones: to check for osteoporosis, tumor.
8. Order exocrine pancreatic function testing (see Tests, GI, p 44).
9. Biopsy
   a) distal duodenum: microscopic examination for cytology, *Giardia lamblia*
   b) rectum: microscopy.
10. Sigmoidoscopy.
11. Measure protein loss
    a) serum concentrations of total protein, transferrin, ceruloplasmin, lymphocyte count
    b) fecal loss of labelled protein (^{51}Cr; p 85).
12. Additional tests may be useful in special cases
    a) liver function
    b) serum cholesterol
    c) duodenal contents, lipid digestion, bile salt content
    d) electrolyte balance
    e) stool Na^+, K^+, Cl^-.

Management: depends on etiology

1. If indicated, correct dehydration, electrolyte imbalance, and/or severe anemia, with parenteral fluids and blood.

2. General treatment:
    a) if infectious: identify organism (bacterial, fungal or parasitic) and use the appropriate therapy (p 158)
    b) if postinfectious, dietary or carbohydrate malabsorption: remove offending food from diet and ensure balanced diet
    c) if endocrinous, metabolic, or hepatic: if possible treat underlying disease and if necessary adjust diet
    d) if due to malnutrition: give well-balanced diet.
3. Specific treatment:
    a) celiac disease: order gluten-free diet
    b) acrodermatitis enteropathica: order zinc supplementation
    c) cystic fibrosis (p 179)
    d) ulcerative colitis: give salicylazosulfapyridine (Azulfidine) po, 500 mg – 4 g/day qid; prednisone; parenteral alimentation (to rest bowel); If toxic megacolon present or if medical therapy fails – surgery (colectomy)
    e) Crohn's disease: Azulfidine, steroids, parenteral alimentation.
    f) Malabsorption (i.e., steatorrhea) due to other causes; medium-chain triglycerides (MCT) may be helpful, either as supplement or as special formula (Portagen, Pregestimil) (p 323); if indicated, give additional vitamins.

LIVER DISEASE

Jaundice in Early Infancy

Classification and causes

A. *Indirect reacting (unconjugated) hyperbilirubinemia*
    1. Hemolytic (overload)
        a) Hemolytic disease of newborn (Rh, ABO, other rare)
        b) Sepsis (early phase)
        c) Congenital spherocytosis
        d) G-6-PD deficiency
        e) Pyruvate kinase deficiency
        f) Vitamin K-analog overdose
        g) Drugs and toxins causing hemolysis
        h) Shunt hyperbilirubinemia

2. Non-hemolytic
   a) Physiologic jaundice:
      more severe; lasts longer in prematures, post-hypoxic neonates, infants of diabetic mothers, and if large hematoma present
   b) Breast-fed babies
   c) Cretinism
   d) Pyloric stenosis (fasting)
   e) Crigler–Najjar syndrome

B. *Direct reacting (conjugated) hyperbilirubinemia*
   1. Congenital extrahepatic biliary atresia
   2. Infections
      a) TORCH (toxoplasmosis, rubella, CMV infection, herpes simplex and other viruses)
      b) Hepatitis A or B
      c) Sepsis (late phase), especially in urinary tract infections
   3. Metabolic
      a) α_1-Antitrypsin deficiency
      b) Galactosemia
      c) Fructosemia
      d) Tyrosinemia
      e) Cystic fibrosis
      f) Niemann–Pick's disease, type A
      g) Byler's disease, Dubin–Johnson's, Rotor's, or Alagille's syndromes
   4. Miscellaneous
      a) Complication of any hemolytic disease
      b) Microcystic disease of liver or kidney
      c) Histiocytosis X
      d) Toxic drug or chemical
   5. Idiopathic: "neonatal hepatitis"

Investigation
1. Note important points in family history:
   a) Any liver disease or jaundice in family?
   b) Any contact with jaundice by any family member?
   c) Transfusion, prenatally to mother, or for major surgery?
   d) Any maternal disease during pregnancy? medication and injections?
   e) Genital or oral herpes in mother during pregnancy?
   f) Ethnic background
   g) Consanguinity of parents?

2. Also, note in history
   a) Time of onset of jaundice
   b) Changes in character and color of urine and stools
   c) Any associated disturbances: GI, respiratory, neurological, etc.
   d) Transfusions, medication, exposure to toxic agents, ear-piercing.
3. During physical examination, note:
   a) Severity of jaundice and character of icteric skin color, sclerae, and mucous membranes (in daylight)
   b) Pruritus?
   c) Petechiae, hemorrhages, ecchymoses, edema, cataracts?
   d) Dilated veins, free fluid?
   e) Liver: size, shape, consistency, edge, surface texture (measure liver size in cm from right costal margin in mid-clavicular line).
4. Order lab investigations
   a) Bile pigment (p 226) (to differentiate between direct/indirect-reacting hyperbilirubinemia and incomplete/complete biliary obstruction)
   — Test blood, urine, stool specimens: without delay or keep refrigerated in dark
   — Stool specimens must not be contaminated with urine
   — Stool and urine should be tested for both bilirubin and urobilin.
   Note. Microbilirubin method inaccurate when bilirubin low.
   b) If hyperbilirubinemia direct-reacting, and bile pigment studies do not prove incomplete obstruction, order Rose Bengal study (see Nuclear Medicine, p 85)
   c) Liver function tests (see p 353, etc.)
   — *Commonly used:*
   Serum bilirubin, total and direct
   Serum alkaline phosphatase
   Serum cholesterol
   Serum protein electrophoresis
   Aspartate aminotransferase (SGOT)
   PT and PTT (if abnormal: test response to vitamin K im)
   BSP when direct-reacting bilirubin normal.
   — *For special purposes:*
   IgG, A, M
   Serum lipoprotein electrophoresis and total lipids
   Plasma clotting factor assays
   Plasma and urinary amino acids.

		Direct reacting		Indirect reacting
		Incomplete obstruction	Complete obstruction	
Color of	stool	normal	pale, putty	normal
Color of	urine	dark	dark	normal
Bilirubin in	stool	+	−	+
	urine	+	+	−
Urobilin in	stool	+	−	+
	urine	+	−	+
Serum bilirubin	direct	+	+	normal
	indirect	+	+	+

226

d)   Investigation for specific disease entities
    Hematology:
        CBC, retic count
        Coombs' test, blood type (infant and mother), maternal antibodies
        Screening for G-6-PD, pyruvate kinase, galactosemia
            Take blood from infant:
        Culture & sensitivities
        Plasma amino acid
        Chromatography
        Pi (protease inhibitor) typing.
            Take blood from mother and infant:
        Toxoplasma CF titer, Sabin—Feldman dye test
        CMV herpes and rubella virus antibodies
        VDRL
    Urine tests (see p 388)
        Bilirubin, urobilin
        Amino acids
        Reducing substances (while infant receives milk)
        Culture & sensitivities
    Miscellaneous
        Skull film for intracranial calcification
        Bone films re: rubella, lues, rickets
        Sweat chloride
        If microcystic disease suspected: IVP
        If rash: skin biopsy, for histiocytosis X
        Liver biopsy: PT, PTT, platelet count (give vitamin K, 5 mg im, day before procedure).

CLASSIFICATION OF HYPERLIPOPROTEINEMIA

Type	Cholesterol	Triglycerides	lipoprotein electrophoresis			
			Chylomicrons	Beta	Pre-Beta	Alpha
Normal	N	N	absent	N	N	N
I	N or ↑	↑↑↑	present	N or ↓	N	N or ↓
II	↑	N or ↑	absent	↑	N	N
III	↑	↑	absent	"Broad-Beta"		N
IV	N or ↑	↑ or ↑↑	absent	N	↑ or ↑↑	N
V	N or ↑	↑ or ↑↑↑	present	N or ↑	↑↑↑	N or ↓

(N = normal, ↑ = increased, ↓ = decreased)

NEPHROLOGY

Acute or Recurrent Urinary Tract Infection
(Cystitis and/or Pyelonephritis)

History
1. Previous urinary infection or unexplained fever
2. Change in urinary frequency; burning, enuresis, day-time wetting, dribbling, abnormal appearance or smell of urine; suppression of voiding/'holding', voiding with labia together
3. Abdominal flank or suprapubic pain
4. Pinworms, constipation, incorrect wiping
5. Use of 'bubble-bath' or salts; nylon pants
6. Family members with kidney or urinary-tract problems.

Physical Examination
Especially:
1. Height and weight percentile
2. Ocular fundi, BP
3. Abdomen: for enlargement of kidney/bladder, costo-vertebral/suprapubic tenderness
4. External genitalia: for congenital anomalies, local inflammation.

Investigation
1. Obtain fresh specimen of midstream urine. If necessary, use suprapubic aspiration* (especially in neonates) or catheterization (p 78). *Note. Suprapubic aspiration should be carried out only by residents who have done it under supervision.
   a) Examine specimen with naked eye for haziness due to bacteria, and confirm under high-power microscope; test for protein, Hb. $\geqslant 5$ WBC/ml (uncentrifuged) is abnormal.
   b) Send specimen to Bacteriology for bacterial count. (Urine infection can occur without pyuria; proof is a bacterial count of $> 10^5$/ml).
   c) If the count is between 10^4 and 10^5/ml, send another specimen for culture.
   d) **Note.** In urine obtained by suprapubic aspiration, probably any count is abnormal.

2. Order radiographic studies for every patient except those with typical acute hemorrhagic cystitis. Include IVP, and probably catheter voiding cystourethrogram (at catheterization, send urine for culture and sensitivities).

Treatment

1. Bedrest while feverish; extra-high fluid intake.
2. Normal diet as soon as tolerated with fluids.
3. Chemotherapy and antibiotics.
   a) *Mild infection:* after obtaining urine for culture, give sulfisoxazole (Gantrisin) (p 413) or suitable antibiotic in therapeutic dose for 10 days.
   b) *Severe infection:* after obtaining urine for culture, give bactericidal antibiotic such as ampicillin (p 407) for 10-14 days. If no improvement in 2 days, change antibiotic to match sensitivity or organism.
4. Urinalysis daily until bacteria/pyuria have disappeared.
5. Follow-up: after cessation of treatment, obtain midstream urine for examination ± culture at approx 1 wk, 6 wk, and 3 mo.

Renal Failure

Definitions

Azotemia: BUN above normal level.

Uremia: A complex of signs and symptoms reflecting dysfunction of organ systems from kidney failure.

Oliguria: Urine output <300 ml/m^2; or 5 - 10 ml/100 cal expended.

Investigation

1. Urine examination

Urine	Pre-renal	Intra-renal
SG*	>1.020	<1.018
(Na$^+$)*	<15 mEq/liter	>20 mEq/liter
sediment	Hyaline & finely granular casts	Renal tubular cells and casts, RBC & RBC casts, Hb casts, coarsely granular casts.
*If diuretics have been given, these values are not useful.		

2. Flat plate abdomen — size of kidneys, ?stones.
3. Complete cessation of urine indicates bilateral obstruction, cortical necrosis, or severe glomerulonephritis.
4. If findings suggest post-renal cause (posterior urethral valves): consult urologist re catheterization.
5. If failure is pre-renal, adequate hydration is mandatory.
   - To check whether failure is pre-renal, give a test dose of an isotonic solution (10 ml/kg).
6. If failure is pre-renal: after re-hydration, furosemide (1 mg/kg, p 441) should increase urine output.

Treatment

1. If failure caused by nephrotoxin, mannitol (0.5 g/kg in 20% soln) may be helpful.
2. *Hyperkalemia*
   a) *Stat* ECG (p 197)
   b) Repeat serum potassium. If K^+ >7.0 mEq/liter:
      i) 10% Ca gluconate 0.5 ml/kg, iv — with ECG monitoring.
      ii) 7.5% $NaHCO_3$, 2-3 mEq/kg (3 ml/kg), iv
      iii) — iv, 1 ml/kg/hr, 50% dextrose (BS 250 mg/100 ml) then 30% dextrose (volume = insensible water loss).
         — addition of insulin (1 U/g glucose) is useful in some cases.
      iv) Kayexalate 1 g/kg, po or in enema (vehicle, 70% sorbitol)
      v) If these measures fail, peritoneal or hemodialysis will be needed.
3. *Acidosis* (p 126)
4. *Hypertension:* remove extracellular fluid if indicated. Antihypertensive therapy, see p 238.
5. *Fluid therapy:* approx. 300 ml/m^2/day + urine output; **or** 20 ml/100 cal expended/day + urine output.

RENAL FAILURE. DRUG THERAPY*: Maintenance-dose Intervals

(*Modified from W. M. Bennett *et al.* JAMA 214:1468, 1970)

Renal failure defined as: Creatinine clearance (ml/m²) =	mild 29-46	moderate 6-29	severe <6

Drug	Normal Renal Status	Renal Failure		
		Mild	Moderate	Severe
acetylsalicylic acid	q4h	q4h	q4 – 6h	q8 – 12h
allopurinol	q8h	q8h	q12h	q12 – 24h
aminophylline	q6h	unchanged	unchanged	unchanged
amphotericin B	q24h	q24h	q24h	q24 – 36h
ampicillin	q6h	q6h	q6h	q8 – 12h
azathioprine	q12h	q12h	q12 – 18h	q12 – 24h
carbenicillin	q4h	q4h	q6 – 12h	q12 – 16h
cephalexin	q6h	q6h	q12h	q18 – 24h
cephaloridine* (avoid if possible)				
codeine	q6h	q6h	q12h	q24 – 36h
cyclophosphamide	q4h	unchanged	unchanged	unchanged
diazoxide	iv boluses	unchanged	unchanged	unchanged
digoxin	q12h	q24h	q24-36h	q36 – 48h
diphenylhydantoin	q8h	unchanged	unchanged	unchanged
erythromycin	q6h	unchanged	unchanged	unchanged
ethacrynic acid	q6h; as needed for diuresis	q6h	q6h	avoid
furosemide*	q6h; as needed for diuresis	unchanged	unchanged	unchanged

232

gentamicin (avoid if possible)	q8h	q8 – 12h	q12 – 24h	q48h
guanethidine	q24h	unchanged	q24 – 36h	q36 – 48h
heparin	q4h	unchanged	unchanged	unchanged
hydralazine	q8h	unchanged		unchanged
insulin, regular	q6h	q6h	q8 – 12h	q12 – 24h
kanamycin	q8h	q24h	q24 – 72h	q72 – 96h
lincomycin	q6h	q6h	q6h	q8 – 12h
mercurials	q24h	q24h	avoid	avoid
methicillin	q4h	q4h	q4h	q8 – 12h
methotrexate	q24h	q24h	q24 – 36h	q36 – 48h
methyldopa	q6h	q6h	q9 – 12h	q12 – 18h
nitrofurantoin	q8h	q8h	q8h	avoid
oxacillin	q6h	q6h	q6h	q8 – 12h
penicillin G	q8h	q8h	q8h	q12h
phenobarbital	q8h	q8h	q8h	q8 – 16h
propranolol	q6h	unchanged	unchanged	unchanged
reserpine	q24h	unchanged	unchanged	unchanged
spironolactone	q6h	q6h	avoid	avoid
streptomycin	q12h	q24h	q24h – 72h	q72 – 96h
sulfisoxazole	q6h	q6h	q8 – 12h	q12 – 24h
thiazides	q12h	q12h	q12h	avoid
ticarcillin: see carbenicillin				
triamterene	q12h	q12h	avoid	avoid
warfarin	q24h	unchanged	unchanged	unchanged

*Combination with furosemide significantly increases toxicity of cephaloridine

KIDNEY DISEASE

Acute Glomerulonephritis

History

Enquire specifically about:

1. Possible hemolytic strep infections in month preceding onset, including scarlet fever, skin infections
2. Edema, hematuria, oliguria
3. Family history of nephritis or deafness
4. Abdominal or joint pains, or rash suggestive of Henoch–Schönlein purpura.

Investigation

1. *Blood*
   a) CBC, smear, ESR
   b) ASO titer (if ASO normal, get antihyaluronidase titer).
   c) Total serum hemolytic complement and $\beta_1 C$ globulin.
   d) Serum for BUN, creatinine; and, if more than slight edema, cholesterol and protein electrophoresis.
   e) If oliguria present: blood for pH, PCO_2, HCO_3^-; Na^+, K^+, Cl^-.
2. *Urinalysis*
   a) Daily at first
   b) When gross hematuria clears, examine fresh am urine at least 3 x wk: SG, protein (using 10% sulfosalicylic acid), Hb, microscopy. Heme or RBC casts are of diagnostic importance.
3. *Throat culture* for hemolytic strep.

Treatment

1. Bedrest until gross hematuria, edema, and hypertension subside (usually <4 wk).
2. Penicillin in therapeutic dosage x 10 days (p 406).
3. Clear fluids (low Na^+ and K^+) until gross hematuria, oliguria, and edema subside; then, Nephritis diet no 1, 2, and 3 – Junior or Senior (p 328), progressively.
4. Record fluid balance until good urinary output.
5. BP: bid at first, more often if elevated.
6. No prophylactic inoculations or vaccinations during convalescence.

Complications

1. *Hypertension*
   Check BP q1-4h, depending on severity or accompanying symptoms of headache, blurred vision, vomiting, convulsions, or papilledema. For details of treatment, see Hypertension (p 238).
2. *Heart failure*
   If hypertension present; treat as above; digitalize, and give other treatment as outlined under Heart Disease (p 200). Furosemide is an effective diuretic.
3. *Anuria or severe oliguria:* see p 230.

Nephrotic Syndrome

History

Enquire specifically for family history of renal disease, allergy, and whether the patient has had any infection, rash, bee-sting, inoculation or vaccination in the month or two preceding onset of the kidney problem. Also, whether recent trimethadone or other drug therapy, or ingestion of/exposure to mercury, gold, bismuth.

Investigation

1. *Blood* for BUN, creatinine, cholesterol, protein, electrophoresis, $\beta_1 C$ globulin and total hemolytic complement.
   – Not essential in all cases is blood for pH, pCO_2, HCO_3^-, Na^+, Cl^-, Ca^{++}, phosphorus, creatinine clearance.
2. *Urinalysis:* daily at first; later, 3 x wk for SG, protein (test with 10% sulfosalicylic acid), Hb, and microscopy.

General Treatment

Except at onset and during severe relapses, patient should lead as normal a life as possible.

1. *Bedrest:* only when disabling edema or severe infection.
2. *Diet:*
   a) protein normal or high unless BUN elevated
   b) sodium low when patient edematous or receiving high doses of steroid
   c) multiple vit supplement especially if appetite poor
   d) restricted fluid intake only if edema severe.

3. *Infection:*
   a) extra concern for upper respiratory-tract infections
   b) nursing care important when patient is edematous – skin breaks down easily, so do not tape for urine collection.
   c) prophylactic antibiotic not usually necessary.

4. *Psychological*
   a) reassurance and encouragement of parents and patient important; always be optimistic
   b) explain clinical course, and expected side-effects of treatment.

5. *Edema*
   a) steroid usually induces diuresis in 8-10 days
   b) if edema severe, combination hydrochlorothiazide (p 443) and spironolactone (p 461) helpful.
   c) Watch serum Na^+ and K^+ levels.

6. If the above measures fail: give trial infusion of salt-poor albumin, given over a few hr; with or without iv furosemide (p 441) at the end of the infusion.

7. Abdominal paracentesis (p 75) is rarely necessary.

Specific Treatment

STEROIDS

1. *To induce remission*
   Prednisone 2 mg/kg/24 hr in 3 or 4 divided doses; maximum usually 60 mg/24 hr, rarely 80 mg/24 hr.
   a) Continue until urine negative for protein x 5 days, or for maximum of 4 wk if proteinuria persists.
   b) If no remission within 28 days: start intermittent therapy at 4 mg/kg (maximum, 120 mg) at breakfast on alternate days for up to 28 days, then reduce.

2. *To maintain remission*
   a) Give up to 2 x daily dose as single dose at breakfast every 2nd day; usual maximum, 100 mg.
   b) Reduce by 10 mg q2-4 to 30 mg, then by 5 mg q2-4 wk, until discontinued.
   c) Teach parents to test first am urine for protein (with Albustix or 10% sulfosalicylic acid) and keep a record of results. Instruct them in recording treatment also.

3. *During relapse* — probable relapse indicated by 2+ or heavier proteinuria for 3 consecutive days, without fever and with no definite relapse evidenced clinically by edema and/or biochemically.
   — Treat as initially to induce remission; subsequent reduction in therapy may be much faster.

IMMUNOSUPPRESSIVE AGENTS

1. *Cyclophosphamide* (p 434) is of proven value in 'minimal change' nephrotic syndrome which has become dependent on or resistant to steroid. Complications may be serious (leukopenia, hemorrhagic cystitis, sterility, etc), and treatment should not be considered without histologic confirmation of diagnosis by renal biopsy and discussion with child's parents about known complications and possibility of unknown ones.
   a) Usual dosage of cyclophosphamide is 2.0-2.5 mg/kg/24 hr
   b) it is combined with intermittent prednisone therapy (given every 2nd day at breakfast)
   c) total duration probably should not exceed 8-12 wk.

2. *Azathioprine* (Imuran) has not proved of value.

COMPLICATIONS

1. Diminished resistance to infection.
2. Hypovolemia — postural hypotension, circulatory collapse, acute renal failure.
3. Protein depletion — osteoporosis, cutaneous striae, muscle wasting, apathy.
4. Increased coagulability of blood — arterial and venous thrombosis, embolism (femoral artery puncture should not be done — it has led to femoral artery thrombosis and gangrene).
5. Reduced renal function — progressive uremia, hypertension, etc.
6. Complications of therapy:
   a) diuretics may deplete Na^+ and/or K^+.
   b) steroids may stunt growth, delay puberty, cause Cushingoid obesity (can be limited by low-calorie diet), hypertension, osteoporosis, aseptic necrosis of bone.
   c) cytotoxic agents — see above.

HYPERTENSION

History
Kidney disease, hematuria, renal trauma, headache, blurred vision, episodic diarrhea, sweating or flushing, recent weight gain, drugs or poisons (contraceptive pill, licorice, etc.).

Family History
Hypertension, heart disease, strokes, diabetes mellitus, neurofibromatosis — and at what age?

Physical Examination
Especially:
1. Height and weight percentiles
2. fundoscopic examination, heart size, signs of heart failure
3. bruit over kidney anteriorly or posteriorly
4. BP — both arms, upright and supine (allow 5 min after change of position), both legs.
5. Liver, spleen, and kidneys palpable? *café-au-lait* spots; virilization?

Useful Investigations
1. serum Na, K, Cl, pH, pCO_2, HCO_3, creatinine; BUN
2. creatinine clearance
3. urine concentration test
4. 24-hr urine for 17-hydroxy- and 17-ketosteroids
5. separate 24-hr urine collection for VMA study (p 400) and/or catecholamines
6. blood sugar, fasting and 2 hr post-prandial
7. rapid-sequence IVP
8. chest film (for heart size)
9. ECG
10. renal arteriogram.

Special Tests
Peripheral-vein renin
1. Normal-sodium diet (3 mEq Na^+/kg body wt/day; maximum, 120 mEq) x 3 days. Then take blood for supine test (after 8 hr or more supine) followed by upright test (after 4 hr upright, fasting).

2. Low-sodium diet (0.3 mEq Na$^+$/kg body wt/day; maximum, 10 mEq) x 3 days. Then take tests as in (1). (See p 238).

3. If indicated, separate renal-vein renin collections can be made while patient is still on low-sodium diet.

4. Procedure for collecting specimens for renin assay:
   a) Alert Clinical Chemistry lab that a renin study is to be done. *Specimens will be accepted on weekdays only.*
   b) Obtain from Clinical Chemistry lab 1 lavender-topped Vacutainer tube (contains EDTA) for each specimen to be collected.
   c) *For each sample,* enter the following details on a Clinical Chemistry requisition:
      i) name of patient
      ii) date
      iii) time
      iv) patient's posture (supine or upright)
      v) patient's diet
      vi) site of sampling.
   d) Each specimen should be 4-5 ml; place on ice immediately after collection.
   e) Specimen and requisition should be delivered to Clinical Chem lab **immediately.**

Isotope renogram and renal scan (p 84).

Diurnal serum cortisol (p 362).

Plasma aldosterone: 3-5 ml of heparinized blood collected on ice (p 354).

Colored photograph of fundus (consult Ophthalmology).

Treatment

Low-NA$^+$ diet
a) Severe restriction (0.5 g Na or less) rarely necessary and may cause hyponatremia if diuretic used.
b) 1.0-2.0 g Na/day should be adequate restriction, or patient may simply avoid salty food and use no salt at table.

During hypertensive crises
1. Diazoxide (Hyperstat) is a rapid, potent antihypertensive. Give 5 mg/kg in a single iv injection over 30 sec; repeat if no effect in 1 hr.

2. Sodium nitroprusside: requires constant monitoring in ICU. 50 mg/liter of 5% dextrose/water (5 mg/ml); infuse at 0.5-8.0 mg/kg/min.

3. Reserpine 0.07 mg/kg, im; maximum 2.5 mg, repeated q12-24 hr (p 459).

4. Methyldopa (p 449) 5 to 10 mg/kg; give iv over 30-60 min. Can be repeated q6-8h. (Available in 5-ml ampules, 50 mg/ml. Dilute in 50 ml 5% dextrose in distilled water.)

Less severe or chronic hypertension

1. Oral diuretic (chlorothiazide, hydrochlorothiazide): can be used as initial medication for mild hypertension or in combination with reserpine.
   a) chlorothiazide (Diuril): 10-20 mg/kg/24 hr, in 3 or 4 divided doses, po
   b) hydrochlorothiazide (Hydro-Diuril): 1-2 mg/kg/ 24 hr, in 3 or 4 divided doses, po.

2. Hydralazine hydrochloride (Apresoline) is more potent than reserpine or diuretics and is often given in combination with reserpine. Give 1 mg/kg/24 hr, in 3 or 4 divided doses; iv, im or po; can be gradually increased to 5 mg/kg/24 hr, maximum 200 mg/ 24 hr. If used in combination with reserpine, give hydralazine 0.15 mg/kg/day, iv or im, as a single dose.

3. Reserpine (Serpasil) po has tranquilizing and mild antihypertensive effect. Starting dose 0.25 mg once daily, often reduced in a few wk to 0.1 mg once daily. Reserpine is usually combined with an oral diuretic or hydralazine.

4. Methyldopa (Aldomet) is more potent than hydralazine and does not affect renal blood flow — but it may cause postural hypotension, drowsiness. Starting dose, 10 mg/kg/24 hr po, in 3 divided doses; then gradually increase. Maximum for **adults,** 3.0 g/24 hr. Aldomet, iv, 20-40 mg/kg/day, divided q6h.

5. Propranolol (Inderal) po 0.5-1.0 mg/kg/day divided q6-8h, see p 457.

6. Guanethidine (Ismelin) is a potent antihypertensive but causes postural hypotension and reduces renal blood flow, GFR, and cerebral blood flow.
   a) Give 0.2 mg/kg once daily, or a lower dose if combined with oral diuretic.
   b) Contraindicated in pheochromocytoma.

7. Bethanidine (Esbaloid) is similar to guanethidine but shorter-acting; causes postural hypotension.
   a) Dosage, see p 424. Can be combined with oral diuretic or methyldopa.
   b) Contraindicated in pheochromocytoma.

Renal Biopsy

1. Child <5 yr: whether closed or open, biopsy is done under general anesthesia by urologist.

2. Child >5 yr: biopsy may be done with local anesthesia by nephrologist.

3. All cases: determine platelet count, PT and PTT.

4. Open surgical biopsy: order ordinary IVP (see Radiology, p 82).

5. Needle biopsy under local anesthetic:
   a) Pre-biopsy sedation: CM3 (see Anesthesia, p 273) 0.1 ml/kg (maximum 1.5 ml) deep im, 1 hr before biopsy.
   b) Nephrologist marks a pattern of spots (using indelible pencil) on the skin over lower pole of kidney.
   c) IVP is taken with a 10-min film in prone position, pad under abdomen, and markers on the spots.

6. After biopsy:
   a) Child remains in bed for 24 hr.
   b) Check pulse and BP q15 min for 2 hr, then pulse q1h overnight.
   c) Save all urine samples for 24 hr — check each for hematuria.
   d) Report any unusual bleeding, pain, or sign of shock.

ENDOCRINOLOGY

DIABETES MELLITUS

Diabetes mellitus can begin abruptly or insidiously, at any age.

Newly Diagnosed Diabetes without Severe Acidosis

Management
If the child is not clinically ill, not vomiting, and not dehydrated, a blood sugar level and urinalysis for sugar and acetone are sufficient to establish the diagnosis.

If the child is acutely ill
1. Order electrolytes, acid–base, and BUN, in addition to blood sugar.
2. Diabetes diet appropriate for age.
3. Give regular (crystalline) insulin 0.25 U/kg body wt, q4-6h depending on sugar response. Intermediate-acting insulin (e.g., Lente) usually can be started the next morning.
4. Begin diabetes protocol.
5. Inform diabetes nurse-practitioner to arrange education programs for parents and child.
6. Do not give parents and child too much detailed information about diet, urine-testing, and insulin routines, until the initial shock of diagnosis has worn off (usually a week or more). *A positive, optimistic attitude is most important.*
7. a) Begin Lente insulin, 1 U per yr of age, the day after admission.
   b) Increase the dose approx. 10% a day until urine is negative for sugar. (Ketonuria may persist for a few days but, unless the child is clinically ill, it is no indication for extra insulin.)
   c) All urine tested should be the second voided that day.
   d) When the urine becomes negative for sugar, measure blood sugar to determine renal threshold.
   e) When 3 or 4 samples are negative for sugar in 1 day, reduce insulin until blood sugar levels fasting and at 16:30 hr are between 100 and 150 mg/dl.
8. Initial control and teaching usually require 10-14 days in hospital.

9. Write 'release slips' for out-of-hospital activities.

Diabetes Diets, see p 328.

Diabetic Ketoacidosis

This is a medical emergency!
1. Persistent ketonuria, even without acidosis, signals impending trouble. Acidosis is usually accompanied by vomiting, abdominal pain, dehydration, and hyperventilation.
2. Mild ketoacidosis: pH <7.3 and bicarbonate <20 mEq/liter.
3. Severe acidosis: pH <7.2, bicarbonate <12 mEq/liter, usually accompanied by hyperventilation.

Management
1. Take blood for sugar, pH, bicarbonate, pCO_2, Na, K, Cl, BUN.
2. Start diabetes ketoacidosis protocol.
3. Most children in severe ketoacidosis are 10% or more dehydrated.
   a) Start iv infusion of either Ringer's lactate or N saline soln, 15-20 ml/kg for at least the first hour, then 10-15 ml/kg/hr until acidosis corrected. A good rough rule for any child >6 yr old is to give 1 liter of fluid in first hr, 1 liter in next 2 hr, and 1 liter in next 3 hr.
4. When the child has voided, add KCl to the iv soln, 3 mEq/kg body wt over 24 hr. (If the initial serum K is <4.0 mEq/liter, K deficit may be severe.)
5. Frequently, evaluate patient's condition and fluid balance — take into account the amounts administered and lost as urine. Use evaluation as guide in calculating fluid and electrolyte replacement necessary after first few hours.
6. *Insulin*
   There are several different dose schedules and routes of administration of insulin for treating diabetic ketoacidosis in children. Although currently popular, continuous iv infusion has no proven advantages over sc administration.

243

If the *subcutaneous route* is used:
a) If acidosis severe, give 0.5 U crystalline insulin/kg body wt — *in addition to* the usual daily dose of insulin and *regardless of when* it was administered.
b) *Milder acidosis:* smaller doses can be given.
c) If blood sugar <300 mg/dl: give the insulin in conjunction with a glucose-containing solution such as 2/3–1/3, or 5% glucose in saline.
d) Subsequent doses of insulin (usually 0.25 U/kg):
   i) Give q4-6h sc, depending on blood-sugar response to initial dose.
   ii) Next day: give the child his usual dose of insulin.

If the *intravenous route* is used:
a) Give 0.1 ml insulin (100 U/ml), diluted in 10 ml of saline then further diluted to 100 ml with saline or Ringer's soln in a Buritrol. (Final concn of insulin = 1 U/10 ml.)
b) Infuse 0.1 U/kg body wt/hr as part of rehydrating solution (e.g., a child weighing 50 kg would receive 5 U insulin/hr — 50 ml of the insulin-containing soln.) This is piggybacked in through the rehydrating iv line and is controlled by an IVAC pump.
c) When blood glucose <300 mg/dl, reduce infusion rate to 0.02 U/kg/hr. Maintain at this rate until next morning, then give Lente insulin. Then increase or decrease the rate according to blood glucose level.

7. *Sodium bicarbonate*
a) Give (as 7.5% solution iv) if pH <7.2 or blood bicarbonate <12 mEq/liter. Calculate the amount by the following formula:
   12 − measured bicarbonate (mEq) x 0.6 x body wt (kg) = amount of bicarbonate (mEq) required to raise blood bicarbonate to 12 mEq/liter.
b) Give half the amount over 15-20 min, and the remainder over the next 1-2 hr.
c) Approx. 4 hr after initiating therapy, recheck acid–base values, blood sugar, electrolytes, BUN. Most children should be out of severe acidosis by 6 hr.

8. *General measures*
a) *As soon as the child is admitted* notify Endocrinology fellow, senior resident, and ward chief. The Endocrinology fellow is responsible for treatment until the child is out of danger.

b) Check and record intake and output. Watch level of consciousness – the child may fall asleep but usually is easily roused. If level of consciousness deteriorates during treatment, assume development of hypoglycemia: take blood for blood sugar, then give 50% glucose, 0.5 g/kg, iv.

c) If child does not void or is incontinent, use condom drainage or (rarely necessary) catheterize briefly.

9. *Continuing care*
   a) When nausea and vomiting controlled, give fluids po.
   b) Next day, if child able to take fluids or diabetes diet, begin Lente insulin.
   c) Discontinue iv infusion when: pH >7.3, bicarbonate >20 mEq/liter, and child is drinking well, fully alert, and conscious.

Complications during Treatment of Ketoacidosis

Hypoglycemia, hypokalemia, alkalosis, slipping back into acidosis, cerebral edema, inadequate fluid intake.
Infection is a common precipitating cause of acidosis. Treat appropriately.

Hypoglycemia

1. Mild: give glucose po in fruit juice, soft drinks, corn syrup.

2. Severe:
   a) Give 50% glucose iv, 0.5 g/kg body wt *stat,* then continue infusion of 10-15% glucose until fluids/food tolerated.
   b) Ensure that all diabetic children have epinephrine or glucagon at home – epinephrine, 0.25 ml of 1:1000 soln sc, or glucagon 1 mg sc, will raise the blood sugar in most children.

Surgery

Consult Diabetes service when child with diabetes mellitus is about to undergo surgery.

1. *Elective.* Admit several days before surgery, to improve control. The fasting blood sugar should be <200 mg/dl, and the urine free of ketone bodies, before surgery.

2. *Minor surgical procedures* (T & A, hernia, etc.).
   a) The operation should be performed between 0800 and 0900 hr.
   b) On morning of operation, give no regular (crystalline) insulin. Give ¼ to ½ the usual dose of Lente, or other intermediate-acting insulin, sc.
   c) Determine blood sugar before operation.

d) Start iv infusion of 1/3 glucose in 2/3 saline soln.
e) Determine blood sugar postop in the recovery room; if blood sugar >250 mg/dl, give extra crystalline insulin.
f) Begin fluids po when child returns to ward. Discontinue iv line when he is drinking well. Give regular insulin, in amounts guided by urine and/or blood sugar levels, q4-6h during the day.
g) Next day, increase Lente insulin to 2/3 to 3/4 of pre-operative dose, depending on clinical condition. Increase diet as tolerated.
h) Discharge home 2-3 days postop (when back on pre-op dose of insulin).

3. *Major surgical procedures:*
   a) to e) as for minor procedures.
   f) Continue extra regular insulin q6-8h, and 1/3 to ½ the dose of Lente insulin, as long as iv administration, suction, etc.
   g) When fluids po started, increase dose of Lente insulin.

4. *Emergency surgical procedures*
   a) Correct dehydration, acidosis, and electrolyte imbalance.
   b) Give additional regular insulin to correct hyperglycemia.
   c) Proceed with surgery when condition stable.

THYROID

See Biochemistry (pp 382, 384, 385) and Nuclear Medicine (p 84).

ADRENAL INSUFFICIENCY

Etiology

1. Commonest cause is congenital adrenal hyperplasia, presenting in the neonatal period with salt wasting and ambiguous genitalia in the female.
2. Next most likely is iatrogenic, from steroid withdrawal after prolonged adrenal suppression. Differential diagnosis includes Addison's disease, adrenal hypoplasia, and hemorrhagic infarction of the adrenal.

Management
Acute phase

1. Venipuncture for serum electrolytes and glucose.
2. Follow immediately with iv infusion of 5% glucose in N saline.

a) 3% saline may be necessary if child has severe hyponatremia.
b) Never give hypotonic saline initially.
c) If hypoglycemia is present, give additional 50% glucose.

3. Infuse hydrocortisone succinate (Solu-Cortef) iv.
   a) initial dose, 25 mg/m² in newborns (including prematures) and 100 mg in others
   b) continue with 100 mg/m²/24 hr, given q6h.

4. If hyponatremia is present: give desoxycortisone acetate (DOCA) in oil, 5 mg/ml. Inject up to 0.2 ml (1 mg) im initially, then increase dosage until serum Na maintained in normal range.
   a) Hypernatremia, edema, and hypertension are signs of overdosage.
   b) Infants: weigh daily.
   c) All patients: measure serum electrolytes daily.

Long-term management

1. To confirm the diagnosis: when condition stabilized, cortisone (but not DOCA) can be discontinued so that serum and urinary steroids can be assayed (pp 356, 362, 370, 393).
   a) Measurements should include
      i) at 0800 hr, serum cortisol, 17-OH progesterone, and androstenedione
      ii) plasma renin
      iii) 24-hr urine for 17-ketosteroids, 17-hydroxycorticoids, and pregnanetriol.
   b) If congenital adrenal hyperplasia suspected: determine karyotype and measure serum testosterone
   c) ACTH stimulation test may be necessary to clinch the diagnosis of adrenal failure.

2. Start oral replacement of cortisone acetate, 20-25 mg/m²/24 hr, given q8h.
   a) If congenital adrenal hyperplasia established: the cortisone is best given in a dose schedule with diurnal rhythm
      i) largest dose at 2400 hr (or as close as possible), to suppress endogenous ACTH
      ii) middle-sized dose at 0800 hr
      iii) smallest dose at 1600 hr
   b) If plasma renin levels indicate mineralocorticoid deficiency: give 9-α-fluorohydrocortisone po
      i) older children, 0.05-0.1 mg/24 hr — but
      ii) neonates and infants: up to 0.25 mg/day may be necessary to suppress plasma renin levels to normal.
   c) If 9-α-fluorohydrocortisone therapy is judged unreliable: DOCA pellets can be implanted.

3. *All patients with adrenal insufficiency should wear an identifying bracelet*, and their parents should be told of the need for 3-fold increases in cortisone dosage at times of infection, surgery, and other stress.

AMBIGUOUS GENITALIA

This condition is a neonatal emergency
The differential diagnosis is best based on the genetic sex (table opposite). A team approach (general pediatrician, urologist, and pediatric endocrinologist) is advocated.

Management

1. Delay birth announcement; do not make arbitrary sex assignment.
2. Get detailed history, for familial disorders of sexual differentiation, maternal exposure to hormones, maternal illness, consanguinity.
3. Careful physical examination for other anomalies.
4. Karyotype (buccal smears for Barr bodies are unreliable neonatally, and inconclusive).
5. Retrograde urethrogram (to define internal genitalia) ± IVP.
6. Hormone studies, 17-OH progesterone, testosterone, LH, FSH, and other tests as indicated.
7. Gonadal biopsy, including laparotomy, may be necessary.
8. Base the sex assignment and parent counseling on the diagnosis and prognosis for the appropriate adult sexual function.
    —   In difficult cases still doubtful after investigation, assignment of female sex is preferable.

HYPOCALCEMIA

1. Defined as total plasma Ca <3.4 mEq/liter; plasma Ca++ <1.4 mEq/liter.
2. Patient asymptomatic but plasma Ca <3.0 mEq/liter: treatment with Ca given iv is indicated.
3. Patient symptomatic and plasma Ca <3.5 mEq/liter: treat with Ca.

Causes

Include tetany of newborn; transient or permanent hypomagnesemia or hypoparathyroidism; pseudohypoparathyroidism; vitamin-D deficiency; steatorrhea; acute or chronic renal insufficiency; alkalosis (normal plasma serum Ca and decreased plasma Ca^{++}).

Ambiguous Genitalia

	Female pseudohermaphrodite	Male pseudohermaphrodite	Mixed gonadal dysgenesis	True hermaphrodite
Karyotype	46XX	46XY	45XO/46XY, 46XY, others	46XX, 46XY, others
Defect	Masculinization	Inadequate masculinization	Inadequate masculinization	Male and female gonads
Gonads	Ovaries	Testes	Testes and streak	Testes and ovary
Müllerian ducts	+	±	±	±
Wolffian ducts	–	±	±	±
Differential diagnosis	1. CAH 2. Transplacental androgen 3. Androgenic tumor	1. Androgen insensitivity 2. Testosterone biosynthetic defect 3. Testicular dysgenesis 4. Nonendocrine developmental defect: a) part of a syndrome b) pseudovaginal perineal hypospadias		

Management with Ca Gluconate iv

1. Administer diluted Ca gluconate by continuous iv.
   a) Starting dose: 0.2 mEq Ca/kg body wt/hr.
      Note. 1 g Ca gluconate contains approx. 5 mEq Ca. Suitable concn = 2% Ca gluconate soln (i.e., 10% Ca gluconate diluted 1:5 with 5% glucose in water). This dilution provides approx. 0.1 mEq Ca/ml (example: starting dose for 10-kg child = 2% Ca gluconate soln, to run at 20 ml/hr).
   b) Adjust infusion rate after 4 hr, and again at 8 hr, to achieve plasma Ca within 4.25-5.0 mEq/liter.
      – Thereafter, maintain plasma Ca according to plasma Ca and P (determine both *at least bid* while Ca infusion is running).

2. When terminating Ca infusion, reduce rate very gradually while monitoring plasma Ca and P.
   Note. Beneficial effects of Ca infusion are transitory unless underlying cause is corrected. Several days' infusion is usually required.

Special notes

1. **Symptomatic hypocalcemia is an emergency**, particularly in infancy. Oral calcium supplements do not usually alleviate symptoms.

2. Be sure iv needle is definitely and securely in scalp vein or large vein of extremity.

3. Watch for evidence, and alter location immediately if infusion is interstitial or vein thrombosed. Addition of 0.1 ml of 1:1,000 U heparin to each 100 ml Ca gluconate soln delays thrombosis.

4. Do not administer Ca gluconate and Na bicarbonate into same iv tubing.

5. Never give Ca im or sc.

6. Acute hypercalcemia
   a) >6.5 mEq/liter causes vomiting and bradycardia.
   b) Very high levels cause cardiac arrest.

7. Hypocalcemia potentiates adverse effects of hypokalemia and digitalis.

8. a) Trousseau test: inflate BP cuff above systolic for 3 min.
   b) Chvostek test: tap gently with reflex hammer above and below zygoma.

Management with Parathyroid Extract

1. Administer parathyroid extract (use Para-Thor-Mone [Lilly], which contains 100 USP U/ml).
   a) Starting dose: 4 USP U/kg body wt im q8h.
   b) Rotate sites — injections may be painful.
2. Determine plasma Ca and P 4 hr after each dose, as basis for prescribing next dose.
3. When dose of parathyroid extract is established that maintains plasma Ca within 4.25-5.0 mEq/liter: check plasma Ca and P bid.
4. When terminating this therapy, gradually reduce size of the 8-hrly doses.

Adjuncts to Management

1. Oral Ca supplements: give 4 mEq Ca/kg body wt q8h.
   a) Ca lactate (1 g yields 10 mEq) given between feedings may be efficacious in neonates.
   b) Ca syrup 20%, Sandoz (contains 5.5 mEq Ca/5 ml).
   c) Ca effervescent tablets, Sandoz (500 mg tablet provides 25 mEq Ca).
2. Aluminum hydroxide: to control hyperphosphatemia (Amphojel liquid provides 60 mg/ml).
   a) Infants: 300 mg, 3-6 times daily (can be added to milk formula).
   b) Children and adults: 900-1,800 mg, 3-6 times daily between meals.

HYPOPARATHYROIDISM

Definition

Parathormone levels constantly <0.03 ng/ml, accompanied by hypocalcemia and elevated phosphorus.

Management

1. Treat symptomatic hypocalcemia (p 248).
2. Permanent hypoparathyroid states: treat with vit D.
   a) If symptomatic hypocalcemia is present: give high-dosage vit D build-up.
   b) Give vit D 8,000 U/kg body wt/day po.
   c) Measure plasma Ca and P each day, as basis for continuing the vit D build-up, until plasma Ca is at or above 4.5 mEq/liter (9 mg/dl) on 2 successive days. Then, discontinue this dosage and start maintenance therapy.

    d)   Maintenance therapy:
vitamin D 2,000 U/kg body wt/day initially; increase/decrease daily dosage 15% according to plasma Ca level at 6 wk , then every 3 mo.

3. Aluminum hydroxide gel and oral Ca supplementation are rarely needed when proper dosage of vit D has been established.

VITAMIN D-DEFICIENCY RICKETS

Definition

Stage 1. Onset at 3-5 mo: convulsions, occasionally tetany, hypocalcemia, normophosphatemia, alkaline phosphatase slightly elevated, no aminoaciduria, minimal radiographic changes.

Stage 2. Onset at 4-12 mo: skeletal signs, normocalcemia, hypophosphatemia, alkaline phosphatase elevated, aminoaciduria, lesions apparent radiographically.

Stage 3. Onset at 5-12 mo: skeletal signs, convulsions, tetany, hypocalcemia, hypophosphatemia, alkaline phosphatase elevated, aminoaciduria, lesions apparent radiographically.

Treatment

1. **Note.** Obtain blood for serum vit D and PTH assays before starting treatment.

2. Treat symptomatic hypocalcemia (p 248).

3. Start vit D concurrently.
    a)   Initially, give 4,000 U (0.1 mg) vit D po daily for 1 mo (therapeutic trial), using high-potency preparation (see below).
    b)   When biochemical and radiographic healing has started, reduce vit D to 400 U/day and give as a multivitamin preparation.

4. If the therapeutic trial evokes no response, investigate for vit D-refractory conditions.

High-potency vitamin-D preparations

1. Radiostol liquid BDH (red label): 100,000 U (2.5 mg) of vit D_2/ml.

2. Radiostol liquid, diluted 1:10 (green label): 10,000 U (0.25 mg) of vit D_2/ml.

1. & 2.   The patient measures the appropriate dose in a tuberculin syringe, and administers it directly into mouth.

3.   Ostoforte capsules, Frosst: 50,000 U (1.25 mg vit D_2/capsule).

HYPOMAGNESEMIA

Definition: plasma Mg^{++} <0.8 mEq/liter.

Management

1.   Acute Mg deficiency: replacement therapy
   a)   Provided urine output is adequate, 0.5 mEq Mg per kg body wt im q12h should increase plasma Mg concn by approx. 1.0 mEq/liter. Use 50% $MgSO_4$ (provides 4 mEq of Mg per liter).
   b)   After 2 doses, check plasma Mg and adjust subsequent doses accordingly.

2.   Maintenance therapy
   a)   Give iv (p 447); **or**
   b)   Give po: 0.6-1.0 mEq Mg per kg body wt/day in divided doses.

Prescribe $MgCl_2$ $6 H_2O$	4.0 g
$MgHC_6H_5O_7$ $5 H_2O$	6.0 g
H_2O to	100 ml

This solution provides 0.8 mEq Mg per ml, but often it is impossible to attain exact dosage with it.

METABOLIC DISORDERS

Diagnosis, see Tests, p 55

Carbohydrate Metabolism

GLUCOSE

Hypoglycemia
The aim of therapy is to maintain glycemia at >40 mg/dl.

Ketotic Hypoglycemia Syndrome
1. Avoid prolonged starvation (give midnight feeds).
2. Increase no. of snacks during infective episodes.

Hyperinsulinism
1. Maintain normoglycemia with glucose iv (3-5 mg/kg/min) *via a dependable infusion site.* (This may require cutdown or central venous line.)
   - **Do not** increase glucose infusion above 6-8 mg/kg/min.
   - Avoid iv bolus injection of glucose.
   If hypoglycemia persists:
2. Add glucagon iv, 0.25-0.5 mg/kg/24 hr.
3. Give diazoxide suspension po (5-15 mg/kg/day); gradually withdraw the glucose and glucagon infusion after 4-5 days.
4. If normoglycemia is not maintained at higher doses of diazoxide, the only alternative is subtotal pancreatectomy.

Note. The efficacy of steroids and the advantages of long-acting epinephrine preparations in addition to the above are debatable.

Metabolic Acidosis
Gluconeogenic Defects
1. Continuous normoglycemia is achieved by 3 meals + 2 snacks during day, *plus* constant nocturnal intragastric glucose infusions.
2. Glucose is administered as a polymer (Polycose), at 3-4 mg/kg/min. In most cases, other biochemical derangements (e.g. acidosis, lipidemia) resolve with this regimen.

*Pyruvate Dehydrogenase Defects and Organic
   Acidurias*
These require complex therapy, involving detailed dietary
manipulation and specific vitamin therapy – different for
each disorder.

Hepatomegaly in Metabolic Disorders

In general terms, no treatment is indicated, as the condition tends to lessen with age.

GALACTOSE

Galactosemia

1. Upon confirmation of diagnosis, institute galactose-
    free diet with protein hydrolysate (Nutramigen) or
    soya-bean milk formula.
2. Later in life, child to avoid milk-containing products.

FRUCTOSE

Hereditary Fructose Intolerance

Upon confirmation of diagnosis, delete all fructose- or
sucrose-containing feeds – seek the assistance of a dietitian.

Amino-acid Metabolism and Transport

Most are autosomal or X-linked recessive diseases.
1. Detection requires a high index of clinical suspicion.
2. Some are treatable with diet or specific high-dose
    vitamin (cofactor) therapy.
Classified in two main groups, metabolic and transport
defects.

METABOLIC DEFECTS (ENZYMOPATHIES)

There are 4 main clinical groups:
   Group 1. Acute Fulminant Illness in Neonates
a) Easily rationalized as due to sepsis, hypoglycemia, or
    acidosis, all of which also may be present.
b) Examples: MSUD, hypervalinemia, urea-cycle disor-
    ders (alkalotic, hyperammonemia), hyperglycinemia.
c) Transient aminoacidopathies are common in neo-
    nates, especially the premature. Increases in phenyl-
    alanine or methionine are common. Elevation is usu-
    ally mild, and should be followed-up to be sure it is
    truly transient.

Group 2. Neurologic Disease

a) Any patient with neurologic signs/symptoms in whom mental retardation or developmental delay has not been diagnosed should be screened (see Tests, p 55).

b) In many, *no* specific clinical signs (e.g., PKU, MSUD).

Group 3. Hyperammonemia

May have persistent or intermittent neonatal or childhood vomiting, migraine, acute encephalopathy, respiratory alkalosis and hyperammonemia, especially during infection, starvation, stress (see Hyperammonemia, p 258).

Group 4. 'Clinical Diagnosis Group'

Clinical diagnosis often possible but requires lab corroboration (see Tests, pp 62, 63):

— cystinosis
— homocystinuria
— tyrosinemia (liver disease, renal Fanconi syndrome)
— iminopeptiduria (chronic otitis, sinusitis, dermatitis, and splenomegaly)
— untreated classical PKU
— Hartnup disease (i.e., pellagra in a well-nourished person)
— diseases with odors (e.g., MSUD, isovaleric acidemia)
— gyrate atrophy of retina (hyperornithinemia)
— tyrosinemia with palmar/plantar keratosis, corneal ulcers, mental retardation (Richner—Hanhart syndrome).

TRANSPORT DEFECTS

The effects are renal, and may be intestinal also. These disorders cause *aminoaciduria* — from defects in tubular reabsorption, or secondary to increased blood levels of amino acid due to a metabolic defect (see above). Detection of aminoaciduria ALWAYS requires blood screen.

Group 1. Generalized Aminoacidurias

a) Due to metabolic or toxic damage to proximal tubules, as part of a renal Fanconi syndrome (e.g. lead [or other heavy metal] intoxication, galactosemia, fructosemia, tyrosinemia, cystinosis, Wilson's disease, Lowe's syndrome, vitamin D-deficiency rickets).

b) Also may be due to generalized hyperaminoacidemia (hyperalimentation, liver disease).

Group 2. Specific Aminoacidurias. See Tests, p 63.

Diagnostic Approach

1. *Transport diseases:* detected by screening urine, because the amino acid is filtered and not well reabsorbed by the kidney.

2. *Most metabolic defects:* the particular amino acids accumulate in blood, and blood screening is preferred because nearly all the filtered amino acid is reabsorbed by the kidney even at high plasma levels (e.g., phenylalanine, branched-chain amino acids).

3. *Some metabolic defects:* screen urine, because the particular amino acid(s) may not be well reabsorbed by the kidney (e.g., homocystine, argininosuccinic acid).

4. **In all cases, both blood and urine should be screened.**
   a) An abnormal urine test result ALWAYS requires a blood screen (e.g., aminoaciduria because of hyperaminoacidemia or a renal transport defect).
   b) Both blood and urine *may* be abnormal, but in different ways; e.g.,
      - homocystinuria: methionine increased in blood, and homocystine increased in urine;
      - tyrosinemia: tyrosine increased in blood, and amino acids increased in urine (Fanconi syndrome).
   c) The same abnormality in both specimens is less likely to be missed in a semiquantitative screen.

Lysosomal Storage

1. Lysosomal hydrolases catabolize macromolecules (mucopolysaccharides, sphingolipids, and oligosaccharides).
   a) Defects in these enzymes lead to storage of one or more compounds in viscera, reticuloendothelial cells, skin, bones, and/or CNS.
   b) Patients may have organomegaly (general or specific) and/or dysmorphic features.
   c) Dysmorphic features are accompanied by radiographically apparent changes.

2. Three classes of lysosomal hydrolase disorders can be identified with screening tests: *oligosaccharidoses, mucopolysaccharidoses,* and *sphingolipidoses.*

3. None of these disorders is treatable, but identification of the specific enzyme defect (see Tests, p 59) is important for genetic counseling and carrier detection.
   Enzyme defects can be determined only in the laboratory.

Clues to which defect(s) to test for can be determined by a combination of:
a) *History.* Fabry's disease and Hunter's syndrome are X-linked. All others are autosomal recessive. Thus, family history is rarely contributory. Consanguinity is common.
b) *Physical examination* can be misleading, but watch for:
   — disproportionate stature: see upper—lower ratio (p 341).
   — short stature
   — coarse hair, thick skin, coarse facies
   — cloudy cornea, retinal cherry-red spot
   — hypertrophy of gums
   — prefrontal bossing
   — chronic chest disease, pulmonary infiltration with poor air entry, clubbing.
c) *Radiology*
   i) Common signs include coarse trabeculation and abnormal modeling of bone.
   ii) Do skeletal survey to check long bones, metacarpals, ribs, spine and skull. Beaking at L_{2-3} is common. Check for Ehrlenmyer-flask deformity of long bones and degenerative arthropathy.

Clinical Laboratory
a) Usual indices — hematology (e.g., bone marrow — foam cells = Niemann—Pick disease, etc.), biochemistry (especially liver & kidney function), neurophysiology, etc.
b) Specific enzyme assays, see Tests (p 60).

Ammonia Metabolism

1. *Hepatic encephalopathy of childhood* (Reye's syndrome)
   See Gastroenterology (p 225).
   Note. In all cases, other causes of hyperammonemia must be ruled out.

2. *Urea-cycle defects*
   Management is complex —
   a) during acute phases, with peritoneal dialysis;
   b) during chronic phases, dietary manipulation to include low-protein diet and supplements of α-keto acid analog.

3. *Transient neonatal hyperammonemia*
   a) Suspect in any newborn who has neurologic depression.
   b) If hyperammonemia is confirmed, institute peritoneal dialysis **immediately.**

GYNECOLOGY

A basic principle of gynecology is categorization by age into:

A. Childhood (premenarchal), and
B. Adolescence (postmenarchal).

VAGINAL BLEEDING

A. Childhood (Premenarchal)

Differential Diagnosis

1. Trauma
   a) Straddle injury
   b) Alleged assault
2. Foreign body
3. Tumor
4. Precocious puberty

Management of Trauma

1. General assessment; note bruises, vital signs; take detailed history, including tetanus immunization.
2. Inspect perineum carefully, in feet-together/knees-apart position.
3. If any perineal laceration or tear (this suggests internal damage): call Gynecology consultant immediately for a careful examination — EUA may be required.
4. If EUA to be done, pre-op orders include:
   a) Hb, Hct, cross-match for 2 units whole blood.
   b) Start iv infusion of '2/3–1/3 soln'.
   c) Radiology: 3 views of abdomen, to check for free air.
   d) Insert Foley catheter, for routine pre-op urinalysis and check for RBC.

Alleged Sexual Assault

1. The dr must obtain and witness a written consent before proceeding with the examination (see also no. 10 below).
2. Record the date, time, and place of examination.
3. Record time elapsed between alleged assault and examination.
4. Let patient relate the episode in her own way.

259

5. Evaluate the body for signs of violence and/or evidence of environment where alleged assault occurred:
   a) Record any bruises, laceration, abrasions, etc.
   b) Illustrate with diagrams whenever possible.
6. Laboratory evaluation: ensure that all specimens are labeled accurately and clearly.
   a) Take 4 vaginal swabs:
      − 3 for sperm-identification by police
      − 1 smeared and sprayed on glass slide (send to HSC Pathology Lab).
   b) With 10 ml distilled water, flush vagina through Foley catheter; give washings to police.
   c) Pubic hairs, fibers, fingernail clippings: give to police.
   d) Take swabs from anus and cervical os, for gonococcus identification.
   e) Take blood for VDRL (p 155).
7. Start VD prophylaxis at initial visit.
8. If suturing is necessary: this must be done under anesthesia in the OR.
9. Follow-up:
   a) Children over 11 yr: refer to Adolescent Clinic.
   b) Children under 11 yr: refer to Medical Clinic, attention Dr D. A. Stewart.
10. For more information, refer to Alleged Sexual Assault procedures manual (available in Emergency).

Management of Vaginal Bleeding not due to Trauma

Foreign body
(In fact, an intra-uterine or intravaginal FB gives rise to serosanguineous foul discharge rather than frank bleeding.) Refer child to Gynecology OPD Clinic.

Tumor
Vaginal bleeding may be due to polyps or a gonadotropin- or estrogen-secreting tumor.
Obtain Gynecology consultation.

Precocious Puberty − isosexual precocious development with menarche

1. Obtain Gynecology consultation.
2. Order:
   a) radiographs: skull; wrists (for bone age)
   b) 24-hr urinary 17-ketosteroids ⎫ see Biochemistry,
   c) serum LH, FSH, and estradiol ⎬ pp 366, 367,
   d) serum T_4 ⎭ 373, 382, 394

VAGINAL BLEEDING

B. Adolescence (Postmenarchal)

Differential Diagnosis

1. Complications of pregnancy
2. Abnormal uterine bleeding
3. Lapse in oral contraception

Complications of Pregnancy

1. Intra-uterine
   a) Labor
   b) Placenta previa
   c) Placenta abruptio
2. Extra-uterine — Ectopic pregnancy

Abnormal Uterine Bleeding

1. Functional (FUB), secondary to anovulatory cycles.
2. Local or systemic pathology (e.g., blood dyscrasia, tumor).
   Management
   a) Classify according to clinical status — mild or severe bleeding.
   b) If Hb <11 g/dl, **or** active exsanguination, management as for any acute hemorrhage:
      - Admit patient, start iv infusion, cross-match, Hb, Hct.
      - Give Premarin in direct iv line, slowly, 40-60 mg, up to q6h x 3 doses.
      - Start therapy with Ortho tablets (5 mg) po, 5 per day initially.
      - Request Gynecology consultation immediately.
3. Lapse in oral contraception — 'forgetting' 1-3 tabs will cause spurious breakthrough bleeding.
   Discontinue tabs for **total** of 5 days; then start new cycle.
   Note. This regimen will not ensure contraception until next regular cycle is established.

ABDOMINAL PAIN

Differential Diagnosis

1. Acute or subacute pelvic inflammatory disease (PID); see Infectious Disease, p 151.
2. Twisted, infarcted, or ruptured ovarian cyst
3. Dysmenorrhea and Mittelschmerz (mid-cycle ovulatory pain)
4. Ectopic pregnancy

} Request Gynecology consult

Pelvic Inflammatory Disease

This is a generalized type of infection, usually extra-uterine and presenting as bilateral lower abdominal tenderness.

Commonly:

1. Previous gonorrheal infection of the lower genital tract
2. High temperature (102-103°F; 39-40°C), WBC = 20- to 30,000/mm^3, and elevated ESR, but non-toxic general appearance.

In acute cases, admission is required for intensive high-dose parenteral antibiotic therapy. The antibiotic of choice initially is penicillin in high dose, combined with gentamicin, iv.

Management

1. Peritonitis regimen:
   a) bed rest in Fowler's position;
   b) oral intake restricted according to degree of ileus.
2. Antibiotics: see above.
3. Acute phase: the clinical response to therapy is quite dramatic, fever and discomfort subsiding within 24-48 hr.

   If the response is slow, reconsider diagnosis.
4. Chronic or mild acute case: Outpatient treatment with antibiotics (ampicillin) po is acceptable.

VULVOVAGINITIS AND VAGINAL DISCHARGE (NON-BLOODY)

A. Infancy and Childhood (Premenarchal)

Causes

1. Neonatal leukorrhea: transient, physiological, and due to maternal estrogens.
2. Nonspecific vaginitis: mixed bacterial flora originating in colon, usually secondary to poor hygiene, etc.
3. Specific vaginitis: gonoccoccal or other.
4. Parasitic vulvovaginal infections: intestinal parasites, most commonly pinworms.
5. Cyclic 'leukorrhea' in premenarchal girls: entirely physiologic.
6. Secondary infection and discharge: foreign body, 'bubble-baths', tumor.
7. Labial agglutination: acquired adherence of labia minora.
   - Never separate by force!
   - Treat conservatively with topical estrogen cream, bid for 2-3 wk.

Management

1. Obtain specimen for culture and sensitivities:
   a) Collect with platinum-wire loop and inject this into transport medium;
      or
   b) Instill transport medium through eye-dropper, and aspirate from vagina.
2. **Do not use** dry cotton swab — irritating.
3. Specimen for pinworms (pp 80, 159).
4. Nonspecific measures
   a) improved hygiene
   b) topical therapy (e.g., vulvovaginal cream/ointment).
5. Stubborn infection.
   In premenarchal girls, topical application of estrogen cream for 10-14 days stimulates the vulvovaginal epithelium to cornify and thicken temporarily, increasing resistance to bacterial invasion.

B. Adolescent Girls (Postmenarchal)

Subject to same vaginal infections as adult females, and management is similar.

1. Physiological leukorrhea: egg-white asymptomatic discharge.
2. Nonspecific vaginitis: discharge with no distinct characteristics.
3. Moniliasis: cheesy, white, pruritic.
   Predisposing factors are tetracycline (e.g., for acne), cortisone, diabetes, pregnancy, oral contraceptives.
   Identification of hyphae and spores in fresh wet preparation;* confirmation by culture.
4. Trichomonas: green, frothy discharge. Motile, flagellated organisms seen in fresh, wet preparation.*
5. Acute gonorrhea affecting lower genital tract: creamy, yellowish discharge.
6. *Haemophilus* vaginitis: greyish, irritating, malodorous discharge.
7. Pediculosis pubis (p 268).
8. Others: sexually transmitted disease (e.g., *Herpes genitalis*).

---

*Fresh wet or hanging-drop preparation — useful for identifying especially trichomonads and occasionally vaginal moniliasis. Place cotton-tipped vaginal swabs in approx. 2 ml N saline in a clean test tube previously warmed by dipping in hot water. Pipet out a drop of the saline soln, place it immediately on a glass slide, and examine it by both low and high power. The highly mobile trichomonad is unmistakable, and hyphae and spores from vaginal moniliasis are sometimes identifiable.

Management

1. a) Vaginal swab for culture and sensitivities (send cotton-tipped applicator in transport medium).
   b) Treatment: see principles of topical therapy, below.
2. If gonorrhea suspected: must take endocervical, urethral, anal, and pharyngeal swabs, and blood for VDRL.

Principles of Topical Therapy

Vulvar Conditions: *A & B.* Children & Adolescents

1. *Acute vulvitis*
   a) Wet dressings (e.g., Domeboro wets, 1:20 to 1:50 soln), Tucks, and sitz baths (warm tub water), tid.

     b)   Bland olive oil for cleansing vulva.

2. *Subacute vulvitis*
- a) Vioform + hydrocortisone ointment; **or**
- b) calamine lotion; **or**
- c) mixture of zinc oxide 15%, talc 15%, glycerine 10%, H_2O.

Apply qs after sitz baths and prn.

Intravaginal Conditions

1. *Nonspecific:* **A & B. Children & Adolescents**
- a) Furacin or Furacin-E vaginal suppositories, bid x 10 days
- b) Vagitrol, AVC, Sultrin (with or without added estrogen), inserted through pediatric applicator, bid x 3 wk
- c) 1:20,000 aqueous Zephiran irrigations (no. 12 Fr catheter), bid.

2. *Moniliasis*

    A.   **Children**
- a) Nystatin suspension (100,000 U/ml): 1 ml po, qid x 10 days. **and**
- b) Nystatin suspension, 1 ml instilled intravaginally (through eye-dropper), qid x 10 days; **Or** Gentian violet, 0.5% aqueous soln, 1 ml instilled intravaginally qhs x 10 nights.

    B.   **Adolescents**
- a) Mycostatin oral tablets (500,000 U/tab): tab 2 po x 10 days. **and**
- b) Mycostatin vaginal tabs (100,000 U/tab): insert 1 tab intravaginally qam and qhs x 14-21 days; **or** Nystatin intravaginal cream, applied qam and qhs x 14-21 days.

3. *Trichomonas*

    A.   **Children:** extremely rare

    B.   **Adolescents:** treat with metronidazole (Flagyl; p 450)

4. *Intestinal Parasites*
See Parasitic disease, p 158

5. *Gonorrhea*
Treat with systemic antibiotic therapy (p 151).

6. *Haemophilus vaginalis*
- a) Apply AVC, Sultrin cream intravaginally.
- b) If persistent, give ampicillin po (p 407).

7. *Pediculosis Pubis*
Treat with Kwellada (see Dermatology, p 268).

DERMATOLOGY

Eczema

General Management
1. Avoid skin irritants (strong soaps, detergents, woollen clothing and toys, cosmetics, dust, and starched bed linen).
2. To prevent scratching: give phenobarbital, or antihistamines po — diphenhydramine HC1 (Benadryl), promethazine HC1 (Phenergan), or hydroxyzine HC1 (Atarax).

Diet
Restrict wheat, eggs, orange juice, cow's milk — efficacious for some children under age 2 but not for older ones.

Local Therapy
1. Crusted lesions. Remove with compresses soaked in warm saline, or Burow's solution (Domeboro; 1 in 40), or by colloidal oatmeal (Aveeno) baths.
2. Acute lesions. Apply steroid lotion or cream qid; e.g., 0.5 − 1% hydrocortisone, or 0.1% β-methasone-17-valerate (Betnovate), or 0.01% fluocinolone acetonide (Synalar).
3. Subacute lesions. Apply steroid cream or ointment qid (0.5 − 1.0% hydrocortisone, or 0.025 − 1% Betnovate, or 0.01% Synalar).
4. Chronic lesions. Apply steroid cream or ointment as above. Addition of 1 − 5% LCD (liquor carbonis detergens) sometimes useful.
5. If lesions appear infected, apply bacitracin or gentamicin cream (0.1%) qid. If infection severe, give systemic penicillin or erythromycin.

Seborrheic Dermatitis

Scalp
1. Daily tar shampoo followed by removal of scales with fine tooth-comb.
2. Then apply steroid lotion or cream (e.g., 1% hydrocortisone, or 0.1% Betnovate, or 0.01% Synalar).

Trunk

1. Daily colloidal oatmeal baths, followed by application of steroid creams or lotions qid and prn (see p 424).
2. In resistant cases, add 1 − 2% precipitated sulfur and/or 1 − 2% salicylic acid to local medications.

Acne

1. No chocolate, cola drinks, or nuts.
2. Keep hair off face.
3. Shampoo scalp daily, and wash skin bid: use household soap or 10% centrimide (Cetavlon).
4. Apply keratolytics locally at night (e.g., Fostex, Persol, Sulfoxyl or Benoxyl lotion). Start with low concn, and increase slowly.
    When acute lesions are under control, remove comedones periodically.
5. If severe, give course of antimicrobial therapy.
    a) Prepubertal child: erythromycin.
    b) Older child − tetracycline.

Pyodermas

1. Wash skin with 2−10% centrimide (Cetavlon).
2. a) Remove crusted lesions with compresses soaked in Burow's solution (1 in 40) or pot. permang. (1 in 20,000), for 10 min qid.
    b) Then apply gentamicin cream or bacitracin ointment locally, qid or prn.
3. If severe: give systemic antibiotics appropriate to results of culture and sensitivity.

Ringworm

Tinea capitis

1. Local therapy: Daily shampoo, then apply tolnaflate (Tinactin) lotion tid.
2. Systemic therapy: Griseofulvin ultrafine for at least 3 mo.
3. Inflammatory lesions: also, apply compresses soaked in Burow's solution (1 in 40) or pot. permang. (1 in 20,000), tid; then apply Tinactin.

Tinea corporis

1. Local therapy: Apply Tinactin lotion tid or half-strength Whitfield's ointment bid.
2. Systemic therapy (if no response to local therapy): Griseofulvin ultrafine for at least 6 wk.

Scabies

Infants

1. Warm soapy bath, followed by local application of 10% sulfur ointment, for 3 consecutive nights.
2. All bedding and clothing to be thoroughly washed before and at end of treatment.

Older Children

1. Hot bath, followed by local application of 20% solution of benzyl benzoate, or 1% γ-benzene-hexachloride (Kwellada), to be left on skin for 24 hr.
2. Then, all bedding and clothing to be thoroughly washed or dry-cleaned.
3. Pruritus may persist for several days — steroid creams locally or antihistamines systemically may help.

Pediculosis

1. Shampoo with 1% solution of Kwellada and remove nits with fine tooth-comb. Repeat weekly if necessary.
   or
2. Apply 20% solution of benzyl benzoate to scalp and leave on overnight.
   or
3. Apply tetralin compound (Cuprex) to scalp and leave on for 4 – 6 hr.

Diaper Dermatitis

Ammoniacal

1. Avoid irritants on diapers (fabric softeners, such as Fleecy, Breezy, or Downy), and rinse out detergents and soaps very thoroughly.
2. Change diaper frequently. Avoid plastic and rubber pants.
3. Apply protective medication (zinc oxide ointment) locally.

Other Causes

Eruptions in diaper area may indicate seborrheic dermatitis or candidiasis. If so, treat primary condition.

Warts

Verrucae Vulgaris

1. Apply mixture of 75% salicylic acid in Vaseline. Leave on for 1 wk, then debride.
2. Repeat until all warty tissue removed.

Verrucae Plantaris

1. Single warts: treat as verrucae vulgaris.
2. Multiple warts (mosaic): soak feet in 4% formaldehyde for 10 – 15 min daily.

Verrucae Plana

Apply peeling agent (Benoxyl lotion, strong; Persol cream, strong), daily or bid.

Condyloma Acuminata

1. Apply 20% solution of podophyllin in tinct. of benzoin compound. Leave on for 4 – 6 hr, then wash off with water.
2. Repeat weekly.

ANESTHESIA

PRE-OPERATIVE PREPARATION OF PATIENTS

1. *All patients must be fasting for 4 hr before surgery.*
2. Patients under 24 mo should be given **clear** fluids 4 hr before surgery.
3. Patients over 24 mo may receive clear fluids 4 hr before surgery but no solid food for 8 hr pre-operatively.
4. Exceptions to the above can be made only after consultation between the anesthetist and physician/surgeon involved.
5. Report of pre-op Hb and urinalysis must be on chart accompanying patient to the OR.
   Effective procedures: Hb should be >10 g/dl.
6. Pre-op medication (p 272) will be ordered by the anesthetist.
7. Sedation for special procedures: see p 273.

Patients on Corticosteroids

Steroid preparation for surgery depends on:
1. Duration and dose.
2. Duration and magnitude of operative procedure.

Management
1. Can vary from no additional administration; to
2. Full preparation:
   Cortisone im night before and morning of surgery, with Solu-Cortef in iv drip during and after surgery (p 432).

Patients on Digoxin

Prescribe usual am dose, but im instead of po (p 436).

Patients on Insulin

See p 245 in Diabetes Mellitus.

Patients on Anticonvulsants

Prescribe usual dosage up to 6 hr pre-op.

271

PRE-OPERATIVE MEDICATION*

Drug	Route	Dose according to Weight	
Atropine	im	1-3 kg	0.1 mg
		3-5 kg	0.15 mg
		5-10 kg	0.2 mg
		10-15 kg	0.3 mg
		15-20 kg	0.4 mg
		> 20 kg	0.6 mg
	iv	Use 2/3 of above amounts	Give 30 – 60 min pre-op
Demerol	im	1.5 mg/kg	Order to nearest 5 mg
Morphine	im	0.2 mg/kg for patients >5 kg (not prescribed for <5 kg)	Order to nearest 1 mg. Give 1 hr pre-op
Pentobarbital	im	2 mg/kg	Order to nearest 10 mg. Give 1 hr pre-op
	pr	3 mg/kg	Order to next lowest 15-mg multiple
Diazepam	po	0.2 – 0.4 mg/kg	1 1/2 hr pre-op

*EXCEPTIONS
1. Infants <1 yr or <10 kg: no sedation.
2. Fever >38°C: no sedation.
3. Eye service: squint correction – no sedation.
4. Neurosurgery: no sedation.

272

Sedation for Special Procedures

CM3 Sedative Mixture

chlorpromazine (Largactil) 6.25 mg
promethazine (Phenergan) 6.25 mg } in 1 ml CM3
meperidine (Demerol)   25 mg

Dose: 0.1 ml/kg by deep im, 1 hr before procedure; maximum, 1.5 ml.

POSTOPERATIVE ANALGESIA

1. Consider effects of pre-op narcotics and anesthetic agents before ordering analgesics.
2. Analgesics are contraindicated in:
   a) hypoxia
   b) raised intracranial pressure
   c) fractures with possible vascular involvement (e.g., fractures around elbow).
3. Routine procedures (e.g., reduction of Colles' fracture) with application of cast:
   a) Give one dose of analgesic only.
   b) The patient must be seen, and the cast checked, before a 2nd dose is ordered.

POSTOPERATIVE ANALGESICS

Drug	Route	Dose according to Weight
Demerol (pethidine; meperidine)	im	1.0-1.5 mg/kg. Order to nearest 5 mg
	iv	0.2 mg/kg. Order to nearest 1 mg
Codeine	im	1.0-1.5 mg/kg. Order to nearest 3 mg
Morphine	im	0.2 mg/kg. Order to nearest 1 mg
Levo-Dromoran*	im	0.04 mg/kg. Order to nearest 0.5 mg.

*Note. Effects last 6-10 hr.
Check patient before re-ordering.

GENERAL SURGERY

Neonatal Abdominal Emergencies

General Considerations
1. *Persistent vomiting represents intestinal obstruction until disproved.*
2. *Most important:*
   a) rectal examination (little finger or thermometer)
   b) prevent hypothermia
   c) Na^+, K^+, Cl^-; blood urea, pH, PCO_2, bicarbonate
   d) group and cross-match 250 ml whole blood
   e) abdominal films, supine and erect
   f) Ba enema usually unnecessary — consult radiologist experienced in like problems
   g) If obstructed: NG suction.
3. *In all cases of suspected/proven obstruction: consult pediatric surgeon early.*

Bleeding from Alimentary Canal

Differential Diagnosis
1. The commonest causes are listed in the table below.
2. If presentation is unusual, consider foreign body (p 281) and systemic hemorrhagic disease.

CAUSES OF BLEEDING FROM THE ALIMENTARY CANAL

Age of patient	Hemorrhage		Possible Cause
	Size	Color	
A.	**Presenting Symptom: Hematemesis**		
Neonate	small	dark	Ingested maternal blood
Infant	small	dark	Pyloric stenosis
Infant	small	dark	Reflux esophagitis
Older child	large	bright	Peptic ulcer (very rare)
Older child	large	bright	Esophageal varices
Older child	large	bright	Acute erosions
Older child	large	bright	'Stress' ulcers
B.	**Presenting symptom: Rectal Bleeding or Melena**		
Neonate	small or large	bright	Enterocolitis
Neonate	small or large	bright	Volvulus
Infant	small	bright	Intussusception, fissure
Infant	large	bright	Tubule duplications
Infant	large	bright or dark	Meckel's diverticulum*

cont'd overleaf

Age of patient	Hemorrhage		Possible Cause
	Size	Color	

B. *(cont'd)*

Presenting symptom: Rectal Bleeding or Melena

Age of patient	Size	Color	Possible Cause
Toddler	small	bright	Anal fissures & prolapse
Toddler	large	bright	Ulcerated Meckel's divertic.*
Older child	small	bright	Polypi
Older child	small	bright	Ulcerated Meckel's divertic.*
Older child	large	bright or dark	Esophageal varices
Older child	large	bright or dark	'Stress' ulcers
Older child	large	bright or dark	Colitis
Older child	large	bright or dark	Crohn's disease

*Technetium scan may be diagnostic.

276

Esophageal Atresia and Tracheo-esophageal Fistula

1. *All neonates:* pass a no. 14 rubber catheter into stomach in delivery room.
   a) If obstruction at about 9 cm from gingival margin, diagnosis is esophageal atresia.
   b) Air in abdomen confirms tracheo-esophageal fistula.
2. *Do not instill Ba or Lipiodol — dangerous.*
3. If unable to pass NG tube, do AP and lateral chest films and consult radiologist.
4. Keep infant upright, with suction to blind upper pouch, until surgery.

H-type Tracheo-esophageal Fistula without Atresia

1. Suspect in "mucousy" neonate with respiratory problems. May have abdominal distention.
2. Also consider in older infant with recurrent chest infections.
3. Diagnosed by radiography and broncho-esophago-scopy.

Diaphragmatic Hernia

1. Respiratory distress is prime consideration. Chest film *stat.* Ventilation usually restricted to one partly collapsed lung.
2. Catheterize umbilical artery at once.
3. Correct metabolic and respiratory acidosis, with bicarbonate (p 163) and assisted ventilation via NT tube (p 167).
4. Proceed to surgery. Watch for contralateral pneumothorax, which can result from too-vigorous 'bagging'.

Omphalocele and Gastroschisis

1. Cover with sterile saline-soaked towel — *never use dry dressings.*
2. Defect usually closed with Silastic sheeting by staged procedure.
3. Special iv feeding required if postoperative ileus prolonged.

Biliary Atresia

Porto-enterostomy at age 4 wk.

INTESTINAL OBSTRUCTION

1. Contrast examination of upper GI tract *nearly always contraindicated.*
2. Seek Radiology consult before ordering any special radiologic investigation.

High Obstruction

General Considerations

1. Usually confined to duodenum — malrotation, atresia, or stenosis (30% have Down's syndrome); annular pancreas, duodenal diaphragm, 'windsock'.
2. *Abdomen not distended.*
3. *Vomiting early.* Regard persistent vomiting (not always bilious) in neonates as due to duodenal obstruction until disproved.
4. Plain abdominal films usually diagnostic — show double bubble.

Hypertrophic Pyloric Stenosis

1. Commonly occurs between 3 and 8 wk.
2. Projectile vomiting (never bile-stained), failure to thrive, constipation; peristalsis visible across epigastrium.
3. Operation should be done *only if the surgeon personally has palpated the 'tumor'.*
4. Radiology rarely required.
5. Hypokalemic alkalosis common. Metabolic correction with iv fluids usually possible in 12 – 24 hr, before pyloromyotomy.
6. Feeding is started 4 – 6 hr postop.

Low Obstruction

(upper jejunum to anus)

1. Abdominal distention and bilious vomiting (latter may be delayed).
2. Meconium plug may indicate fibrocystic disease or Hirschsprung's disease.

Volvulus

1. Always associated with malrotation (± duodenal obstruction).

2. Suspect if blood pr, abdominal distention, and profound shock.
3. Malrotation diagnosed by Ba enema.
4. *Delay in diagnosis* → gangrene of entire small bowel → death.

Intussusception

1. Characteristically, healthy child in apparent pain, with episodes of spasmodic crying. Mass and rectal bleeding not always apparent.
2. If intussusception considered:
   a) consult surgeon
   b) group & cross-match blood and advise OR of possible need
   c) have Ba enema done (*surgical resident must be in attendance*). Ba enema reduction must show free reflux into terminal ileum.
3. Then observe child for up to 24 hr. If intussusception not reduced hydrostatically (Ba enema), surgical reduction or resection is necessary.
4. *If acute 'surgical abdomen' or long-standing advanced obstruction:* proceed to surgery without prior Ba enema.

Polypi (other than familial polyposis)

1. No malignant potential.
2. Main problem = bleeding; occasionally, intussusception.
3. Demonstration of polyps requires special radiologic techniques. Consult radiologist.
4. a) If readily reached with sigmoidoscope: remove.
   b) If higher: follow-up with serial air-contrast enemas every 1-2 yr.
5. Laparotomy or colonoscopy indicated only if (very rare) uncontrollable bleeding.

Hirschsprung's disease

1. The typical narrowed segment is rarely demonstrated by Ba enema in the neonate.
2. Look for retained Ba on 24-hr film.
3. Rectal biopsy mandatory.
4. Surgery: transverse colostomy in newborn; definitive surgery after 6 mo.

Rectal Prolapse

Commoner in children who have fibrocystic disease or meningomyelocele.

Imperforate Anus

1. *Low-type*
   a) Usually with recto-cutaneous fistula.
   b) Requires perineal operation.
2. *High-type*
   a) Commoner in males.
   b) Fistula to urinary tract.
   c) Surgery: colostomy as newborn; 'pull-through' operation after 6 mo.
   d) Always do IVP to rule out associated renal abnormality.

Pneumoperitoneum

1. Abdominal distention.
2. Intraperitoneal free air is visible on ordinary AP and lateral supine films, but a R lateral decubitus (AP cross table, R side up) — or, if the infant is fit enough, an upright AP film — may be necessary to show air/fluid levels.
3. May be secondary to meconium ileus, bowel atresia, Hirschsprung's disease, necrotizing enterocolitis, perforation of stomach.

Necrotizing Enterocolitis (p 171)

1. Abdominal distention, vomiting, blood pr.
2. Radiograph: *air in bowel wall ± in biliary tree.* Repeat q4-6h to exclude pneumoperitoneum.
3. Treatment: NG suction, fluids iv, antibiotics (p 168).
4. **Assess hourly:** if no improvement or if deterioration or perforation, proceed to surgery.

Abdominal Masses

1. Up to 3 yr of age: regard as Wilms' tumor or neuroblastoma until disproved. Other possibilities include benign renal cyst, obstructive uropathy.
2. Minimal handling of mass. Request consult with pediatric surgeon at once: the younger the infant when investigated, the better the prognosis.
3. Investigations include plain films, IVP, skeletal survey, arteriography, bone marrow, and VMA assay.
4. Early surgery indicated.

Inguinal and Scrotal Problems

Inguinal Hernia
1. Should be surgically corrected when diagnosed. (High incidence of strangulation and incarceration <1 yr.)
2. Do not prescribe truss.
3. Remember to check hernial orifices.
4. Bilateral hernia commoner in young child.
5. Surgery as outpatient up to 5 yr of age.

Hydrocele
1. <1 yr: repair if very tense or communicates with peritoneal cavity.
2. >1 yr: repair when convenient.

Undescended Testes (see also GU surgery, pp 248, 300)
1. Important to distinguish from retractile testes that can be brought into scrotum.
2. Should be 'brought down' by 4 – 6 yr, to lessen possibility of infertility and malignant change.

Torsion of Testicle or Appendix Epiploica
1. Sudden onset of testicular pain; swollen, tender, discolored scrotum, and testis may be elevated.
2. Epididymo-orchitis rare under 10 yr.
3. Emergency surgical exploration nearly always necessary.
4. If operation required, do contralateral orchidopexy.

MISCELLANEOUS CONDITIONS

Foreign Bodies (FB)

1. If ingestion or aspiration of FB is suspected, obtain AP and lateral chest and abdominal films.
2. Esophagogram may be needed.
3. FB in esophagus or tracheobronchial tree: endoscopy required.
4. Most FB that pass the pylorus cause no further difficulty.
5. Long sharp objects or large jagged objects: laparotomy.
6. FB in soft tissue: best removed under general anesthesia, using an image intensifier.

Cervical Swellings

Torticollis (Sternomastoid Tumor)
Physiotherapy should begin by age 6 wk.

Thyroglossal Cyst
1. Midline cyst or sinus. Moves upward on swallowing or protrusion of tongue.
2. Surgical excision indicated.

Branchial-cleft Cyst
1. Lump or sinus at anterior border of sternocleido-mastoid muscle. May open into pharynx or external auditory meatus.
2. Surgical excision indicated.

Umbilical Hernia
1. Usually disappears by 2 − 3 yr. Surgery may be considered after 2 yr if significant hernia persists.
2. Strangulation of hernia extremely rare in childhood.

Umbilical discharge
1. From granuloma due to local infection in neonates **or** poor local hygiene in older children.
2. Persistence of omphalomesenteric duct or urachus, with discharge of feces or urine, requires surgical correction. (Uncommon)

INFECTIONS

Local

Suppurative Lymphadenitis
1. Most commonly in cervical and inguinal regions.
2. If fluctuation present: incision and drainage.
3. If induration alone, and/or lymphangitis: heat locally and cloxacillin systematically (p 408) will resolve it or bring it to a "head".

Perianal Abscess
1. Common in infancy.
2. Start drainage at once — avoid fistula formation.

Anal Fistula
Once established, surgical excision is necessary.

Ischiorectal Abscess
1. Rectal exam aids diagnosis.
2. Drainage required.

Pilonidal Disease
1. Painful swelling between buttocks over sacrum.
2. May drain spontaneously.
3. Abscess or sinus requires surgical attention.

General

Appendicitis
1. Localized R lower quadrant tenderness or peritonitis represents appendicitis until disproved.
2. If in doubt, admit and re-assess frequently.
3. Perforation before diagnosis is common in children <5 yr.
4. Antibiotic therapy often indicated.

Peritonitis
1. Most commonly due to perforated gut, especially acute appendicitis.
2. Primary peritonitis occasionally in girls and in children who have nephrotic syndrome.

NEUROSURGERY

UNDIAGNOSED COMA
(See Table opposite)

1. Child in coma but with no evidence of meningismus or lateralized neurologic signs:
   a) The coma most probably originates from metabolic, toxic, or endocrine factors. Initial investigations are basically biochemical.
   b) Occasionally, sequel to (unwitnessed) seizure.
2. Coma and meningismus but not focal neurologic features: etiology usually hemorrhage or bacterial meningitis.
   — LP distinguishes the two, and in particular identifies the micro-organism in meningitis.
3. Coma and lateralized neurologic findings, especially if intracranial hypertension is present: probably a surgical lesion, which demands carefully scheduled investigation.

RAPID DIAGNOSTIC ASSESSMENT OF COMA

Clues			Answer	Investigations/Treatment required
Consciousness?	Meningismus?	Lateralizing neurologic signs?		
Coma	No	No	Metabolic, toxic, or endocrine; or postconvulsive	Biochemical, hematologic
Coma	Yes	No	Meningitis or subarachnoid hemorrhage	Lumbar puncture. (First, assess optic fundi, etc., re increased ICP)
Coma	No	Yes	Lateralized intracranial lesion, usually surgical	Specific neuroradiologic evaluation and/or surgery

HEAD INJURIES

Management

1. ***Examine carefully*** upon admission, and every 15 min − 2 hr (depending on patient's state), to ascertain:
    a) State of consciousness (response to stimuli)
    b) Size and reactivity of pupils
    c) Rate and character of respirations
    d) Pulse
    e) BP

2. ***General state***
    a) *Unconscious:* always maintain a clear airway.
    b) *Unconscious or vomiting:* place in semiprone position.
    c) *Excessive nasopharyngeal secretions:* insert and maintain nasal airway; keep suction available at all times.

3. ***Hypovolemic shock:*** seldom due to head injury alone; never due to closed injury.
    a) Search for bleeding elsewhere.
    b) Treat shock: give colloid fluids and blood iv.

4. ***Coma developing after lucid interval,*** accompanied by unilateral dilated pupil, facial paralysis, and hemiparesis: indicates formation of intracranial hematoma.
    This is an emergency: obtain CT immediately and/or exploratory burr holes.

5. ***If clinical state deteriorating and emergency treatment required:*** do not waste time getting plain skull radiographs taken.

6. **Do not perform LP.**

Treatment

General
1. Fluids: switch from iv to oral intake (or NG tube) as soon as possible.

Pharmacologic

1. Cerebral edema: can be temporarily controlled with mannitol: give 20% solution (Osmitrol), 1.5-2.0 g/kg iv, over 20-30 min.
   Mannitol: indwelling urethral catheter is mandatory (to deal with profound diuresis).

2. Prolonged cerebral edema: steroid therapy is useful. Give dexamethasone (Decadron), 1 to 4 mg, q6h.

3. Patient on high doses of Decadron, particularly if ICP raised: institute prophylaxis with Maalox and gastric diet, to prevent bleeding GU or DU.

4. **Do not give** ASA to deal with fever in any neurosurgical patient (because of its interference with normal clotting).
   Acetaminophen (p 417) can be used, in addition to other cooling methods.

5. If patient is restless, give chlorpromazine (p 430) to prevent shivering and settle him.

6. MORPHINE IS CONTRAINDICATED IN **ALL** HEAD-INJURY PATIENTS

7. Post-traumatic seizure soon after head injury is common. Unless the seizure is prolonged, anticonvulsant therapy is not required.

8. Compound brain wound: place sterile pressure dressing, start prophylactic antibiotics, obtain plain films of skull, and take patient to OR as soon as possible.

9. Neurologic deficits: order physiotherapy to start as soon as possible.

CONGENITAL CNS DEFECTS

Hydrocephalus

1. **All** patients whose head is enlarged should have transillumination.

2. CT scanning is the first investigation.

3. Consider isotopic CSF scan next.

4. If ventricular puncture is required: do subdural taps first.

5. CSF shunts.
   a) Most shunting systems drain CSF from a lateral ventricle to the peritoneal cavity (VP shunt) or right cardiac atrium (VA shunt). These systems can be used for obstructive or communicating hydrocephalus.
   b) The less-common lumboperitoneal (LP) shunt is used only in patients with communicating hydrocephalus.

6. Ventricle-originating systems have three components:
   a) ventricular catheter; which is secured to
   b) small sc plastic reservoir ('pump') beneath scalp in posterior parietal region; which is joined to
   c) descending, or peritoneal (or atrial) end.
7. Shunt patency can be determined by depressing the sc pump.
   a) If depression is difficult, the distal end of the system may be at fault.
   b) If the pump depresses easily but fails to refill, the proximal or ventricular catheter may be malfunctioning.
8. Radio-opaque shunts: if obstruction is suspected, obtain radiographs.
9. All shunts: if blockage is suspected, a shunt scan may be needed to delineate site of block.

Myelomeningocele

1. Open myelomeningocele
   a) Infant should be nursed on Bradford frame.
   b) Dress myelomeningocele with perforated Saran wrap, and gauze soaked in solution of aqueous Zephiran 1:20,000. Change dressings every 4 hr.
   c) Dressings must be kept wet at all times.
2. Weeping myelomeningocele
   a) On admission, take swab for culture and sensitivities.
   b) If patient is to be treated, defect should be closed within 24 hr of birth.
3. Notify spina bifida co-ordinator as well as personnel from GU surgery, Orthopedic Surgery, Physiotherapy, and Occupational Therapy.
4. Follow-up after discharge is arranged through Spina Bifida Clinic, O.C.C.C.

Craniosynostosis

1. Obtain bone scan of skull.
2. If patient has had a craniectomy:
   a) Watch carefully for loss of blood (falling Hb) into wound postop.
   b) Obtain Hb estimation in the immediate postop period and at 24 hr postop.
   c) Keep the iv running for at least 24 hr postop, in case transfusion needed.

INTRACRANIAL MASS LESIONS

1. All patients whose history suggests this:
    a) Obtain skull film and CT.
    b) Depending on location of mass: obtain definitive studies (e.g., regional tomograms, cerebral arteriography, ventriculography, air encephalography).
2. Sellar/parasellar lesions: neuroendocrine assessment essential.
3. Visual and oculomotor disorders: neuro-ophthalmologic assessment essential.

Brain Tumor

1. Pre-operatively, particularly if sellar lesion and/or raised ICP: steroids.
2. After intracranial supratentorial surgery, particularly if brain was retracted: institute prophylaxis with Dilantin.

Brain Abscess

1. Consider brain abscess if intracranial mass in patient with cyanotic heart or chronic ear disease, frontal sinusitis, septicemia, lung sepsis, or penetrating brain wound.
2. If suspected brain abscess presents **very early** as focus of nonsuppurative encephalitis:
    a) Treatment can be attempted with appropriate antibiotics.
    b) Efficacy of treatment can be judged by serial CT scans.
3. Brain abscess in non-vital area (e.g., cerebellum): treat by surgical excision.
4. Brain abscess in vital area: treat by aspiration and instillation of antibiotics.
5. Chronic brain abscesses
    a) In cerebellum, either frontal lobe, or non-dominant temporal lobe: treat by excision.
    b) Otherwise, treat by repeated aspiration through burr-hole, followed by instillation of antibiotics and Steripaque.
6. Anticonvulsant therapy is usually required.

SPINAL-CORD LESIONS

Congenital

1. Cutaneous stigmata of spina bifida occulta (hairy tuft, dimple, lipoma and angioma) and progressive neurologic defect in legs and/or bladder:
   a) Obtain contrast myelogram in both prone and supine positions, for lesions such as diastematomyelia, tethered cord, neurenteric cyst, intraspinal meningocele, intraspinal lipoma, dermoid, teratoma.
   b) If syrinx is suspected, obtain air myelogram.
2. Scoliosis and congenital spinal defects: investigate as above, *before* the spine is surgically straightened.

Acquired

1. a) Painful scoliosis usually indicates intraspinal mass.
   b) Progressive loss of neurologic function in limbs, particularly if spine and/or root pain also, always indicates intraspinal mass.
   c) Obtain plain spine film and myelogram.
2. Suspected traumatic lesions of spine: move child very carefully, with traction applied to head and feet. Such a lesion must be considered in every unconscious child who has a head injury.
3. If myelogram indicates AV malformation: obtain spinal-cord angiogram.

INTRACRANIAL HEMORRHAGE

Subarachnoid and Intracerebral Hemorrhage

Any child who, previously well, suddenly has severe headache and neck stiffness and progressive neurologic deterioration, probably has subarachnoid hemorrhage from a ruptured intracranial aneurysm or AV malformation, or hemorrhage into a cerebral neoplasm.

1. Don't waste time on routine investigation.
2. Institute emergency resuscitative measures if required (p 467), and consult Neurosurgery.
3. CT scanning and cerebral angiography are mandatory.

Chronic Subdural Hematoma and Effusions

Any infant who has sustained head trauma or has bacterial meningitis and in whom the head enlarges, sutures split, and fontanel is full, requires:

1. Skull radiographs
2. Brain scan
3. Diagnostic subdural taps
4. Daily therapeutic subdural taps: may remove sufficient fluid. If, after 5-7 days, fluid volumes do not diminish: indication for surgical exploration and drainage.

BIRTH TRAUMA

1. Traumatic subarachnoid hemorrhage: observe infant closely, for development of communicating hydrocephalus.

2. Obtain CT scan.

3. Signs of increased ICP, small pupils, and respiratory problems: investigate for posterior-fossa hematoma.

4. Infant born by breech delivery who has limb weakness and poor body-temperature control: probably, damaged cervical cord. Obtain a myelogram.

CARDIAC SURGERY

Pre-operative Preparation

1. Diet and activity as usual unless specific restrictions indicated.
2. Give ascorbic acid and multiple vitamin preparations.
3. Give cardiac drugs as before admission. In most cases, give patient's regular dose of digoxin im on day of surgery; stop propranolol 24 hr before surgery.
4. Record height and weight on chart.
5. 'Pump' cases: order Hb, WBC count and smear, PTT, PT, platelet count and urinalysis.
6. PA *and lateral* chest films and ECG unless already taken in previous 2 wk.
7. Blood type and cross-match 2 days before operation. See table (below) for approx. amounts.
8. Resident should:
   a) Include record of liver size, in history
   b) Recheck for respiratory infection the afternoon before operation
   c) Enquire about history of bleeding tendency
   d) Enquire about antibiotic hypersensitivity.
9. Older child: ask physiotherapist to instruct in arm and breathing exercises (p 97).
10. Shave chest, and upper arm and axilla if necessary.
11. Order chest scrubbed with antibacterial soln nightly x 3 nights pre-op. If extracorporeal circulation to be used: axilla and groin, also, to be shaved and scrubbed.
12. Give prophylactic antibiotics before going to OR, in the OR, and x 5 days postop.

BLOOD REQUIREMENTS FOR CARDIAC SURGERY

1. *Closed heart surgery*
   Order 20 ml/kg body wt (*not less than 500 ml*).
   Cyanotic child: order 2 units of plasma also (p 26).
2. *Open heart surgery*
   Newborn to 2 yr: 2 units heparinized and 3 units CPD blood
   >2 yr: 6 units CPD blood
   Cyanotic child: order 2 additional units
3. *Pump cases* — check with anesthetist regarding:
   a) fresh frozen plasma
   b) platelet concentrate

Postoperative Care

1. Keep patient flat unless otherwise ordered (Glenn procedure, sitting).
2. Give humidified O_2 (40% to 60%) continuously according to blood gases. Monitor frequently.
3. Monitor and record:
   a) temp, pulse, resp rate, and BP – q 15-30 min until stabilized, then q1h x 24 hr, then q2h.
   b) ECG and central venous pressure – also left atrial pressure, if line present.
4. Suction airway prn.
5. Turn q1h (side/back/side) day 1 postop, then turn q2h at night.
   a) Encourage deep breathing and coughing each time turned.
   b) Except in open-heart or hypothermia cases, have patient sit up to cough q2h.
   c) If unconscious: **nurse on side** – not back.
6. Maintain continuous closed (underwater) drainage with suction at 15 cm water pressure.
7. Make sure Blood Bank has adequate amount of blood products at all times.
   a) Give blood iv to replace loss in drainage until drainage is serosanguineous.
   b) If loss is large, replace serosanguineous losses with plasma.
8. If left atrial catheter present: remove it before chest drains. After removing LA catheter, *and before removing chest drains:* obtain plain chest film.
9. Sedation: alternately, each hr, meperidine (pethidine) 0.2 mg/kg, and diazepam 0.04 mg/kg up to 0.2 mg/kg, iv.
10. If digoxin received pre-op, reinstitute this day 1 postop.
11. Antibiotics as indicated (p 407) iv, x 5 days.
12. Record fluid intake and output on balance sheet until well established on oral intake.
13. Give continuous infusion 5% glucose in 0.2% NaCl, *slowly,* as ordered. Give maintenance KCl in iv.
14. After profound hypothermia: give $MgSO_4$ iv 1 mEq/kg/day x 2 days.

15. Fluids:
    a) If no abdominal distention, fluids po.
       - sips of clear fluids for first 24 hr
       - then fluids as tolerated
       - full diet, ascorbic acid, and multiple-vita-
         min tablets, when tolerated.
    b) If distention, nurse may insert NG tube and
       aspirate by gentle suction. Replace loss iv.
16. Plain chest film evening of and morning after opera-
    tion.
17. Hb, Hct, electrolytes (Na^+, K^+, Cl^-), Ca, BUN: fre-
    quently. Arterial blood gases (pH, pCO_2, pO_2, HCO_3)
    as indicated.
18. Weigh daily.

Postoperative Complications

Chest (atelectasis, pneumonia)
1. Moist atmosphere; turn frequently; encourage deep-
   breathing and coughing. Order clapping and postural
   drainage by physiotherapist (p 97).
2. Tracheal suction prn.
3. Chest film to monitor.
4. Antibiotics.
5. Assisted ventilation if necessary.

Bleeding Tendency and Hemorrhage
1. Check blood balance calculations after operation.
2. If PT and PTT prolonged, give fresh frozen plasma.
3. If bleeding continues, consult hematologist.
4. Check platelet count.

Cerebral Irritation/Edema
1. Phenobarbital (p 454) im, or diazepam (p 436) iv, by
   weight.
2. Consider mannitol (p 136).
3. Steroids: Decadron iv q6h.

Cardiac Complications
1. *Congestive failure* (hepatomegaly, gallop rhythm);
   p 200.

2. *Arrhythmias.*
   a) One person (usually cardiology fellow) should be responsible for this management — especially during the first few critical days, it is undesirable to have several individuals frequently adjusting drugs and the pacemaker.
   b) Pharmacologic treatment of arrhythmias should not be started without ECG diagnosis (p 200).

3. *Heart block*
   a) In OR: if complete block, pacemaker with intracardiac wire electrodes.
   b) Outside OR: if in danger of block, monitor continuously.
   c) Insert percutaneous wires if necessary (equipment available in ICU):
      – #18 needle (long), bipolar pacing catheter, connecting clips
      – steel wires with straight needles on one end, curved needles on other end.
   d) Maintain pulse rate >120/min in neonates and >70 min in older children.
      – If patient on pacemaker, do not attempt weaning for 2 – 3 days.
   e) Keep a syringe of isoproterenol (0.02 mg in 10 ml diluent) at hand, in case needed to stimulate cardiac action.

4. *Low-output cardiac failure*
   a) Ensure adequate blood volume.
   b) Exclude arrhythmia.
   c) If pacemaker available, pace heart at optimal rate.
   d) Give inotropic drugs, particularly digoxin (1 mg in 250 ml iv) or Isoproterenol (0.02 mg in 10 ml diluent iv) over 5 – 10 min.
      – Monitor effect on ECG.
   e) **Watch urine output, serum K^+, and BUN.**
      – **If renal shutdown occurs:** consult nephrologist immediately (consider dialysis), withhold digoxin, and take blood sample for digoxin level (p 365).

Discharge Routine

1. Repeat chest film and ECG 1 – 2 days before discharge.
2. Advise parents regarding:
   a) level of activity
   b) prophylaxis against infective endocarditis
   c) medications
   d) follow-up appointment.

GENITOURINARY SURGERY

Injuries to Urinary Tract

Extravasation of urine requires repair of the rupture or diversion of the urinary stream. Drainage of the area, also, may be needed.

Injury to Bulbous/Penile Urethra
Straddle type of injury

Urethra may be damaged distal to external sphincter. Blood usually appears at meatus shortly after injury, before voiding.

1. **Do not** ask patient to void.
2. **Do not** try to pass a catheter. (Only a urologist should attempt catheterization, and may request retrograde urethrogram first.)
3. Cystotomy probably required, to divert urine.
4. If child has already voided: characteristic swelling, limited by attachment of Colles fascia, may be apparent.

Injury to Pelvis, with Suspected Rupture of Bladder/Prostatic Urethra

Blunt upper abdominal trauma may rupture a full bladder and/or damage a kidney.

1. If patient is unconscious or has multiple injuries:
   a) Request IVP immediately.
   b) Next, cystogram may be needed.
2. If large hematoma palpable pr: **do not** ask patient to void.
3. If patient cannot void: pass small catheter; obtain specimen, leave catheter indwelling.
4. Gross/microscopic blood in voided/catheter specimen: bladder may be ruptured
   a) Request cystogram — to be done by Radiology staff.

Suspected Rupture of Kidney(s)

1. The degree of injury is not necessarily reflected by the degree of hematuria.
2. Ruptured kidney: urine usually contains blood, gross or microscopic.
3. Renal pedicle tear: urine may be clear.

296

Management

1. Chart BP and pulse, and measure girth of abdomen, on admission and q15 min until stable.
2. Type and cross-match blood; start iv fluids; treat shock (hypovolemic) in standard manner.
3. Assess associated injuries and institute appropriate initial treatment.
4. Request emergency IVP.
5. Assess normalcy of uninjured kidney, assess degree of damage to injured side, detect extravasation.
   Note. Abnormal kidneys are more prone to injury.
6. Consult staff surgeon as soon as possible:
   a) Uncontrolled bleeding may necessitate early exploration, but initial management is usually conservative.
   b) Major renal injury (defined on IVP) may indicate need for arteriography.
7. Keep a sample of each voiding, properly labeled (to assess increased/decreasing bleeding). Rack them consecutively for comparison.
8. Order absolute bed rest until urine clear.

Note. Major injuries may hemorrhage for up to 3 wk.

NEUROGENIC BLADDER

Routine Investigation

Neurogenic bladder, whether due to congenital, degenerative, or traumatic cord lesions, may severely damage the upper urinary tract.

Continuing follow-up investigation is necessary, by a urologist with pediatric experience.

The objectives of urologic care and follow-up are:
1. To preserve integrity and function of upper urinary tract.
2. To attain socially acceptable control of urination.

Investigation Protocol

1. Urine culture and sensitivity every 1-2 mo.
2. IVP at least once a year.
3. Catheter cinecystogram (CCC) during the initial investigation, and repeated if IVP indicates need.
4. Urodynamic studies (if child will co-operate)
5. Hb, WBC, differential
6. BUN and creatinine

7. Bladder chart:
    a) frequency of voiding
    b) frequency of incontinence
    c) amount of urine, and whether voided or expressed
8. Enema 24 h (to keep rectum empty)
    This routine will indicate:
    a) Whether cystoscopy is required
    b) The frequency of follow-up needed
    c) Management of bladder: expression, double voiding, timed voiding, intermittent catheterization
    d) When urinary diversion is necessary
    e) How incontinence will be managed.

Expression and Voiding Routines

A. Bladder expression is applicable if the external sphincter has some activity but its resistance is lower than normal.
B. Bladder expression not possible in the newborn, the reflex bladder in upper-motor-neuron disease, and megabladder (urethral resistance usually high).

    Purpose of expression:
1. To reduce residual urine and thus help to minimize infection.
2. To provide dry periods during which bladder is filled against urethral resistance. With proper balance this may permit dryness throughout the day.

Expression is best performed by having the patient strain, as if at stool; this increases intra-abdominal pressure, forcing bladder to empty.

This cannot be accomplished in the very young, who require drainage by intermittent suprapubic pressure on the flaccid abdomen (continuous pressure is less effective than intermittent pressure). Start pressure near the umbilicus, and direct it toward the retropubic area.

    Double or Triple Voiding
For children with megacysts who have no outflow obstruction or other surgically correctable lesion: double or triple voiding within a few minutes may greatly reduce residual urine over single acts of micturition, and may be the only treatment necessary for dryness and freedom from urinary tract infection.

PARAPLEGIA

Bowel Routine

In neurogenic bladder there is defective sensation and inefficient emptying of the bladder. Fecal impaction, also, may occur, as the lower bowel is affected in the same way as the lower urinary tract.

Bowel training, with daily enema, will prevent impaction and fecal soiling.

CHRONIC URINARY OBSTRUCTION

Ureteral or bladder-outlet obstruction after urine is sterile: corrective surgery is indicated.

Suspected Obstruction

1. Immediately, do BUN, urinalysis, and culture of midstream urine
2. Unless BUN is too high, order IVP. Delayed film (up to 2 or 3 hr) yields maximal information.

MASS IN RENAL AREA

This is a surgical emergency.

If Wilms' tumor is suspected:

1. On admission, examine very carefully and record your findings.
2. Attach a "Do Not Examine" sign to the bed and notify the staff surgeon.
3. The following investigations should be done as soon as possible:
   1. Urinalysis
   2. BUN & creatinine
   3. CBC
   4. IVP
   5. PA and lateral chest films
   6. Spot test of urine for VMA *stat,* followed by urine collection for VMA (p 400)
   7. Liver function tests
   8. CT scan
      Arteriography
      Skeletal survey } may be indicated
      Bone marrow

URINARY TRACT INFECTION

1. *Males:* Urine normally sterile, and infection usually indicates anatomical urinary tract abnormality.
   a) Investigation should include IVP and CCC.
   b) Obtain Urology consult – may do cystoscopy.

2. *Females:* The short female urethra predisposes the lower urinary tract to infection. Functional constipation, vaginal voiding, interrupted or repressed voiding, pinworms, poor perineal hygiene, and congenital predisposition to pathological vaginal flora add to the problem. (Up to 0.3% of schoolgirls have a GU infection in any 1 yr.)

   Persistent or recurrent lower UTI, or UTI with systemic effects (e.g., high fever) demand full investigation (IVP, CCC, and possibly cystoscopy).

CRYPTORCHIDISM

1. If bilateral or with hypospadias: suspect intersex.

2. Undescended testis: must differentiate from retractile testis (by careful manipulation). If no associated hernia: surgeon may wait until 3 yr for testis to descend before considering surgery. (If not descended by 3 yr, unlikely to do so.) Gonadotropins are used in selected cases to determine need for surgery, or to aid in surgical treatment.

HYPOSPADIAS

1. If mild and uncomplicated: consultation may be delayed.

2. Severe degree: obtain Urology consult in newborn period. Check adequacy of urinary meatus (watch infant void) immediately after birth. Do not circumcize. The treatment of hypospadias is extremely involved and should be left to the discretion of consultant urologist.

CIRCUMCISION

1. Newborn: One should ask why? – rather than why not? But one should consider parental request.

2. Infants: Adequacy of the preputial opening should be checked by extending the prepuce, not by retracting it. (Retraction may not be possible, because of adhesions, until 6 mo to 4 yr of age.

3. Before 2 yr (while child is in diapers): circumcision predisposes to meatal stenosis.

4. Older child: Recurrent balanitis or infection are indications for circumcision.

ORTHOPEDIC SURGERY

Osteomyelitis and Septic Arthritis

Most commonly hematogenous origin, but other foci possible (e.g., boils). Other causes: neonatal umbilical infection; infected cut-down; rarely open fractures or penetrating injuries.

Pathogenesis

Bacteria (usually staph; occasionally strep, pneumococci, or *H. influenzae*) lodge in metaphyseal area of long bone of growing child, creating focus of osteomyelitis; area of 'cellulitis' develops in overlying soft tissues; pus forms subperiosteally; underlying bone dies (sequestrum).

If in metaphyseal area within joint (e.g., hip), acute septic arthritis develops and pus rapidly destroys articular cartilage.

No specific radiographic changes for 10 days.

Diagnosis

1. Clinical suspicion
2. WBC count and ESR elevated.
3. Blood culture positive.
4. Radiographs — early soft-tissue swelling and joint effusions.
5. Nucleotide scan reveals 'hot spots'.
6. Aspiration of pus diagnostic — *but negative aspiration does not rule out osteomyelitis or septic arthritis.* Send aspirate for culture, do Gram stain also.

    Special Note
    A neonate who cries when hip or leg is moved, especially if thigh is swollen, and who is not feeding well, may have acute septic hip. Usually, temp normal but total WBC count increased.

    This is an emergency: seek verification by aspiration of hip joint.

Treatment

1. Pain relief — analgesics and splinting.
2. Hydration.
3. Start antibiotic therapy immediately (after taking blood for culture): cloxacillin 300 mg/kg/day iv q6h.

4. Adjust antibiotic in accordance with sensitivity report on blood culture (within 36 hr):
   a) *Staph. aureus:* cloxacillin 300 mg/kg/day

      or

      cephalothin (Keflin) 200 mg/kg/day q6h.
   b) *H. influenzae:* ampicillin 400 mg/kg/day q6h

      or

      chloramphenicol 100 mg/kg/day q6h – if cultures show resistance to ampicillin, or if child was taking ampicillin without clinical response before admission.
   c) *Pseudomonas:* gentamicin 5 mg/kg/day q8h **or** antibiotic indicated by sensitivities.
      Consult Infectious Diseases; order bi-weekly serum gentamicin determinations.
   d) **Neonates:** ampicillin 400 mg/kg/day q6h, **plus** gentamicin 5 mg/kg/day q12h, for first week of life; then, gentamicin 7.5 mg/kg/day q8h. Order bi-weekly serum gentamicin determinations.
5. Continue antibiotic(s) for up to 6 wk (minimum, 3 wk), depending on weekly ESR and daily clinical evaluation.
   Note: iv administration of antibiotics provides more reliable blood levels.
6. Antibiotics alone of value only in very early cases (symptoms for 2-3 days) and if condition improves dramatically within 36 hr.
7. If patient seen late, if pus suspected/confirmed, or if condition in early case is not improving after 36 hr of antibiotics: immediate surgical exploration indicated, setting up continuous intramedullary irrigation system.

Club Feet

a) Start cast treatment as soon as possible in newborns' nursery.
b) Change cast weekly until correction obtained.

Metatarsus Varus

a) In newborn, often positional.
b) If deformity persists beyond 2 mo, serial casts needed – usually, 4 cast changes at 2-wk intervals.

Congenital Dislocation of Hip

Check for Ortolani's sign at birth, at time of discharge, and at each well-baby examination until infant walks:

1. Place baby supine on firm surface.
2. Flex his hips to 90°, abduct to 45°.
3. Hold thigh with thumb in groin, middle finger on greater trochanter.
4. Press forward with middle finger and back with thumb.
5. If femoral head displaces, there is dislocation.
6. If dislocation suspected, obtain radiograph (**Note:** failure to demonstrate instability of hip radiographically does not rule out dislocation).
7. Orthopedic consult is mandatory.
8. Treatment: Frejke pillow or abduction casts, or (occasionally, in late cases) osteotomy.

Cerebral Palsy: Orthopedic Problems

Every child who is mentally retarded or has cerebral palsy should have a hip examination.

1. Place child supine on firm surface
2. Abduct hips with hips and knees extended
3. If each hip does not abduct 45° (90° combined), the hips are tight
4. Obtain hip films and request orthopedic consultation

Note. Tight hips, if not treated, always lead to dislocation, scoliosis, difficult nursing, and poor sitting.

Scoliosis

Hereditary type (usually in girls) begins at age 9 to 14 yr. May show as asymmetry of hips or pelvis, posterior chest-wall asymmetry (rib hump when child bends forward), or one shoulder higher.

1. Stand child (in minimal clothing) with back facing examiner
2. Have child bend forward to touch knees.
3. Sight along child's spine: prominence on one side of spine indicates scoliosis.
4. Seek radiographic confirmation (standing scoliosis film at 3 ft FFD).
5. Obtain orthopedic consultation.
6. Spinal deviation >15° is likely to worsen until growth ceases.
7. For lesser scoliosis, follow-up with films every 3 mo.
8. Curve >40° may need surgical correction.

Back Pain

Back pain in children is seldom psychological.
If persistent/recurrent, obtain orthopedic consultation.

Hip Problems

1. Acute hip problems due to swollen or inflamed capsule (e.g., acute synovitis, septic arthritis) result in:
   a) early unilateral loss of internal rotation (tested with hip and knee flexed at 90°)
   b) loss of full hip abduction, and
   c) hip flexion deformity (Thomas test).

All of these occur also in acute slipped femoral epiphysis (in children 9-14 yr) and Legg–Perthes' disease (4-10 yr).

2. Hip pain is usually referred to the knee. In any child who has knee pain:
   a) examine hip carefully
   b) order radiographs of hips in AP and frog views.
3. Always examine both hips passively, simultaneously: this reveals any restriction of movement of the affected joint.

Legg–Calvé–Perthes' Disease

Osteochondrosis of femoral head

1. Begins as a painless limp; may be bilateral.
2. Early diagnosis established radiologically. Differentiate from epiphyseal dysplasia by films of wrists and knees.
3. Treatment is by orthopedic surgeon (special splint, and osteotomy may be necessary).

Osgood–Schlatter's Disease

Osteochondritis of epiphysis of tibial tuberosity

1. Restrict vigorous exercise (cycling, soccer, volleyball, tennis, basketball). Quiet exercise (swimming and walking) allowed.
2. Child to have elastic bandage on affected limb during daytime for 3 wk.
3. If condition severe: cylinder walking cast may be necessary.
4. **Do not** instill steroids at site.
5. Condition clears when growth ceases.

Slipped Femoral Epiphysis

Occurs in obese (rarely in thin) boys.

1. Pain commonly referred diffusely to knee.
2. Early diagnosis established radiologically. Can be missed if AP view only — need frog or lateral view.
3. All cases: obtain orthopedic consult immediately — pinning essential, as soon as possible.

PLASTIC SURGERY

General

1. History. When relevant, include questioning about congenital defects in family.
2. Lesion
    a) Sketch of defect; complete the pre-op chart.
    b) Photographs, pre-op and postop.
3. Operation notes
    a) Immediately after operation, write a short note on chart. Include sketch of technique.
    b) Dictate operation note (p 16).
4. Dressings
    a) the first ones are removed/replaced by resident; subsequently, as arranged with nurse.
    b) donor sites: dressings are soaked off at 10 days.
5. Removal of sutures
    a) face and hands, at 5-7 days.
    b) palate, as ordered by surgeon.
    c) elsewhere, at 7-10 days.
6. Progress notes
    a) write up at least q3 days
    b) note infection, viability of flaps, percentage 'take' of grafts, healing of donor site, suture removal, etc.

Specific Cases

Cleft Lip and Palate
1. General, as above.
2. Sketch to include measurements of width and degree of cleft (lip, alveolus, palate) and degree of nasal deformity.

Facial Disproportion
1. General, as above.
2. Request anthropometric and stereophotogrammetric measurements.
3. Record the type of operation planned (decided by craniofacial team).

Abrasions

1. General, as above.
2. Cleanse adjacent skin and infiltrate wound with 1% Xylocaine.
3. Scrub area, to remove embedded dirt and prevent tattooing.

Lacerations

1. General, as above.
2. Cleanse adjacent skin and infiltrate area with 1% Xylocaine.
3. Flush with N saline only.
4. Close wound in layers, using 4/0 or 5/0 catgut or Dexon.
5. Close skin, using nylon or polyethylene:
   a) child <8 yr, 5/0 or 6/0
   b) 8 yr or older, 4/0.

Hand lacerations
   - Examine and test flexor and extensor tendons, nerves, intrinsic muscles, joints, bones.
   - If any damaged, or diagnosis in doubt, call Plastic Surgery resident.

Facial lacerations
   - Of free borders of mouth, nose, eyelids, ears: **consult Plastic Surgery Resident**
   - Involving eye: **consult Ophthalmology resident.**

Wringer Injuries

1. General, as above.
2. a) Examine for nonviability of skin, underlying hematoma/edema, pain on active/passive movement, altered nerve sensation or function.
   b) **If any positive, call Plastic Surgery resident.** Otherwise, wrap limb in bulky occlusion dressing and elevate.
   c) Re-examine next day.

Nasal and Facial Fractures

1. General, as above.
2. Examine for
   a) pain on deep palpation or chewing
   b) areas of anesthesia
   c) crepitus, malocclusion
   d) subconjunctival hemorrhage, eye movement, visual acuity.
3. **Note.** Radiograph may be reported as negative. Check film. If in doubt, rely on clinical findings/suspicions.
4. If nasal septal or auricular hematoma, drain it *stat*.

Thermal Burns

Record degree and area.

Outpatient management is usually appropriate for:
   a) child <2 yr with 1° or 2° burns of <6% of body area.
   b) child >2 yr with 1° or 2° burns of <10% body area.
   c) child with any burn of face, hands, buttocks, perineum — *if approved by Plastic Surgery resident.*

   Outpatient treatment
1st degree: none except analgesic (p 417, 433).
2nd degree: (except face): occlusive dressing, analgesic.
   a) Record medical and burn history.
   b) Draw diagram in chart, noting size, position, depth of burn.
   c) Check tetanus immunization (p 146).
   d) Give analgesic.
   e) Cleanse area of burn with Cetavlon (Ayerst).
   f) Debride broken blisters and loose epidermis — leave intact blisters alone.
   g) Dry the area, and apply one layer of Sofratulle. Cover with bulky bandage of gauze, then a pad, and finally a Kling bandage.
   h) Re-examine in Clinic in 5-7 days.

Admit any child with burn as listed here:
a) 2° or 3° burn of 10% or more of body area.
b) child under 2 yr, with 2° or 3° burn of 6% or more of body area
c) flame burn, whatever the size, acquired while child in enclosed space (*see p 308*)
d) 2° or 3° burn of critical areas (perineum, hands, feet, etc).

307

FLAME BURNS OR EXPLOSIONS when the patient was in an enclosed space:
a)   determine blood gases *stat*
b)   obtain chest radiograph
c)   discuss with staff surgeon on call.

Inpatient management (all types of burns)

1.   On admission
a)   Notify *stat* the Burns Unit (8E), Plastic Surgery Resident on call, and staff surgeon on call.
b)   Transfer patient to Burns Unit *stat* (don't wait to start iv line or change dressings).
c)   Do not give analgesic.

2.   After admission
a)   Take burn history, and calculate size and degree.
b)   Take blood for Hb, serum electrolytes, proteins, BUN.
c)   Burns >10% body area: start saline iv infusion, by cutdown at ankle unless contraindicated.
d)   Analgesic: codeine in small doses iv (p 433) only if necessary — never routinely.
e)   Insert urinary catheter.
f)   Record size, depth, area of burn. Complete medical history.

3.   **Fluid replacement**
a)   Record input and output hourly (see table, p 310).
b)   Order npo for 24 hr
c)   *To replace burn loss:*
i)   give saline **or** Ringer's lactate soln: % area burned x kg body wt x 0.75 ml; **plus** colloid: % area burned x kg body wt x 0.25 mg. (Administration of calculated amounts to be complete by 8 hr after burning.)
ii)   repeat these amounts over the next 16 hr, and again over the following 24 hr.
d)   *Maintenance:* give 5% dextrose in water, in amount appropriate to age, for 24 hr (p 118).
Note. This fluids formula is only a guide. Modify according to urine output/hr, Hb q4h, serum electrolytes and BUN q9-12h, and patient's general condition.

4.   **Treatment of burn**
a)   Take swabs for culture and sensitivity, from nose, throat, perineum, unburned skin, and area of burnt skin.
b)   Cleanse burned areas with Cetavlon; debride broken blisters and loose epidermis.
c)   Treat topically according to regimen established by staff surgeon on call.

5. Antibiotics: order only according to regimen established by staff surgeon on call.

6. Tetanus immunization: complete if this is necessary.

7. Diet (see Nutrition, pp 315, 328-9)

    a)   Child with 2° burns of <10% body surface: routine ward diet.

    b)   Child with 3° burns requiring grafting, or with burns of 10% body surface or more:

        — diet to contain more calories than normal for age; at least 25% of total calories as protein.

        — multiple-vitamin capsules, 1 daily

        — prophylactic ferrous sulfate supplement daily (p 445)

        — fluids *ad lib.*

Burn Patient: Urine Output in Relation to Age

Urine output per hr	Up to 2 mo	2 mo to 1 yr	1-3 yr	3-5 yr	5-8 yr	8-14 yr
Average	10-18 ml	15-22 ml	20-25 ml	25-30 ml	25-40 ml	25-50 ml
Maximal permissible range	5-20 ml	7-30 ml	10-35 ml	10-45 ml	15-50 ml	15-60 ml

NUTRITION

BREAST MILK

Feeding of breast milk is encouraged.
The mother's expressed breast milk is stored on the ward
— not pasteurized if to be used within 48 hr.

BREAST-FEEDING

It is the responsibility of the attending physician to discuss with the mother, early in her pregnancy, whether she
wishes to breast-feed. This decision should be based on a
thorough consideration of the factors outlined below.
Furthermore, any mother who is breast-feeding must
receive continual counseling and support from her attending physician, who may also recommend that she seek
information from public-health and community agencies
(including La Leche League). *Care must be taken to ensure that the infant thrives.*

Advantages

1. Nutritionally complete
   - Fe: high availability
   - contains vitamin D (but supplement required)
   - contains fluorine (but supplement required un-
     less infant receives supplemental feeds of fluori-
     dated water).
2. Low renal solute load.
3. Easily digested
   - casein: lactalbumin = 30:70
   - fat: ideal blend; adequate essential fatty acids
4. Sterile.
5. Anti-infective functions (lactoferrin, lysozymes, secretory IgA, bifidus factor, macrophages).
6. Readily available.
7. Cheaper than commercial feedings.
8. Unmonitored volume: less risk of overfeeding than
   with commercial preparations.
9. Promotes maternal/infant bonding.

Precautions/Contraindications

1. Unsuccessful if mother or father opposed.

2. Mother must be counseled re adequate daily diet (poor nutritional status is likely to decrease milk volume).
3. Maternal drug use (including alcohol, cigarettes) must be discussed.
4. Serious chronic illness (e.g., neoplastic disease) in mother: usually = contraindication for breast-feeding.
5. Specific inborn errors in the infant (e.g., galactosemia, phenylketonuria).
6. Moderate or severe neonatal jaundice or Rh/ABO incompatibility = indications to cease breastfeeding.

Establishing Initial Schedule
1. Begin as soon as possible post partum.
2. Begin with short sucking time (approx. 3-5 min at each breast), increase gradually to maximum 15 min at each breast.
3. Begin feedings with alternate breasts, to ensure complete emptying of both at alternate feedings.
4. Flexible feeding schedule essential for first 2-3 wk (some babies feed q2-3 h during the day at this time).

Breast and Nipple Care
1. Painful nipples: can be prevented by adequate prenatal care, correct feeding position, and prevention of engorgement.
2. Inverted nipples: rare — most are 'pseudo-inverted', which can be corrected by exercising during last trimester.
3. Hygiene: cleansing of nipples with cooled boiled water is sufficient. Use of soap should be avoided (it may aggravate cracking of skin in nipple area).
4. Dry, cracked nipples: treat with lanolin cream.
   If abscess occurs: breastfeeding may be discontinued until condition clears — but sucking infant is best form of drainage. Systemic antibiotics, and/or incision and drainage, may be necessary.

BOTTLE-FEEDING

Preparations of Modified Cows' Milk

If the mother cannot or chooses not to breastfeed, *commercially prepared infant formulas* are the best alternative to human milk.
Commercial formulas are in various forms (Table A).

TABLE A

Form	Preparation	Relative Cost	Advantages/Disadvantages
Powder	Normal dilution: 1 Tbsp (9 g) powder to 60 ml water	Least expensive	More difficult to mix. Possible to over-concentrate formula if measurements not level (e.g., rounded Tbsp).
Liquid concentrate	Normal dilution: equal volumes of concentrate & water	More expensive	Fewer problems with preparation.
Ready-to-feed	No dilution required: ready to pour into bottles	Most expensive	Costly. Convenient (e.g, when travelling)

313

If no commercial formula is available, modified cows' milk can be used – *preferably evaporated whole cows' milk:*
- the protein is more readily digested (result of heat-processing)
- already sterilized (ordinary whole cows' milk would have to be heat-treated).

Note. Condensed milk is not equal to evaporated milk and **should not be used** for infant feeding.

Preparing evaporated-milk formulas (see Table B)

Problems Associated with Bottle Feeding

1. Poor technique
   - improper sterilization
   - errors in dilution
2. 'Night-bottle syndrome' – putting the child to sleep with a bottle.
   - May lead to oral and dental complications.
3. Over-feeding: forcing the infant to empty the bottle regardless of appetite.

Formula Selection

1. Calculate caloric requirement based on infant's developmental age, and ideal weight and height, according to the Dietary Standards* for Canada (Table C).
2. Select appropriate formula to meet infant's nutritional needs (Table D, pt I).
3. Check whether formula meets protein and fluid requirements (150–180 ml/kg/day, in total volume not exceeding 1200 ml/day).
4. Consider supplementation if formula does not meet infant's recommended daily nutrient intake (Table E).

Definition of Dietary Standard: The daily amounts of energy and essential nutrients considered *adequate* (not necessarily ideal), on the basis of scientific data, to meet the physiological needs of healthy members of a population. Recommended nutrient intakes exceed minimal requirements of most persons but are not formulated to meet therapeutic needs.

ORDERING FORMULAS AND DIETS

1. Breast milk (see p 311).
2. Bottle feeds (Table D, pt I).
3. Infants/children 6 mo and older:
    Various textures of foods are available. Select the one appropriate to the patient's age:

Texture	Developmental Age
Strained	6-9 mo
Junior	9-12 mo
Minced	12-24 mo
Diced	2-5 yr
Sliced	6 yr and older

4. Notify the Selective Menu Office (ext. 1318, 2419) of the formula or diet suitable for the individual patient. Use computer *Formula/Diet Order Sheet* or *Special Formula/Diet Prescription.*
5. Table F shows sample meal patterns for infants.

Special Formulas/Diets

1. Special metabolic diets: contact nutritionist in Clinical Investigation Unit (ext. 1766).
2. All special formulas (Table D, pt II) and special diets (Table G) must have the authorization of the appropriate dietitian/nutritionist.
3. All patients discharged on special diet or formula: patient/parents should be instructed beforehand by a dietitian/nutritionist.

TABLE B

Age	Infant's body wt (lb)	Infant's body wt (g)	Each Feeding — Evap. whole milk (fl oz)		Boiled water (fl oz)	Corn syrup/sugar (tsp)	Per 24 hr — Evap. whole milk (fl oz)		Boiled water (fl oz)	Corn syrup/sugar (Tbsp)	No. of feeds
1-2 wk*	6-7	2720-3175	1	:	2	1	6	:	12	1	6
3-4 wk	8	3630	1.5	:	2	1	8	:	14	1½	6
1-2 mo	9-10	4080-4535	2	:	3	1½	10	:	15	2	5
3-6 mo	12-15	5445-6805	3.5	:	4	1½	14	:	18	2	4
>6 mo	16+	7255+	5	:	5	0	15	:	15	0	3

*This dilution can be used up to 6 mo.

TABLE C. DIETARY STANDARDS FOR CANADA, 1975
(Recommended daily nutrient intake, revised 1975)

PART I

Age	Sex	Weight (kg)	Height (cm)	Energy[a] kcal/kg	kJ/kg[b]	Protein (g)
0-6 mo	both	6	–	117	489.5	kg x 2.2 (2.0)[c]
7-11 mo	both	9	–	108	451.9	kg x 1.4
1-3 yr	both	13	90	107	447.7	22
4-6 yr	both	19	110	95	397.5	27
7-9 yr	M	27	129	81	338.9	33
7-9 yr	F	27	128	74	309.6	33
10-12 yr	M	36	144	70	292.9	41
10-12 yr	F	38	145	60	251.0	40
13-15 yr	M	51	162	55	230.1	52
13-15 yr	F	49	159	45	188.3	43
16-18 yr	M	64	172	50	209.2	54
16-18 yr	F	54	161	40	167.4	43
During pregancy				+300[d]	1255.2[d]	+20
While lactating				+500	2092.0	+24

[a] Recommendations assume characteristic activity pattern for each age group.
[b] 1 kilocalorie = 4.184 kilojoules.
[c] Recommended protein intake: 2.2 g/kg body wt for infants age 0-2 mo and 2.0 g/kg body wt for those age 3-5 mo. Protein recommended for infants 0-11 mo assumes consumption of breast milk or protein of equivalent quality.
[d] Increased energy intake recommended during 2nd and 3rd trimesters. An increase of 100 kcal (418.4 kJ) per day is recommended during 1st trimester.

TABLE C. PART II

Water-soluble Vitamins

Age	Sex	Thiamine (mg)	Niacin (NE)[e]	Riboflavin (mg)	Vitamin B$_6$[f] (mg)	Folate[g] (µg)	Vitamin B$_{12}$ (µg)	Vitamin C (mg)
0-6 mo	both	0.3	5	0.4	0.3	40	0.3	20[h]
7-11 mo	both	0.5	6	0.6	0.4	60	0.3	20
1-3 yr	both	0.7	9	0.8	0.8	100	0.9	20
4-6 yr	both	0.9	12	1.1	1.3	100	1.5	20
7-9 yr	M	1.1	14	1.3	1.0	100	1.5	30
	F	1.0	13	1.2	1.4	100	1.5	30
10-12 yr	M	1.2	17	1.5	1.8	100	3.0	30
	F	1.1	15	1.4	1.5	100	3.0	30
13-15 yr	M	1.4	19	1.7	2.0	200	3.0	30
	F	1.1	15	1.4	1.5	200	3.0	30
16-18 yr	M	1.6	21	2.0	2.0	200	3.0	30
	F	1.1	14	1.3	1.5	200	3.0	30
During pregnancy		+0.2	+2	+0.3	+0.5	+50	+1.0	+20
While lactating		+0.4	+7	+0.6	+0.6	+50	+0.5	+30

[e] 1 NE (niacin equivalent) = 1 mg of niacin or 60 mg of tryptophan.
[f] Based on estimated average daily protein intake of Canadians.
[g] Free folate.
[h] It may be prudent to give considerably higher levels to infants during the first week of life, to guard against neo-natal tyrosinemia.

TABLE C. PART III

Fat-soluble Vitamins

Age	Sex	Vitamin A (RE)[i]	Vitamin D (μg cholecalciferol)[j]	Vitamin E (mg d-α-tocopherol)
0-6 mo	both	400	10	3
7-11 mo	both	400	10	3
1-3 yr	both	400	10	4
4-6 yr	both	500	5	5
7-9 yr	both	700	2.5[k]	6
10-12 yr	both	800	2.5	7
13-15 yr	M	1000	2.5	9
13-15 yr	F	800	2.5	7
16-18 yr	M	1000	2.5	10
16-18 yr	F	800	2.5	6
During pregnancy		+100	+2.5	+1
While lactating		+400	+2.5	+2

[i] 1RE (retinol equivalent) corresponds to 1 μg retinol (3.33 U) or 6 μg B-carotene (10 U).
[j] One μg cholecalciferol is equivalent to 1 μg ergocalciferol (40 U vitamin-D activity).
[k] Most older children (7-18 yr) receive vitamin D from irradiation but dietary intake of 2.5 μg daily is recommended. Daily intake recommended for those confined indoors or otherwise deprived of sunlight for extended periods is 5.0 μg.

TABLE C. PART IV

		Minerals					
Age	Sex	Calcium (mg)	Phosphorus (mg)	Magnesium (mg)	Iodine (µg)	Iron (mg)	Zinc (mg)
0-6 mo[l]	both	500	250	50	35	7	4
7-11 mo	both	500	400	50	50	7	5
1-3 yr	both	500	500	75	70	8	5
4-6 yr	both	500	500	100	90	9	6
7-9 yr	M	700	700	150	110	10	7
	F	700	700	150	100	10	7
10-12 yr	M	900	900	175	130	11	8
	F	1000	1000	200	120	11	9
13-15 yr	M	1200	1200	250	140	13	10
	F	800	800	250	110	14	10
16-18 yr	M	1000	1000	300	160	14	12
	F	700	700	250	110	14	11
During pregnancy		+500	+500	+25	+15	+1[m]	+3
While lactating		+500	+500	+75	+25	+1[m]	+7

l The intake of breast-fed infants is considered adequate even if it is less than recommended.
m The recommended intake of 15 mg daily during pregnancy and lactation assumes the presence of adequate stores of iron. If inadequacy of Fe stores suspected, additional iron (supplement) is recommended.

TABLE D. COMPOSITION OF FORMULAS

Due to changes in formulation, all data subject to change.

Liquid Feedings – unless otherwise specified 100 ml, normal dilution	ENERGY (kcal)	(kJ)	Pro (g)	Fat (g)	CHO (g)	Ca (mg)	P (mg)	Fe (mg)	Na (mg)	Na (mEq)	K (mg)	K (mEq)
PART I: STANDARD												
Enfalac	67	280	1.5	3.7	7.0	57	45	0.2	23	1.0	47	1.2
Enfalac with iron	67	280	1.5	3.7	7.0	57	45	1.3	23	1.0	47	1.2
Milk, cows' whole	65	272	3.5	3.5	4.9	118	93	trace	50	2.2	144	3.7
Milk, cows' 2%	50	209	3.3	1.9	4.8	122	95	0.1	50	2.2	154	3.9
Milk, human	70	293	1.0	4.4	6.9	32	14	trace	17	0.7	51	1.3
Milk, cows' skimmed	36	151	3.6	0.1	5.1	121	95	0.0	52	2.3	145	3.7
SMA	67	280	1.5	3.6	7.2	44	33	1.3	15	0.7	56	1.4
Similac	68	285	1.5	3.6	7.2	52	39	0.1	22	1.0	65	1.7
Similac with iron	68	285	1.5	3.6	7.2	52	39	1.2	22	1.0	65	1.7

Liquid Feedings – unless otherwise specified 100 ml, normal dilution	ENERGY (kcal)	(kJ)	Pro (g)	Fat (g)	CHO (g)	Ca (mg)	P (mg)	Fe (mg)	Na (mg)	(mEq)	K (mg)	(mEq)
PART II: SPECIAL												
CHO-free with 7% CHO	67	280	1.8	3.5	7.0	90	69	0.9	37	1.6	89	2.2
Cutter Formula 2 (per 100 g)	100	418	3.8	4.0	12.1	100	90	1.5	45	2.0	150	3.8
Ensure (per 100 g)	106	444	3.7	3.7	14.5	50	50	0.9	70	3.0	120	3.1
Flexical (per 100 g)	100	418	2.2	3.4	15.5	50	45	0.5	35	1.5	150	3.8
Goats' milk	67	289	3.6	4.1	4.5	134	111	0.1	50	2.2	204	5.2
Isocal (per 100 g)	106	444	3.4	4.4	13.2	60	50	0.9	53	2.3	132	3.4
Isomil	67	280	2.0	3.6	6.8	70	50	1.2	30	1.3	71	1.8
Lofenalac	67	280	2.2	2.6	8.6	63	48	1.3	47	2.0	105	2.7
Meat-base formula* (lamb – 7% CHO)	67	280	1.9	3.4	7.2	1.0*	19	0.3	23	1.0	23	0.6
Meritene Liquid (per 100 g)	102	427	6.1	3.4	11.6	127	127	1.5	93	4.0	169	4.3
Nutramigen	67	280	2.2	2.6	8.6	63	48	1.3	32	1.4	105	2.7
Portagen	67	280	2.3	3.2	7.6	71	54	1.2	42	1.8	103	2.7
Precision Isotonic (per 100 g, normal dilution)	84	351	2.5	2.6	12.7	57	57	1.0	67	2.7	84	2.2

Precision L.R. Diet (per 100 g, normal dilution)	97	406	2.1	0.1	22.0	41	41	0.9	61	2.7	77	2.0
Precision High Nitrogen (per 100 g, normal dilution)	93	389	3.9	0.0	19.2	25	25	0.5	87	3.8	81	2.0
Pregestimil	68	280	2.2	2.8	8.7	63	48	1.3	32	1.3	94	2.4
Prosobee	68	280	2.5	3.4	6.8	95	69	1.3	52	2.2	91	2.3
Similac PM 60/40	68	285	1.5	3.4	7.2	33	17	0.2	15	0.7	57	1.4
Soyalac	68	285	2.1	4.0	5.9	40	36	1.1	30	1.3	69	1.7
Sustacal (per 100 g)	100	418	6.1	2.3	13.9	152	135	1.7	109	4.7	175	4.5
Sustagen (per 100 g, normal dilution)	148	619	9.0	1.3	24.9	352	311	1.3	161	7	456	11.7
Vivonex: High Nitrogen (per 100 g, normal dilution)	90	377	3.7	0.1	18.9	24	24	0.3	69	3	63	1.6
Vivonex: Standard (per 100 g, normal dilution)	90	377	1.8	1	20.3	40	40	0.5	77	3.3	105	2.7

*800 mg Ca (as Ca carbonate) should be added to total daily amount of this formula.

323

TABLE E. NUTRITION SUPPLEMENTS

Due to changes in formulation, all data subject to change.

Supplement	Energy (kcal)	Energy (kJ)	Pro (g)	Fat (g)	Cho (g)	Ca (mg)	P (mg)	Fe (mg)	Na (mg)	Na (mEq)	K (mg)	K (mEq)
Amin-Aid (per 100 g, normal dilution)	172	720	1.7	6.1	27.7	10	8.0	0.0	12	0.5	20	0.5
Caloreen powder (per 100 g)	384	1607	0.0	0.0	96	0.0	0.0	0.0	2.0	0.1	4.0	0.1
Casilan powder (per 100 g)	380	1590	90	1.8	0.0	1200	800	N/A	80	3.5	10	0.3

Controlyte powder (per 100 g)	504	2109	0.1	24	72	4	8.0	0.0	15	0.7	4.0	0.1
MCT oil (per 100 g)	792	3314	0.0	97 (MCT 97% LCT 3%)	0.0	0.0	0.0	0.0	0.0	0.0	0.0	0.0
Polycose liquid (per 100 ml soln)	200	838	0.0	0.0	50	N/A	N/A	0.0	62	2.7	—	—
Polycose powder (per 100 g)	376	1573	0.0	0.0	94	13.4	4.8	0.4	110	4.8	5.0	0.1

TABLE F. SAMPLE MEAL PATTERN FOR INFANT FEEDING

Feeding	3 mo	6 mo	9-12 mo	12-24 mo
1	5-6 oz milk (breast or formula)	6-8 oz milk	2-4 oz juice (undiluted). 2-4 Tbsp dry infants' cereal mixed with milk (undiluted). Dry whole-wheat toast. 1 Tbsp meat or ½-1 egg yolk (mashed). 6-8 oz milk.	3-4 oz juice. 3-4 Tbsp infants' cereal mixed with milk or ¼ cup cooked cereal. Whole-wheat bread or toast with butter or margarine. 6-8 oz milk.
2	1-2 Tbsp infants' cereal made with milk. 5-6 oz milk (breast or formula).	2 oz juice (diluted 2:1). 4-6 Tbsp infants' cereal made with milk. 4-6 oz milk.		
3	5-6 oz milk (breast or formula)	1-2 tsp pureed meat. 2-4 Tbsp pureed vegetables. 6-8 oz formula or whole milk.	2-4 Tbsp meat or meat alternatives. 2-4 Tbsp vegetables (home prepared). 2-4 Tbsp mashed fruit. Dry whole-wheat toast. 6-8 oz milk.	Chopped, tender meat or boned fish, alone or in sandwich. (Meat alternatives can be substituted). Progress from 3-4 Tbsp vegetables (cooked and cut up) to vegetables served raw. Progress from 3-4 Tbsp cut-up fruit to 1/3-⅔ of whole fruit. Whole-wheat bread with butter or margarine. 6-8 oz milk.

4	1-2 Tbsp infants' cereal made with milk. 5-6 oz milk (breast or formula)	4-6 Tbsp infants' cereal made with milk. 2-4 Tbsp pureed fruit. 6-8 oz milk.	2-4 Tbsp infants' cereal made with milk. 3-4 Tbsp mashed fruit or fruit pudding. Dry whole-wheat toast. 6-8 oz milk.	Meat and vegetables, as at lunch. Progress from 3-4 Tbsp cut-up fruit to 1/3-½ of a whole fruit, or ¼ cup milk pudding, custard, yogurt, or ice cream. Whole-wheat bread with butter or margarine. 6-8 oz milk.
5	5-6 oz milk (breast or formula). *Discontinue when infant is sleeping through the night.*			

TABLE G

Types of dietary control available* *excluding* special metabolic diets (C.I.U.)

Cardiac system	Endocrine/ Exocrine system	Gastro-intestinal system	Neuro-logical system	Renal system	Allergy	Testing	Psychiatric disorders
Controlled fat &/or CHO (for hyperlipemia)	Controlled fat &/or CHO (for hyperlipemia)	For CHO intolerance	Ketogenic diet	Controlled Ca	Egg-free	Fat-balance study	Individual modification (for eating disorders)
Controlled Na	Controlled Ca	Controlled fat	Mechanical soft	Controlled potassium	Milk-free	Fat-free supper	MAO
Modified caloric content	Diabetes diets	Controlled protein	Modified caloric content	Controlled protein	Wheat-free	Red-meat-free	
Tube-feedings	High in Pro, Cal, or sat. fat	Controlled Na	Tube-feedings	Controlled Na	Rowe elimination diets	Renin study	

328

Immune deficiency	Gastric diets		Modified caloric content		
Modified caloric content	Gluten-free		Tube-feedings		
Tube-feedings	Modified residue				
	Mechanical soft				
	Tube-feedings				
	Wired jaw				

*Any of the above diets may be administered in combination, depending on individual patient's needs.

329

TECHNIQUES FOR INTRODUCING FOODS

(Table H)

The methods used to introduce new foods can determine a child's lifelong food habits. Instruct parent(s) as follows.

1. Introduce one new food at a time.
2. *Begin the meal* with the new food.
3. Give a small amount (1 tsp) initially and increase up to a few Tbsp as the infant becomes accustomed to it.
4. Offer new foods when the infant is in good spirits and feeling hungry.
5. Don't show *your* dislike of certain foods. Offer the new food in a casual matter-of-fact way, expecting him to like it.
6. Don't force him to eat, and don't show disappointment if he resists the food — try again the next day.
7. Don't add fat, salt, or sweetening to any food for an infant. (An infant's taste buds are sensitive enough to allow him to enjoy subtle natural flavors.)
8. Allow a few days to elapse before introducing another new food. (If the child has an allergy to the last new food, this is readily identified.)

CANADA'S FOOD GUIDE

— A daily plan designed to help people of all ages choose their food wisely.

Milk and Milk Products
Children up to 11 yr: 2-3 servings
Adolescents: 3-4 servings
Pregnant and nursing women: 3-4 servings
Other adults: 2 servings.

Meat and Alternatives
2 servings

Fruits and Vegetables
4-5 servings — include at least 2 vegetables.

Bread and Cereals
3-4 servings (whole grain or enriched).

BETWEEN-MEAL SNACKS

Some children cannot eat large amounts at one meal, and others engage in such high activity that they need between-meal snacks. For older infants, offer light nutritious snacks.

Remember: the child may only be thirsty, not hungry; if so, plain water will do.

Careful selection is crucial: 'empty-calorie' snacks can lead to poor dental health, tendency to obesity, poor appetite at meal time, and poor food habits.

TABLE H. INTRODUCING THE FIRST FOODS

From a purely nutritional standpoint, solids are not needed before 6 mo; in practice, however, social pressures encourage their earlier introduction.

Age (mo)	Food	Why introduce
1-3	Human milk or formula (fortified with vitamin D source). Vitamin C source.	Meet infant's nutritive needs until 3 mo of age.
3-4	Fe-enriched infant cereal.	Infant's iron reserves last only 3 mo; and milk is a poor source of iron. The cereal aids development and training of the 'swallowing' reflex, now evolving.
4-5	Pureed vegetables. Pureed fruits.	Provide vitamins, minerals, calories; introduce new food flavors; start to set basis for good eating habits. Introduce vegetables first (to reduce chance of developing a 'sweet tooth').

6-7	Bread. Whole undiluted milk.	Encourages chewing when teeth erupt.
6-8	Pureed meats. Egg yolks. Cottage cheese.	Infant requires extra nutrients (protein, vitamins, iron) for rapid growth. (Egg white not offered until 12 mo, to avoid development of allergy.)
8	Mashed 'family' vegetables.	Introduce food texture other than pureed.
8-10	Chewy finger-foods.	Encourage chewing, co-ordination, independence.

GROWTH & DEVELOPMENT

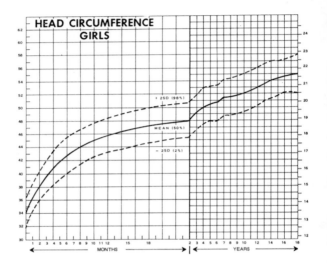

FONTANELS

Anterior: closes at 8-18 mo; > 2 yr is abnormal
Posterior: closes about end of 2nd mo

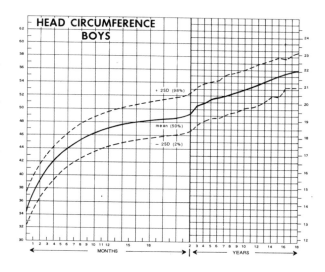

HEAD CIRCUMFERENCE
BOYS

+ 2SD (98%)

mean (50%)

− 2SD (2%)

MONTHS

YEARS

FONTANELS

Anterior: closes at 8-18 mo; >2 yr is abnormal
Posterior: closes about end of 2nd mo

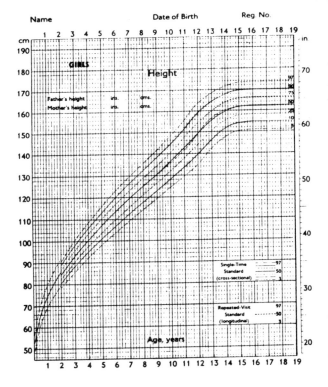

Name   Date of Birth   Reg. No.

GIRLS   Height

Father's height   ins.   cms.
Mother's height   ins.   cms.

Single-Time   97
Standard   50
(cross-sectional)   3

Repeated-Visit   97
Standard   50
(longitudinal)   3

Age, years

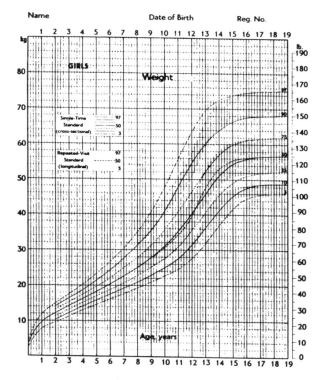

Name   Date of Birth   Reg. No.

GIRLS

Weight

Single-Time
Standard   97
(cross-sectional) 50
                3

Repeated-Visit 97
Standard   50
(longitudinal) 3

Age, years

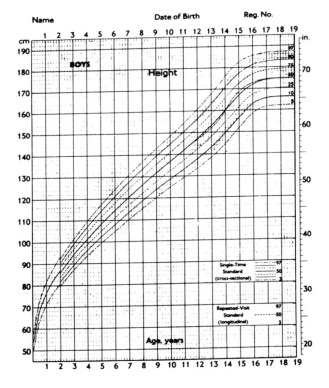

Name · Date of Birth · Reg. No.

BOYS

Height

Age, years

Single-Time
Standard
(cross-sectional)

Repeated-Visit
Standard
(longitudinal)

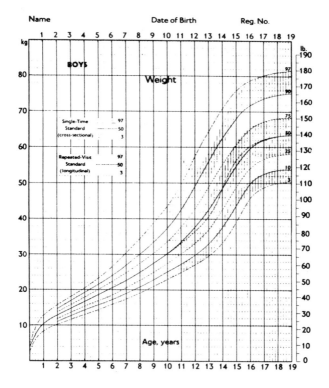

Name   Date of Birth   Reg. No.

BOYS

Weight

Single-Time   97
Standard   50
(cross-sectional)   3

Repeated-Visit   97
Standard   50
(longitudinal)   3

Age, years

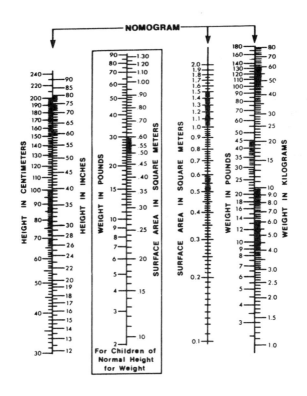

**NOMOGRAM FOR CALCULATION
OF SURFACE AREA**

340

TOOTH ERUPTION (AVERAGE)*

Deciduous (20)	mo
Central incisor	6-8
Lateral incisor	8-10
Cuspid	16-20
First molar	12-16
Second molar	20-30

Permanent (32)	yr
Central incisor	6-7
Lateral incisor	7-8
Cuspid	10-11
First premolar	10-11
Second premolar	10-12
First molar	6-7
Second molar	11-14
Third molar	18-21

*First, second, third, and pre- refer to position in mouth — not in time.

NORMAL U/L VALUES*
IN MALES & FEMALES

AGE		U/L		AGE	U/L	
		M	F	(yr)	M	F
Birth		1.69	1.73	7	1.10	1.09
mo	3	1.65	1.66	8	1.06	1.05
	6	1.61	1.60	9	1.03	1.02
	12	1.54	1.52	10	1.02	1.01
	18	1.51	1.47	11	0.99	1.00
Yr	2	1.44	1.42	12	0.98	0.99
	3	1.33	1.32	13	0.98	0.99
	4	1.27	1.25	14	0.97	0.99
	5	1.21	1.14	15	0.97	1.00
	6	1.14	1.13	16	0.97	1.00

*U=crown to symphysis pubis
L=symphysis pubis to heel

NORMAL VALUES FOR VITAL SIGNS

Age	Pulse/min	Respirations/min
Newborn	85-190	30-50
1-12 mo	115-190	decreasing to 35
1-3 yr	100-190	decreasing to 30
3-5 yr	55-145	25-30
5-8 yr.	70-145	25-30
>8 yr	55-115	20-35

RESTING BLOOD PRESSURE (ARM)

Mean Values (Boys/Girls), mm Hg, for 90th percentile

Age	Systolic	Diastolic	
0-5 mo	96	62	supine
6-11 mo	118	70	
2-5 yr	110	75	
6-7 yr	112	76	
8-9 yr	118	78	
10-11 yr	126	82	seated*
12-13 yr	130	84	
14-15 yr	136	85	
16-17 yr	140	87	

*Based on data from report by National Heart, Lung, and Blood Institute's 1977 Task Force on blood pressure control in children.

THE HOSPITAL FOR SICK CHILDREN
DEVELOPMENTAL CLINIC

PSYCHOMOTOR DEVELOPMENT SCREENING TEST

Patient Name:
Birth Date: _____ Sex: _____ History No: _____
Address:
Phone:
Date: _____ Tested By: _____

INSTRUCTIONS:

1. This is a simple test to help you evaluate the Developmental Age of a child. The purpose is to determine whether Development is in the broad range of normal and if not whether the child should be referred for a more precise assessment.
2. Start with scoring (+) or (−) at one level below the child's age. Go as high as the child may have successes.
3. Supplement your own observations by questioning the mother. Score as (+) successes reported by the mother even if these are not observed by you.
4. Under "Remarks":
   a) Note problem areas in development and behaviour reported by the mother.
   b) Note activity level, alertness, mood, attention span, unusual behaviour.
   c) State your own impressions of, and predictions about, the child.
5. Items indicate performance in one of the following areas: (M) Motor, (A) Adaptive, (L) Language, (PS) Personal-Social
6. Materials needed; Red Wool yarn, one inch wooden blocks, crayons and paper, a rubber ball, a picture vocabulary.

AGE	SCORE		PSYCHOMOTOR DEVELOPMENT SCREENING TEST
4 Weeks		M	Rotates head when placed in prone position
		A	Responds to sound by changing activity
		A	Focuses eyes on bright object (red wool yarn—stethoscope) and follows it for a short distance
		PS	Interest in examiner (focuses eyes for a while on examiner's face − activity deminishes)

Remarks:

8 Weeks		M	Holds head erect briefly in pull-to-sit (pull by the hands until the child is in sitting position)
		M	Holds head 45° up in prone position (child raises head and shoulders off crib level)
		A	Follows object with his eyes past midline
		L	Vocalizes single vowels −"AH" "EH" "UH"
		PS	Social smile (smiles at the approach of mother or examiner)

Remarks:

16 Weeks		M	Raises self up on hands in prone position
		M	Reaches for toys − grasps toy actively if it is near his hand
		A	Follows object with eyes through 180° horizontally and vertically
		L	Coos and laughs
		PS	Recognizes mother (responds promptly and more to her than to other persons)

Remarks:

24 Weeks		M	Raises legs in extension in supine position and touches feet with hands
		M	Rolls over both ways
		A	Approaches and grasps objects in the midline, brings other hand to the object
		L	Babbles
		PS	Aware and/or apprehensive of strangers

Remarks

36 Weeks		M	Sits unsupported 5−10'
		M	Crawls on abdomen
		A	Plays with two toys simultaneously
		L	Vocalizes "mama" − "dada", non-meaningfully
		PS	Responds to pick up gesture

Remarks:

44 Weeks		
	M	Creeps on hands and knees and pulls self up to stand
	M	Grasps small objects (piece of paper — bread crumbs) with thumb and index finger
	A	Imitates behaviour: speech sounds, clapping hands, waving bye-bye
	A	Matches two toys together — places one object into another
	L	Vocalizes "mama" — "dada" and another word, meaningfully

Remarks:

12 Months		
	M	Walks if one hand is held
	A	Attempts to pile two blocks after is shown how
	L·	Imitates words—has two words plus "mama" and "dada"—baby word count if used consistently for a certain object
	L	Responds to simple orders accompanied by gestures: "give me", "no-no" etc.
	PS	Attempts to feed himself with his fingers

Remarks:

18 Months		
	M	Walks well, begins to run
	M	Climbs on furniture
	A	Piles 3 — 4 Blocks
	L	Follows simple directions — no gestures "give me", "give to", "come here"
	L	Vocabulary of ten words
	PS	Attempts to feed himself with spoon

Remarks:

2 Years		
	M	Walks up and down stairs alone (one step at a time—does not need to hold on to the rail)
	M	Kicks ball without being shown how
	A	Imitates vertical and circular strokes
	L	Combines 2—3 words together
	PS	Names and identifies objects and parts (at least 4) of own body
	PS	Imitates domestic activities, (sweeping, dusting, washing)

Remarks:

3 Years		
	M	Jumps down from a small chair
	M	Balances on one foot briefly
	A	Copies circle and imitates cross with crayon
	L	Asks "what" questions
	L	Knows name, sex and age
	PS	Puts on shoes, and simple pieces of clothing
	PS	Co-operates in play with peers

Remarks:

4 Years		
	M	Stands on one foot for 6—10 seconds
	M	Walks heel to toe
	A	Copies cross
	A	Draws a two-part man
	L	Names fourteen or more of the Stanford-Binet picture vocabulary
	L	Recognizes and names three or more colors
	PS	Separates from mother easily — plays specific role in games

Remarks:

IMMUNIZATION SCHEDULES FOR INFANTS AND CHILDREN IN ONTARIO

SCHEDULE I — Using inactivated polio vaccine (Salk type)

2 mo	DPT + POLIO	1 ml
4 mo	DPT + POLIO	1 ml
6 mo	DPT + POLIO	1 ml
10 mo	IC TUBERCULIN SKIN TEST	
15 mo	LIVE FURTHER ATTENUATED MEASLES VACCINE*	
16 to 18 mo	DPT + POLIO	1 ml
4 to 6 yr	DPT + POLIO (School entry)	1 ml
11 to 12 yr	DT + POLIO	1 ml
	Rubella vaccine for females not previously immunized	
16 to 18 yr	DT + POLIO (for recall doses only)	0.5 ml
	or Td + inactivated polio vaccine	1 ml

Preparations:

DPT + P Combined diphtheria toxoid, pertussis vaccine, tetanus toxoid with inactivated polio vaccine.

DT + P Combined diphtheria and tetanus toxoid with inactivated polio vaccine (reduced diphtheria toxoid content).

Td Combined tetanus and diphtheria toxoids, adult type.

*May be given at 15 mo or thereafter as measles-rubella or measles-mumps-rubella combined vaccines.

Routine smallpox vaccination is not recommended.

NOTE: Children and adults travelling outside Canada who have received immunization with inactivated vaccine (Salk) are advised to take at least one dose of Trivalent live oral polio vaccine (Sabin).

SCHEDULE II — Using Trivalent Oral Polio Vaccine
(Sabin type)

2 mo	DPT 1 ml + TRIVALENT OPV
4 mo	DPT 1 ml + TRIVALENT OPV
6 mo	DPT 1 ml + TRIVALENT OPV
10 mo	IC TUBERCULIN SKIN TEST
15 mo	LIVE FURTHER ATTENUATED MEASLES VACCINE*
16 to 18 mo	DPT 1 ml + TRIVALENT OPV
4 to 6 yr	DPT 1 ml + TRIVALENT OPV (School entry)
11 to 12 yr	Td ADULT TYPE 1 ml or DT 0.5 ml; + TRIVALENT OPV; + Rubella vaccine for females not previously immunized.
16 to 18 yr	Td ADULT TYPE 1 ml or DT 0.5 ml; + TRIVALENT OPV

Preparations: *see* p 345

*May be given at 15 mo or thereafter as measles-rubella or measles-mumps-rubella combined vaccines

Routine smallpox vaccination is not recommended.

For details see "Immunization and Related Procedures". A Guide for Physicians in Ontario. Committee on Public Health, Ontario Medical Assoc., 1979.

IMMUNIZATION FOR FOREIGN TRAVEL

There are two main categories of immunization for travel abroad, (1) those required to enter certain countries, or to return to this country, and include only smallpox, yellow fever and cholera, (2) those recommended on the basis of the likelihood of exposure and include diphtheria, tetanus, measles, pertussis, polio, typhoid and typhus. In the event of long visits to certain areas, BCG, plague and rabies immunization should be considered. In addition, immune serum globulin (gamma globulin) is recommended if exposure to hepatitis is a distinct possibility, as is drug prophylaxis for malaria for visitors to certain parts of the world.

Required Vaccinations: – Smallpox, Yellow Fever, Cholera.
The requirements, which are specified by each country are
related to health conditions in the country of departure
and also to conditions in any country through which the
traveller passes (and disembarks) en route. The World
Health Organisation publishes annually a booklet – Vaccination Certificate Requirements for International Travel
– and updates this during the year through notifications
to national health agencies.

Epidemiology Service, Ontario Ministry of Health, dis-
tributes the national Health and Welfare Weekly Quarantin-
able Diseases Report which lists countries currently infected and endemic for smallpox cholera, yellow fever
and plague.

Questions on required vaccinations will receive consideration by a phone call to The Quarantine Service Medical
Officer, National Health and Welfare, Malton, Ontario.

Other sources of detailed information on prophylaxis for
these diseases include the report of the Committee on
Control of Infectious Diseases of The American Academy
of Pediatrics and Immunization Information for International Travel, published by The Department of Health,
Education, and Welfare, U.S. Public Health Service. (Publication 384.)

QUARANTINE REGULATIONS

Under the Public Health Act
Department of Health of Ontario

Disease	Placard	Isolation Period for Patient	Quarantine Period for Contacts
Diphtheria	Yes	2 successive negative cultures after 10 days; or if negative culture cannot be obtained, one culture must be negative on virulence test	One negative culture after contact is broken
Poliomyelitis	Yes	7 days after onset	7 days after last exposure
Meningococcal meningitis including meningococcemia	Yes	From onset of disease until 48 hr. after start of appropriate specific treatment	None
Smallpox	Yes	Until crusts have disappeared, and all lesions healed (minimum 21 days)	16 days after last contact (unless immune)
Whooping cough	No	21 days after onset	Same as patient (none if 12 yr. or over)
Measles	No	7 days after appearance of rash	None

348

Disease			
Rubella (German measles)	No	5 days after appearance of rash	None
Chickenpox [p 27]	No	Until the lesions are healed (Minimum 7 days)	None
Mumps	No	Until salivary glands are normal	None
Infectious hepatitis & Serum hepatitis	No	During 1st 2 weeks of illness and for at least one week after onset of jaundice.	None
Scarlet fever and streptococcal sore throat	No	Isolation may be terminated after 48 hr. of treatment with adequate and effective antimicrobial therapy provided such therapy is continued for 10 days. In the absence of adequate and effective antimicrobial therapy from the onset of the disease, (a) for 7 days thereafter; or (b) until the patient has no 1) sore throat or 2) oral, nasal, or aural discharges, whichever period is the longer.	None

349

BIOCHEMISTRY

Many of the 'reference values' (normal ranges) have not been determined at HSC, but are taken from the literature (e.g., *Pediatric Clinical Chemistry,* ed by S. Meites. Am. Assoc.Clin.Chem., 1977). Values were selected taking into account the similarity of the method to the one in use at HSC. These values may be inappropriate for other institutions.

References were selected by members of the Biochemistry Dept and time has not allowed their checking by staff in the appropriate specialties. The citation of references does not imply endorsement by The Hospital for Sick Children of their authors' ideas, conclusions, or treatment protocols.

Comments on the 'purpose' of tests relate to pediatric patients.

Note. Blood volumes stated are the MINIMUM required for analysis (see next page).

351

BLOOD

ALL BLOOD VOLUMES STATED ARE THE MINI-MUM REQUIRED FOR ANALYSIS. The laboratory prefers considerably more blood where possible, as separation and handling are *much more difficult* with small volumes. Amounts close to the minimum should be sent only from infants or after an unsuccessful venipuncture. Unless otherwise stated, the concentrations and activities of constituents (mg/dl, U/liter etc.) relate to values in plasma or serum obtained from the blood.

ACETAMINOPHEN (Tylenol; Paracetamol)
3 ml clotted blood. Take sample *stat*.

Purpose: Toxicology

Nomogram (p 488) relates plasma level and time after ingestion to the probable severity of hepatic damage. Take 2nd sample 3-4 h later, to determine rate of clearance. ($T_{1/2}$ = 2.0 to 2.5 in adults; slow clearance, with $T_{1/2} > 4$ h, suggests liver damage.)

Take blood for liver function tests including prothrombin time daily for 5 days after ingestion. (BMJ 2:478, 1978; Pediatrics 62, suppl:898, 1978).

ACID − BASE (blood gases)   0.4 ml heparinized blood
Ref values   (Postgrad Med 64(6):163, 1978; Med Clin N Am 62: 1223, 1978)

	pH (arterial)	*pH (venous)*
Newborn	7.33 − 7.49	− −
1 day	7.25 − 7.43	
2 d − adult	7.35 − 7.45	7.32 − 7.42
	pCO_2 (arterial)	*pCO_2 (venous)*
Birth − 2 yr	26 − 41 mm Hg	− −
2 yr − adult	33 − 46 mm Hg	40 − 50 mm Hg
(*Breathing room air) *pO_2 *(arterial)*		*pO_2 *(venous)*
Newborn	65 − 76 mm Hg	− −
Child − adult	80 − 100 mm Hg	25 − 47
	Actual Bicarbonate	*Base Excess*
Newborn	17 − 24 mmol/liter	-10 − -2 mmol/l
2 mo − 2 yr	16 − 24 mmol/liter	-7 − 0 mmol/l
Child	18 − 25 mmol/liter	-3 − +3 mmol/l
Adult	18 − 29 mmol/liter	

BLOOD

ACID PHOSPHATASE
2 ml clotted blood

Purpose
Aid to diagnosis of Gaucher's disease

Ref values (p-npp at 37°C)	Newborn	7 – 20 U/liter
	2 – 13 yr	6 – 15 U/liter
	> 13 yr	up to 11 U/liter

ACTH
By arrangement with Chemistry (special plastic tubes). 20 ml heparinized blood: take at 0900 h (on ice). **Sample is unstable: send stat – must be centrifuged in the cold immediately.**

Purpose (Rarely indicated)
1. Diagnosis and follow-up of patients with Cushing's disease (pituitary ACTH-producing tumor).
2. Evaluation of patients with melanin hyperpigmentation.

Ref value
0900 hr (diurnal variation) – children and adults: <100 pg/ml.

Note
ACTH is very high (up to 400 pg/ml) during day 1 of life; as adrenals mature, value decreases to ref value within a few weeks. For adequate interpretation of test, cortisol should be measured in same sample. In Cushing's disease, ACTH may be inappropriately high normal or slightly elevated even in presence of a high cortisol.

ACTH-STIMULATION TEST
See p 51

ALANINE AMINOTRANSFERASE (ALT), (was SGPT)
1.0 ml clotted blood

Purpose
Diagnosis of hepatobiliary disease

Ref values (at 30°C, no pyridoxal)
< 1 yr	< 35 U/liter
1 yr – adult	< 25 U/liter

ALBUMIN
0.3 ml clotted blood (sufficient for total protein and electrophoresis also, if required)

Ref values	0 – 1 yr	3.2-4.8 g/dl
	Child & adult	3.3-5.8 g/dl

BLOOD

ALCOHOL
See TOXICOLOGY, p 383

ALDOSTERONE
4 ml blood (clotted or heparinized)
1. Request Na^+ & K^+ on same sample
2. 24-hr urine collection for Na^+ excretion (p 399).

Note
Rarely indicated — less useful test than urine aldosterone, and varies widely over short periods (depends upon time of day, posture, Na^+ and K^+ intake). To demonstrate hyperaldosteronism in hypokalemic hypertension, give K^+ therapy until K^+ is in normal range before aldosterone is measured. Diuretics (e.g., furosemide, spironolactone) and several other drugs (especially purgatives, liquorice derivatives such as carbenoxolone) should be discontinued (if possible) for 3 wk before assessment. Indicate any drugs the patient may still be taking.

Ref values (BMJ 4:316, 1975)

<1 yr	Free diet; varied time of day	6 – 105 ng/dl
1 – 4 yr	Free diet; varied time of day	<34 ng/dl
5 – 15 yr	Free diet; varied time of day	<22 ng/dl
>15 yr	Normal salt; ambulant; at noon	8 – 15 ng/dl
>15 yr	Low-salt diet	20 – 44 ng/dl

ALKALINE PHOSPHATASE
0.2 ml clotted blood

Purpose
Diagnosis of liver and bone disease

Ref values (p-npp at 30°C)

Males		Females		
<1 yr	145-480	<1 yr	155-440	U/liter
1-8 yr	145-320	1-2 yr	155-415	U/liter
8-11 yr	150-380	2-8 yr	155-340	U/liter
12-15 yr	165-500	8-13 yr	135-400	U/liter
15-17 yr	90-365	13-15 yr	80-320	U/liter
17-19 yr	70-175	15-18 yr	45-120	U/liter
>19 yr	55-125	>18 yr	30-90	U/liter

BLOOD

ALKALINE PHOSPHATASE ISOENZYMES
0.3 ml clotted blood
Measured by electrophoresis.

Purpose
(Rarely indicated)

Ref values
See report form

ALPHA-FETOPROTEIN
2 ml clotted blood

Purpose
Tumor marker, especially gonadal germ-cell (J Urol 119:759, 1978; Lancet 2:1042, 1978) or primary hepatic tumor.

Ref values
Very high at birth. (Adult normal <5 ng/ml) Also raised during rapid liver regeneration: e.g., after acute hepatitis.

AMINO ACIDS, QUANTITATIVE
1.0 ml heparinized blood on ice, sent **stat** to Chemistry.

Purpose
1. Further investigation of abnormal amino-acid screen.
2. Monitoring known amino-acid disorder.

Ref values
See report form.

AMINO ACIDS, SCREEN
1.0 ml heparinized blood on ice, sent **stat** to Chemistry.

Purpose
Genetic metabolic screen.

AMINOPHYLLINE
See THEOPHYLLINE, p 381

BLOOD

AMMONIUM
By arrangement with Chemistry. 1 ml heparinized blood on ice, sent **stat.**

Purpose
1. Diagnosis of Reye's syndrome
2. Investigation of metabolic disorders that may cause encephalopathy or increase the anion gap.

Ref values

Newborn	up to 200 μmol/liter
Child & adult	up to 100 μmol/liter

AMYLASE
0.3 ml of clotted or heparinized blood

Purpose
Diagnosis of pancreatitis (J Ped 91:211, 1977) and pancreatic trauma.

Ref values
<1 yr, poorly defined; lower than in older children
1 yr — adult 60-160 Somogyi units/dl

ANDROSTENEDIONE
2 ml clotted blood

Purpose
Until puberty in females, and from about 5 mo until puberty in males, androstenedione may be considered an "adrenal-specific" androgen.

Ref values (guide only; poorly defined in children)

Males	1 – 5 mo	<80 ng/dl
	5 mo to adrenarche*	<45 ng/dl
	Adult	60 – 230 ng/dl
Females	Birth – adrenarche*	<45 ng/dl
	Adult	50 – 330 ng/dl

(values are higher during the luteal phase of the cycle than during the follicular phase, but should still be within this range).

Note
*At adrenarche, adrenal androgens start to increase in preparation for puberty; adrenarche occurs as early as 7 or 8 yr in girls and 2 yr later in boys. During adrenarche and puberty, androstenedione increases to adult levels.

BLOOD

ANTICONVULSANT DRUGS

0.2 ml heparinized or clotted blood, for one or all of the following drugs.

Take blood immediately before oral ingestion, or at least 1 hr after end of iv infusion.

	Therapeutic Level	Given po: Time taken to achieve stable level
Carbamazepine (Tegretol)	4 — 10 mg/liter	2 — 4 days
Ethosuximide (Zarontin)	40 — 100 mg/liter	7 days
Phenobarbital	15 — 35 mg/liter	14 — 21 days
Phenytoin (Dilantin)	5 — 20 mg/liter	5 — 15 days
Primidone* (Mysoline)	5 — 12 mg/liter	14 — 21 days

Primidone* is converted to phenobarbital *in vivo;* therefore, both drugs should be measured.

Note

1. **Toxic manifestations**
    a) Ethosuximide:
       — gastric upset
       — loss of appetitie
       — sedation
    b) Other agents:
       — nystagmus
       — unsteady gait
       — somnolence

2. **Oral therapy.** As serum levels become stable only after some weeks, frequent monitoring is unnecessary if toxicity is absent.

α_1-ANTITRYPSIN

1.0 ml clotted blood

Purpose

To assess possible deficiency in patients with liver disease or emphysema.
State diagnosis on requisition.

Ref value

75 — 130% of pooled normal.

See **Note,** p 358.

BLOOD

α_1-ANTITRYPSIN (cont'd)

Note

Usually, only samples with subnormal values are phenotyped. However, since α_1AT is an acute-phase reactant protein, MZ individuals may at times have normal values. If requisition gives sufficient information and there is an indication for typing, this will be done.

Type MM = normal; MS = normal variant (8% of population); MZ = heterozygous for deficiency (<2% of population); ZZ = homozygous for deficiency.

ARGININE TOLERANCE TEST
See p 48 and GROWTH HORMONE (p 370)

ASPARTATE AMINOTRANSFERASE
(AST: *was* SGOT): 0.3 ml clotted blood

Purpose

Diagnosis of cardiac and hepatobiliary disease.

Ref values		
(30°C, "optimized",	<1 yr	<67 U/liter
no pyridoxal)	1 – 10 yr	<30 U/liter
	11 – 20 yr	<25 U/liter

β_1C GLOBULIN
See C_3, p 359

BARBITURATES
See ANTICONVULSANT DRUGS (p 357) and/or TOXICOLOGY (p 383)

BICARBONATE (actual)
See ACID–BASE, p 352

BILIRUBIN – DIRECT
0.5 ml heparinized blood

Ref value

1 mo – adult	0-0.4 mg/dl

BLOOD

BILIRUBIN – TOTAL
0.3 ml blood (see GREINER GROUP OF TESTS, p 369)

Ref values	*Premature*	*Term*
Birth – 1 day	1 – 6 mg/dl*	2 – 6 mg/dl
1 – 2 days	6 – 8 mg/dl*	6 – 7 mg/dl
3 – 5 days	10 – 15 mg/dl*	4 – 12 mg/dl*
1 mo – adult	<1.0 mg/dl	

*Low birth weight increases risk of kernicterus. Approximate guide for exchange transfusion: 8 mg/dl in 800 g infant, 10 mg/dl in 1000 g infant, 12 mg/dl in 1200 g infant, etc., until 20 mg/dl for infant 2 kg and over.

BLOOD GASES
See ACID–BASE, p 352

BLOOD UREA NITROGEN
See UREA NITROGEN, p 386

BROMIDES
See TOXICOLOGY, p 383

BROMSULPHTHALEIN (BSP TEST)
See p 225

Ref value
Adult: at 45 min, retention of <5% of dose

C_3 COMPLEMENT (β_1C GLOBULIN)
1 ml clotted blood

Purpose
Investigation of complement status in immune complex diseases, especially SLE or glomerulonephritis (Clin Chem 24:7, 1978).

Ref value
100-200 mg/dl

C_4 COMPLEMENT
1 ml clotted blood

Purpose
As for C_3

Ref values
20-40 mg/dl

BLOOD

CALCITONIN
　　12 ml heparinized blood

Purpose
　　(Rarely indicated)
　　Aid to diagnosis of medullary thyroid cancer or
　　multiple endocrine adenomatosis.

CALCIUM
　　0.3 ml heparinized blood (see GREINER GROUP OF
　　TESTS, p 369) J Pediatr 88:1 (also 177), 1976

Ref values
Premature: Birth − 7 days	6.0 − 10.0 mg/dl
Term: Birth − 7 days	7.0 − 12.0 mg/dl
Child	9.0 − 11.0 mg/dl
Adult	8.5 − 10.5 mg/dl

CALCIUM − IONIZED
　　Contact Dr I.C. Radde, ext 1758

CARBAMAZEPINE (Tegretol)
　　See ANTICONVULSANT DRUGS, p 357

CARBOXYHEMOGLOBIN
　　0.5 ml heparinized blood

Purpose
　　Toxicology

CARCINO-EMBRYONIC ANTIGEN (CEA)
　　2 ml blood in EDTA tube (purple-topped Vacutainer)

Purpose
　　Pancreatic/gastro-intestinal tumor marker (not specific)

Ref value
　　Adult: <4 ng/ml

CAROTENE (precursor of Vitamin A)
　　0.5 ml clotted blood

Purpose
　　Indirect measure of intestinal absorption (of lipid-
　　soluble substances).

Ref value
　　50 − 200 μg/dl

BLOOD

CERULOPLASMIN
Contact Dr A. Sass-Kortsak, ext 1753

CHLORDIAZEPOXIDE
See TOXICOLOGY, p 383

CHLORIDE
0.3 ml heparinized blood: see GREINER GROUP OF TESTS, p 369

Ref values

Premature infants	95 – 110 mEq/liter
Term infants	96 – 106 mEq/liter
Children	99 – 111 mEq/liter
Adults	98 – 106 mEq/liter

CHOLESTEROL
0.2 ml clotted or heparinized blood
Neonates and infants: take sample before feed
Older children: after 12 h fast

Ref values

<3 months	up to 175 mg/dl
3 mo – 2 yr	up to 190 mg/dl
2 – 17 yr	115 – 205 mg/dl

Note. Range not established at HSC for current enzymatic method.

CHOLINESTERASE/PSEUDOCHOLINESTERASE
8 ml clotted blood

Purpose
Investigation of prolonged apnea after succinyldicholine (Scoline)

Ref values

Cholinesterase	620 – 1370 U/liter
Dibucaine no.	77 – 83 (heterozygote, 45-70; homozygote, 15-30)
Fluoride no.	56 – 68
Chloride no.	4 – 15
Scoline no.	87 – 92

CHORIONIC GONADOTROPIN
See HUMAN CHORIONIC GONADOTROPIN, p 370

BLOOD

COMPLEMENT
    See C$_3$, C$_4$, p 359

COMPOUND 'S'
    Not measured. See URINE 11-DEOXYCORTISOL, p 392

COPPER
    Contact Dr A. Sass-Kortsak, ext 1753

COPROPORPHYRIN
    See PORPHYRINS, p 376

CORTISOL
    0.3 ml clotted or heparinized blood

Purpose
    Investigation of adrenal glucocorticoid production

Ref values
    Poorly defined during first weeks of life.
    Children aged 1 − 17 yr in hospital:
        0800-0900 h 7 − 27 μg/dl
        2000 h   1 − 11 μg/dl*
    *<50% of the 0800 h value in 88% of cases
    Healthy adults 0800 h 7 − 19 μg/dl

Note
1. Diurnal variation of cortisol is present in many at an early age but may not develop until about 1 yr.
2. In children with Cushing's disease, values may be normal but diurnal variation may be absent.
3. Some patients with congenital adrenal hyperplasia or tumor may have steroids other than cortisol which cross-react in the assay − these patients, too, may have poor diurnal variation. Stress and shock may raise cortisol into abnormal range.
4. In suspected adrenal hypofunction, an ACTH stimulation test (p 51) is of value.

BLOOD

CREATINE KINASE (CPK)
0.2 ml clotted blood

Purpose

Diagnosis of diseases of muscle, or confirmation of myocardial damage or infarction

Ref values

Males		Females	
11 days – 1 yr	<170	11 days – 1 yr	<170 U/liter
1 – 12 yr	<110	1 – 6 yr	<100 U/liter
13 – 14 yr	<130	7 – 14 yr	<90 U/liter
15 – 16 yr	<250	15 – 16 yr	<75 U/liter
17 – 19 yr	<190	17 – 19 yr	<70 U/liter

CREATINE KINASE ISOENZYMES (CPK ISOENZYMES)
0.3 ml clotted blood

Purpose

(Rarely of value.) Measured by electrophoresis. Reported as CK_{MB} isoenzyme (heart) present or absent. Normally not detectable.

CREATININE
0.5 ml clotted or heparinized blood

Ref values

< 5 yr	<0.5 mg/dl
5 – < 6 yr	<0.6 mg/dl
6 – < 7 yr	<0.7 mg/dl
7 – < 8 yr	<0.8 mg/dl
8 – < 9 yr	<0.9 mg/dl
9 – <10 yr	<1.0 mg/dl
10+ yr	<1.2 mg/dl

Note

Excess blood ketoacids (e.g., diabetic ketoacidosis) interfere with the assay and give falsely high results.

BLOOD

CREATININE CLEARANCE

1. Timed urine collection (e.g., 24 hr)
2. 0.5 ml clotted or heparinized blood taken during urine collection
3. On requisition, state height & weight.

Ref values
Note that ref values are less well defined for clearance than for plasma creatinine

Age	Clearance (ml/min/1.73 m^2)	
Prem infant, day 3	10-23	Arch Dis Childh 49:79, 1974
Term infant, day 1	10-30 ⎫	Ibid 48:717, 1973
Term infant, day 6	15-90 ⎭	
6 mo – 2 yr comparable to adult (when corrected for surface area)		Pediatrics 58:259, 1976

	male	female	
0-9 yr	30-134	43-135 ⎫	Nouv Presse Med p. 2690,
10-19 yr	71-139	68-148 ⎭	17 Sept., 1977

Note
Some suggest that a ratio such as:

$$\frac{0.43 \times \text{height (cm)}}{\text{plasma creatinine (mg/dl)} - 0.14} \text{ (ml/min/1.73 m}^2\text{)},$$

in which the 0.14 corrects for nonspecific chromogens, may be closer to the true GFR (corrected for surface area) than the creatinine clearance. See Arch Dis Childh 51:875, 1976; Postgrad Med J 54:302, 1978.

CRYOGLOBULINS

By arrangement only. 3 ml blood taken in 37°C syringe, maintained at 37°C until delivered stat to Chemistry.

Purpose
(Rarely indicated.) Investigation of symptoms of hyperviscosity syndrome after exposure to cold. Normally, these immunoglobulins are not detectable.

BLOOD

11-DEOXYCORTISOL
> Not measured. See URINE 11-DEOXYCORTISOL,
> p 392

DEXAMETHASONE SUPPRESSION TEST
> See p 51
> Urine metabolites are *usually* measured, unless there
> are *specific* abnormalities in blood.

DIAZEPAM
> See TOXICOLOGY, p 383

DIGOXIN
> 0.5 ml clotted blood
> Take blood 6-8 h after last digoxin dose.
> Note. This assay cannot be done on blood of patients
> treated with digitoxin.

Ref values (JAMA 239: 2594, 1978)

<0.5 ng/ml	'underdigitalized'
0.5 − 2.5 ng/ml	'optimal'
2.5 − 3.0 ng/ml	'overlap'
>3.0 ng/ml	'overdigitalized' (toxic)

Note

1. The serum concentration above which 'toxicity' becomes more likely is not clearly defined and varies between individuals. In some studies, digoxin above 2.5 ng/ml or above 2.0 ng/ml was potentially toxic.
2. Premature and low-birth-weight infants appear to tolerate higher levels (but may not necessarily benefit from them). (Pediatrics 59:902, 1977; J Pediatr 93:652, 1978)
3. Renal clearance of digoxin is immature in the first 3 mo of life, and in patients with renal disease.
4. In adults, hypomagnesemia or hypo- or hyperkalemia may predispose to digoxin toxicity even when the serum digoxin is 'optimal' (Q J Med, NS 47:111, 1978).

BLOOD

DILANTIN (PHENYTOIN)
See ANTICONVULSANT DRUGS, p 357

DRUG SCREEN
See TOXICOLOGY, p 383

ELECTROLYTES
See sodium (p 379), potassium, (p 377), chloride (p 361).
0.3 ml heparinized blood.

ELECTROPHORESIS
See ALBUMIN (p 353) AND GLOBULINS (p 369)
0.3 ml clotted blood

ESTRADIOL
10 ml clotted blood

Purpose
Assessment of precocious puberty, pubertal stage; investigation of abnormal breast development in boys, ovarian function in girls.

Ref values (Am J Dis Child 132: 704, 1978)
Males: Poorly defined. Levels fall from about 10 ng/dl at birth to <2 ng/dl at 1 yr.
1 yr − adrenarche:* <2 ng/dl
Puberty: rising to adult level (<7 ng/dl)
Females: Birth − adrenarche:* as males.
Adrenarche through puberty: rising to adult levels, correlating with pubertal stage and phase of cycle.
Adult: Follicular phase 4 − 15 ng/dl
Luteal phase 10 − 40 ng/dl
Treated with synthetic estrogens <7 ng/dl

*At adrenarche, adrenal steroids start to increase in preparation for puberty.

These changes occur as early as 7 or 8 yr in girls and 1 to 2 yr later in boys. In adult females, most of the estradiol is produced by the ovaries.

ETHCHLORVYNOL
See TOXICOLOGY, p 383

ETHOSUXIMIDE (ZARONTIN)
See ANTICONVULSANT DRUGS, p 357

BLOOD

ETHYL ALCOHOL
See TOXICOLOGY, p 383

F.E.P.
See FREE ERYTHROCYTE PROTOPORPHYRIN, p 368

FERRITIN
Contact Hematology (ext 2104)

FETOPROTEIN (α-)
See ALPHA-FETOPROTEIN, p 355

FOLLICLE-STIMULATING HORMONE (FSH)
3 ml clotted blood

Purpose
Assessment of primary or secondary amenorrhea or dysmenorrhea, investigation of delayed or precocious puberty; and after LHRH stimulation (p 50) is a guide to pubertal stage.

Ref values
Males

0 – 4 mo	<30 (most below 12 U/liter)
4 mo – 2 yr	<5 U/liter
2 – 11 yr	<7 U/liter
11 yr – adult	<14 U/liter

Females

0 – 6 mo	<75 U/liter
6 mo – 2 yr	<15 (most below 10 U/liter)
2 – 10 yr	<7 U/liter

Puberty – rising to adult level (<18 U/liter)‡
(‡Includes follicular and luteal values but excludes ovulatory values [that reach 25 U/liter].)

Note

1. FSH is secreted episodically in pre- and post-pubertal subjects. Values obtained on the same normal individual on the same or different days may vary widely within the normal range.
2. For values after LHRH, see p 50 and Horm Res 8:171, 1977.

BLOOD

FREE ERYTHROCYTE PORPHYRIN (F.E.P.)
0.5 ml heparinized blood. See also PORPHYRINS, p 376

Purpose

Diagnosis of lead poisoning. (Heme is synthesized from protoporphyrin IX and iron by ferrochetalase, an enzyme readily poisoned by lead.)

In lead poisoning (also iron-deficiency and other anemias), protoporphyrin accumulates in the erythrocytes.

Ref values

up to 80 μg/100 ml of RBC

FRUCTOSE-TOLERANCE TEST
See p 59

GALACTOSEMIA SCREENING TEST *see also* Tests, Metabolic Function, p 59
0.2 ml heparinized blood.
Note. Child should have had no blood transfusion in previous 3 mo.

Purpose

Qualitative test of RBC galactose-1- phosphate uridyl transferase (in galactosemia, the enzyme is absent).

If test is abnormal, assay to quantify the enzyme is indicated.

GALACTOSE-1-PHOSPHATE URIDYL TRANSFERASE
1.0 ml heparinized blood.
Child should have had no transfusion in previous 3 mo.

Purpose

Evaluation of galactosemia screening test, or study of families with known galactosemic member(s).

Ref values

Normal*	17 – 28 U/g Hb
Galactosemia heterozygote*	8 – 12 U/g Hb
Galactosemia homozygote	0 – 3 U/g Hb

*'Duarte' variant enzyme (a normal variant) may distort these ranges (see report form).

GASES
See ACID–BASE, p 124–7, 125 (nomogram), 352

BLOOD

GLOBULIN, $\beta_1 C$
   See C_3, p 359

GLOBULINS (by electrophoresis)
   0.3 ml clotted blood. (Sufficient for albumin and total protein also)

Ref values (at HSC)

α_1	....	0.1 – 0.3 g/dl
α_2	Birth – 6 mo	0.2 – 0.7 g/dl
	>6 mo	0.4 – 1.1 g/dl
β	Birth – 6 mo	0.3 – 0.6 g/dl
	>6 mo	0.3 – 1.2 g/dl
γ	Birth	0.6 – 1.2 g/dl
	1 – 6 mo	0.2 – 0.7 g/dl
	6 mo – 2 yr	0.2 – 0.9 g/dl
	>2 yr	0.4 – 1.4 g/dl

GLUCOSE
   0.3 ml heparinized blood (see GREINER GROUP OF TESTS, below)

Ref values (fasting)

Premature infant	over 20 mg/dl
Term infant	over 30 mg/dl
Child <3 yr	40 – 90 mg/dl
Child >3 yr	50 – 110 mg/dl
Adolescent – adult	60 – 110 mg/dl

GLUCOSE-TOLERANCE TEST
   See p 53

GLUTETHIMIDE
   See TOXICOLOGY, p 383

GONADOTROPINS
   See FSH (p 367) and LH (p 373)

GREINER GROUP OF TESTS
   0.3 ml heparinized blood.

Note

   The Greiner Chemistry Analyzer is selective (i.e., it does not perform 6 analyses when only 1 has been requested, and it costs 6 times as much to perform 6 analyses). However, for *operational* reasons, the amount of blood required to perform one or all of the following analyses is the same: sodium, potassium, chloride, urea nitrogen (BUN), glucose, calcium, phosphorus, total bilirubin.

BLOOD

GROWTH HORMONE
3 ml clotted blood (sufficient also for insulin and glucose as part of stimulation test)

Purpose
Differential diagnosis of short stature (Postgrad Med 62(6):81, 1977) or slow growth, or evaluation of pituitary function.

Ref value
After stimulation (by exercise, arginine, or insulin; see p 48), peak level should exceed 5 ng/ml.
Random samples have little diagnostic value.

HEMOGLOBIN (PLASMA): HEMOLYSIS
3 ml heparinized blood

Ref value Up to 3 mg/dl

HUMAN CHORIONIC GONADOTROPIN, β SUBUNIT (HCG-Beta)
2 ml clotted blood to Chemistry.

Purpose
Diagnosis and therapeutic monitoring of certain tumors, especially gonadal germ-cell (Lancet 2:1042, 1978), hepatoblastoma.

Ref value
Normal adult: <5 mU/ml.

17-HYDROXYPROGESTERONE
3 ml clotted or heparinized blood

Purpose
Diagnosis and management of congenital adrenal hyperplasia (J Ped 88:766, 1976; J CEM 46:98, 1978).

Cord blood is unsatisfactory, and blood should not be taken for assay during the first 24 h of life. *Elevated values* (up to 40 nmol/:) occasionally in very sick neonates (stress/ACTH-mediated — cortisol >40 μg/dl), congenital adrenal hyperplasia (untreated) over 60 nmol/l and congenital adrenal hyperplasia (inadequately treated) over 30 nmol/l

Ref value
<10 nmol/liter (in most children 1-8 yr old, <4 nmol/liter).
HSC normal range (pre-1979), <15 nmol/liter
Conversion factors: ng/ml x 3 = nmol/liter
ng/dl x 0.03 = nmol/liter.

BLOOD

25-HYDROXYVITAMIN D
2 ml heparinized blood. Contact Dr G. Jones, ext 2476.

Ref values (at HSC)
Winter, 8 – 24 ng/ml
Summer, 10 – 33 ng/ml
Values exceeding these are *not diagnostic* of vitamin-D toxicity. Values below these are *not diagnostic* of deficiency. (Arch Int Med 138:836, 1978; Ann Int Med 89:966, 1978).

IMMUNOGLOBULINS
0.3 ml clotted blood

Purpose
To assess deficiency, or evaluate autoimmune disease or certain liver or GI conditions

Ref values (at HSC)

	IgG	IgA	IgM
0 – 6 mo	150 – 470	20 – 130	30 – 60 mg/dl
6 mo – 1 yr	140 – 1030	20 – 130	30 – 160 mg/dl
1 – 2 yr	280 – 960	20 – 110	30 – 150 mg/dl
2 – 5 yr	370 – 1500	30 – 200	20 – 220 mg/dl
5 – 10 yr	440 – 1550	50 – 230	30 – 170 mg/dl
>10 yr	450 – 1440	40 – 240	40 – 200 mg/dl
Adult	500 – 1200	50 – 350	30 – 230 mg/dl

INSULIN
1 ml clotted blood

Purpose
1. Differential diagnosis of repeated episodes of hypoglycemia.
2. Confirmation and assessment of response to arginine/glucose in tests of growth-hormone stimulation.
3. Insulin levels are not needed to interpret GTT for diabetes mellitus.

Ref value
Fasting: <25 mU/liter (may be higher in obese patients)
(New method: range not fully established)

BLOOD

INSULIN ANTIBODIES
20 ml heparinized blood.

Purpose
To evaluate insulin resistance in diabetes.

INSULIN-TOLERANCE TEST
See p 49; and GROWTH HORMONE, p 47, 370

IONIZED CALCIUM
Contact Dr. I.C. Radde, ext 1758

IRON
0.5 ml heparinized blood

Purpose
Assessment of anemia or iron toxicity.

Ref values

Newborn	110 − 270 μg/dl
4 mo − 1 yr	30 − 70 μg/dl
>1 yr	50 − 150 μg/dl
Toxicity (1 yr and older)	>400 μg/dl

IRON-BINDING CAPACITY (IBC)
0.5 ml heparinized blood.

Ref values

Newborn	60 − 175 μg/dl
1 yr	250 − 400 μg/dl

LACTATE
Contact Dr B. Robinson, ext 2376

Ref value
1 − 2 mmol/liter

LACTATE DEHYDROGENASE (LDH)
2 ml clotted blood.

Purpose
(Rarely indicated.) Nonspecific test.

BLOOD

LACTOSE-TOLERANCE TEST
　　See p 44

LEAD
　　0.5 ml heparinized blood. Send to Chemistry in syringe (to avoid contamination).

Ref value
　　$0 - 30$ μg/dl blood (J Pediatr 93:709, 1978)

LIPOPROTEINS
　　5 ml blood in EDTA tube (purple-topped Vacutainer). Take blood after 12-hr fast when practicable or, from neonates and infants, before feeding. Measured by electrophoresis — descriptive report.

LUTEINIZING HORMONE (LH)
　　3 ml clotted blood

Purpose
　　As FSH, p 367

Ref values (units adapted to 2nd IRP, U/liter = mU/ml)

Males		Females	
$0 - 3$ mo	<45	$1 - 6$ mo	<40 U/liter
4 mo $- 2$ yr	<13	6 mo $- 2$ yr	<14 U/liter
$2 - 6$ yr	<10	$2 - 8$ yr	<12 U/liter
$6 - 10$ yr	<14	$8 - 12$ yr	3-25 U/liter
Rising through puberty to adult values			
Adult	<30	Adult	<90*U/liter

*Includes follicular and luteal values but ovulatory values (that reach 200 U/liter) are excluded.

MAGNESIUM
　　0.5 ml heparinized blood

Ref values
Newborn	$1.5 - 2.3$ mEq/liter
Children	$1.4 - 1.9$ mEq/liter
Adults	$1.3 - 2.0$ mEq/liter

MEPROBAMATE
　　See TOXICOLOGY, p 383

MERCURY
　　See URINE MERCURY, p 394

BLOOD

METHAQUALONE
See TOXICOLOGY, p 383

METHEMOGLOBIN
5 ml heparinized blood. *Sample is unstable.*

Purpose
Diagnosis of methemoglobin reductase deficiency, methemoglobinemia, and evaluation of cyanosis after exposure to certain drugs and chemicals.

Ref value
$0 - 3\%$ of total Hb

METHYL ALCOHOL
See TOXICOLOGY, p 383

METHYPRYLON
See TOXICOLOGY, p 383

MYOGLOBIN
Rapid clearance from blood; see URINE MYOGLOBIN, p 395

MYSOLINE (PRIMIDONE)
See ANTICONVULSANT DRUGS, p 357

5'-NUCLEOTIDASE
1 ml clotted blood

Purpose
Diagnosis of hepatobiliary disease.
Relatively age-independent in children, unlike alkaline phosphatase (Arch Dis Childh 46:842, 1971).

Ref value
$0 - 14$ U/liter

OSMOLALITY
0.6 ml heparinized blood

Ref values
275-295 mOsm/kg water (may be lower in first 5 days of life).

pH; and pCO_2, pO_2
See ACID–BASE, p 352

PARACETAMOL
See ACETAMINOPHEN, p 352

BLOOD

PARATHYROID HORMONE (PTH)
7 ml heparinized blood sent **STAT** to Chemistry.

Purpose
1. Diagnosis of hyperparathyroidism or multiple endocrine adenopathies.
2. PTH is of little value in the diagnosis of hypoparathyroidism if Ca is normal.

Ref value
0 − 0.25 ng/ml

PHENOBARBITAL
See ANTICONVULSANT DRUGS, p 357

PHENYLALANINE
0.3 ml heparinized blood (preferably fasting) on ice, sent **STAT** to Chemistry.

Purpose
Diagnosis and monitoring of phenylketonuria.

Ref value
<0.11 μmol/ml

PHENYLALANINE/TYROSINE RATIO
0.3 ml heparinized blood (preferably fasting) on ice, sent **STAT** to Chemistry.

Purpose
Determination of heterozygosity for phenylketonuria.

Ref values
Normal ratio	<1.0
Equivocal	$1.0 - 1.2$
Hetero-/homozygote	>1.2

PHENYTOIN (DILANTIN)
See ANTICONVULSANT DRUGS, p 357

BLOOD

PHOSPHORUS (Inorganic)
    0.3 ml heparinized blood (see GREINER GROUP OF TESTS, p 369)

Ref values*

Birth – 1 mo	5.0 – 9.5 mg/dl
1 – 4 mo	4.8 – 8.1 mg/dl
4 mo – 1 yr	4.0 – 6.8 mg/dl
1 – 4 yr	3.6 – 6.5 mg/dl
4 – 8 yr	3.6 – 5.6 mg/dl
9 – 14 yr	3.3 – 5.3 mg/dl
15 yr+	2.7 – 4.7 mg/dl

    *Reported values vary widely, especially during first month of life (Am J Clin Path 69:24, 1978). May depend upon method of collection – capillary samples include some tissue fluid.

PI – type
    See α_1-ANTITRYPSIN, p 357

PORPHYRINS
    0.5 ml heparinized blood (see also FEP, p 368)

Purpose
    Serum/plasma porphyrins are never indicated.
    Request RBC porphyrins (FEP) only:
1. As adjunct to blood lead in diagnosis of lead poisoning.
2. In diagnosis of either congenital erythropoietic porphyria (early presentation, severe skin photosensitivity, anemia) or erythrohepatic protoporphyria (increased skin photosensitivity, no anemia, presenting in childhood onward).
Neither porphyria presents witn acute abdominal pain or neurologic features. For such patients, see URINE and FECAL porphyrins (pp 397 & 402).

Note   Further quantification of specific RBC porphyrins (copro-, uro-, proto-) is labor-intensive and of limited value. Direct measurement of RBC enzymes associated with porphyrin synthesis (Lancet 2:699, 1977) is still under development (April, 1979).

BLOOD

POTASSIUM
0.3 ml heparinized blood (See GREINER GROUP OF TESTS, p 369)

Ref values

Premature infants	4.5 – 7.2 mEq/liter
Term infants	5.0 – 7.7 mEq/liter
2 days – 2 wk	4.0 – 6.4 mEq/liter
2 wk – 3 mo	4.0 – 6.2 mEq/liter
3 mo – 1 yr	3.7 – 5.6 mEq/liter
1 – 16 yr	3.5 – 5.2 mEq/liter

PRIMIDONE (MYSOLINE)
See ANTICONVULSANT DRUGS, p 357

PROLACTIN
2 ml clotted blood

Purpose
Detection of pituitary tumors, investigation of galactorrhea or amenorrhea; assessment of pituitary function after TRH stimulation (p 50).

Ref values
1. Prolactin level very high at birth (mean, 280 ng/ml); falls to a mean of around 75 ng/ml at 4 wk; mean is within adult range by 12 or 20 wk (pre-term infants).
   Prepubertal children: Some reports state values slightly lower than in adults, and a rise to adult levels during puberty. Others report little difference between values for children and adults.
2. Adult range 0 – 30 ng/ml
3. Prolactin may also be elevated in hypothyroidism (stimulated by TRH) and renal disease, and in patients treated with certain drugs (e.g., phenothiazines, metoclopramide, methyldopa, estrogens) or for other reasons (Lancet 2:1245, 1978).

PROLONGED GLUCOSE TOLERANCE TEST
See p 53 and GROWTH HORMONE (p 370), *or* HYPOGLYCEMIA TEST: PROLONGED GTT

PROTEIN
See TOTAL PROTEIN (p 383), ALBUMIN (p 353), GLOBULINS (p 369)

BLOOD

PROTOPORPHYRIN
See PORPHYRINS, p 376

PROTOPORPHYRIN, FREE ERYTHROCYTE
See FREE ERYTHROCYTE PORPHYRIN, p 368

PSEUDOCHOLINESTERASE
See CHOLINESTERASE, p 361

PYRUVATE
Contact Dr B Robinson, ext 2376

Ref value
0.08 – 0.15 mmol/liter (venous)

RBC FEP
See FREE ERYTHROCYTE PORPHYRIN, p 368

RBC COPROPORPHYRIN
RBC PROTOPORPHYRIN } See PORPHYRINS, p 376

BLOOD

RENIN

4 ml blood in EDTA tube (purple-topped Vacutainer). Place tube in ice and send to Chemistry **STAT.**

Purpose
1. Monitoring adequacy of mineralocorticoid therapy in salt-losing congenital adrenal hyperplasia, Addison's disease, etc.
2. Differential diagnosis of hypertension. If possible, antihypertensive therapy should be stopped 3 wk before blood is taken.

Note

Normal values vary with method, Na^+ intake, time of day, posture, and age. The following are a guide only.

Ref values

	Plasma renin activity (ng/ml/h) (Normal salt intake; 9 a.m., supine, after 1-12 hr rest)
<3 mo	Wide range; values as high as 48 (particularly high in premature infants)
3 mo – 1 yr	<15 these ranges can be used for
1 – 4 yr	<10 ambulant patients, also
4 – 15 yr	< 6
Adult	< 2 (<4 at 1200 h, ambulant)

Renal-vein renins

If the renin value from one renal vein exceeds 1.5 X value in blood from contralateral vein: in >80-90% of cases, suggests a correctable lesion (BMJ 2:168, 1978).

SALICYLATE

1 ml heparinized blood.
For interpretation, see nomogram on p 485

SODIUM

0.3 ml heparinized blood (SEE GREINER GROUP OF TESTS, p 369)

Ref values

Premature infants	132 – 140 mEq/liter
Term infants	133 – 142 mEq/liter
Children	135 – 143 mEq/liter
Adults	135 – 145 mEq/liter

BLOOD

SGOT
    See ASPARTATE AMINOTRANSFERASE, p 358

SGPT
    See ALANINE AMINOTRANSFERASE, p 353

TEGRETOL (CARBAMAZEPINE)
    See ANTICONVULSANT DRUGS, p 357

TESTOSTERONE
    6 ml clotted blood

Purpose
    Assessment of precocious puberty, virilization, hirsutism, or menstrual irregularities, or (after HCG stimulation; p 54) investigation of cryptorchism.

Note
    The normal range below is a guide only. Many early studies of testosterone in children used competitive protein binding or RIA with chromatography and are not directly applicable to RIA in untreated serum

Ref values

Males

1 – 15 days	<190 ng/dl
1 – 3 mo	<350 ng/dl
3 – 5 mo	<200 ng/dl
5 – 7 mo	< 60 ng/dl
7 mo – start of puberty	< 30 ng/dl

During puberty: increases to adult values, the level relating to pubertal stage or bone age rather than chronological age.
Adult   350 – 1100 ng/dl

Females

Birth – start of puberty	<30 ng/dl
Puberty – see above	
Adult	20 – 70 ng/dl*

*May rise as high as 95 ng/dl during treatment with estrogens or progesterone. On average, levels are higher during the luteal phase of the cycle than the follicular phase.
During puberty: in girls experiencing anovulatory cycles, levels are higher but should still be within the above range.

BLOOD

THEOPHYLLINE

0.3 ml clotted or heparinized blood, taken before giving next dose.

Ref value

Therapeutic range: 5 – 20 mg/liter

THYROID ANTIBODIES

2 ml clotted blood

Purpose

Investigation of goiter, thyroid nodules, and confirmed hyper-/hypothyroidism. Normally, antithyroglobulin and antimicrosomal antibodies are absent.

THYROID-STIMULATING HORMONE (TSH)

1 ml clotted blood

Purpose

Detection of primary hypothyroidism.

After TRH stimulation (p 50) may be used in investigation of hypothalmic–pituitary function or to confirm hyperthyroidism.

Ref values

Usually <30 mU/liter in cord blood, but rises shortly after birth to peak value (may be as high as 50 mU/liter). Because of these rapid changes, TSH can be interpreted only in cord blood or in children over 4 days old.

Children older than 4 days, and adults: 10 mU/liter ($\equiv \mu$U/ml).

BLOOD

THYROXINE (T_4)
0.3 ml clotted blood

Purpose
  Diagnosis of thyroid disorders

Ref values
  0 − 3 days: levels rise shortly after birth to peak at 24 hr, then fall to 9 − 22 μg/dl at 3 days.

  Premature infants: much lower values (the more premature, the lower the value; J Pediatr 92:963, 1978).

4 days − 3 wk	8 − 19 μg/dl
3 wk − 2 mo	7 − 16 μg/dl
2 mo − 1 yr	5 − 14 μg/dl
1 yr − childhood	5 − 13 μg/dl
Adult	4 − 12 μg/dl

Note

1. *Spuriously low T_4 values:*
   a) During treatment with anticonvulsant drugs, especially diphenylhydantoin (Epilepsia 19:323, 1978).
   b) Congenital absence of thyroxine-binding globulin (TBG) − approx. 1:3000 − 14,000 of population (J Pediatr 90:264, 1977). Free T_4 (non-protein-bound) is likely to be normal. To investigate further, check TSH and T_3RU.

2. *Spuriously high T_4 values:* in patients treated with estrogens. (Check with T_3RU, p 385)

THYROXINE-BINDING GLOBULIN (TBG)
0.5 ml clotted blood

Purpose
  Confirmation of TBG deficiency suggested by abnormally low T_4 and high T_3RU in euthyroid patient.

Ref value
  10 − 28 μg/ml (adults).
  Children: slightly higher (but range ill-defined).

BLOOD

TOTAL PROTEIN
0.3 ml clotted blood (sufficient for albumin and electrophoresis, also, if required).

Ref values

0 – 6 mo	4.5 – 7.0 g/dl
6 mo – 2 yr	5.4 – 7.5 g/dl
Children & adults	5.3 – 8.5 g/dl

TOXICOLOGY (DRUG SCREEN)
8 ml clotted blood. Please indicate any substances likely to be present.

1. Qualitative tests are performed at Addicton Research Foundation as a screen (where necessary) for the following:
   barbiturates (phenobarbital: available at HSC during normal hours; see Anticonvulsant drugs, p 357)
   ethyl alcohol
   glutethimide
   iso-propyl alcohol
   meprobamate
   methaqualone
   methyl alcohol
   methyprylon
2. Salicylate: at HSC (24-hr service)
3. The following assays are labor-intensive and will be performed only upon specific request (e.g., for patient known to have had access to drug):
   bromides
   chlordiazepoxide
   diazepam
   ethchlorvynol

Note
See also TOXICOLOGY, URINE, p 399

TRH STIMULATION
See p 50

TRIGLYCERIDES
3 ml clotted or heparinized blood.

Take after 12-hr fast (where practicable); neonates and infants, before feeding.

Ref values

0 – 9 yr	30 – 100 mg/dl
10 – 19 yr	30 – 140 mg/dl

BLOOD

TRIIODOTHYRONINE (T_3) – Do not confuse with
T_3RU

0.3 ml clotted blood

Purpose

Further investigation of hyperthyroidism, detection
of T_3 toxicosis (Am J Dis Childh 132:374, 1978), and
monitoring thyroid replacement therapy in the *problem* patient.

Because of assay sensitivity, T_3 is of limited value in
hypothyroidism.

Ref values

0 – 3 days	T_3 rises rapidly after birth, from <70 ng/dl to 50 – 350 ng/dl at 3 days.
6 days – 1 yr	90 – 300 ng/dl
1 yr – childhood	90 – 270 ng/dl
Adults	90 – 220 ng/dl

Note

Spuriously low/high T_3 may be due to changes in
TBG concn or drug effects: see comments under T_4,
p 382

BLOOD

TRIIODOTHYRONINE RESIN-UPTAKE TEST (T_3RU)
Do not confuse with T_3
1 ml clotted blood

Purpose

Further investigation of abnormal thyroxine (T_4) results (*see* p 382).

At HSC this assay is done only on specific request and if the T_4 on the sample is <7 μg/dl or >11 μg/dl.

Note

No established method for reporting results; therefore, published values confusing. ('Normal mean' can be about 30% by one convention and 100% by another, and 'reduced' binding sites for T_3/T_4 may be indicated by higher or lower percentages.)

Ref values (at HSC)

Children 22 – 32%
Adults   25 – 35%

Note

In this test, a synthetic resin and T_3/T_4 binding proteins from the patient's serum compete for radioactive T_3 in a test tube.

1. T_3RU >32% indicates *fewer available* binding sites in serum, as in hyperthyroidism (sites occupied by T_4) or deficiency or thyroxine-binding globulin (TBG).

2. T_3RU <22% indicates *more available* binding sites in serum, as in hypothyroidism (little T_4 produced by thyroid to occupy available sites), estrogen therapy, or pregnancy (more TBG produced by liver).

3. Children have higher serum TBG concentrations; therefore their T_3RU values are lower than adults'.

TYLENOL
See ACETAMINOPHEN, p 352

BLOOD

UREA NITROGEN (BUN)
0.3 ml heparinized blood (see GREINER GROUP OF TESTS, p 369)

Ref values

Newborn	8 – 28 mg/dl
1 – 2 yr	5 – 15 mg/dl
2 – 16 yr	8 – 20 mg/dl

URIC ACID
0.2 ml heparinized blood

Purpose

Diagnosis of hyperuricemia: primary (e.g., gout or Lesch–Nyhan syndrome); or secondary to rapidly growing malignancy, excessive tissue breakdown (e.g., psoriasis, tissue damage, treatment of malignant tumor), or reduced excretion (e.g., acidosis or thiazide diuretics).

Ref values

Child, or adult female	2.0 – 6.0 mg/dl
Adult male	3.0 – 7.0 mg/dl

UROPORPHYRIN
See PORPHYRINS, p 376

VITAMIN A
0.5 ml clotted blood (fasting).

Purpose

Assessment of deficiency; otherwise, see CAROTENE (p 360)

Ref value

20 – 60 μg/dl

VITAMIN D
See 25-HYDROXYVITAMIN D, p 371 (Vitamin D, also, may be available in special circumstances)

VITAMIN E
Contact Haematology, ext 2104

BLOOD

XYLOSE TEST
0.6 ml heparinized or clotted blood.

Purpose
Investigation of intestinal absorption of xylose. See also p 44

Note
At either 30 or 60 min after a dose of 14.5 g/m^2, plasma xylose over 20 or 25 mg/dl suggests normal absorption. (Still a rather controversial field; see Arch Dis Childh 53: 420, 1978; J Pediatr 92:725, 1978; J Pediatr 92:729, 1978.)

ZARONTIN (ETHOSUXIMIDE)
See ANTICONVULSANT DRUGS, p 357

ZINC
0.5 ml heparinized* blood

Purpose
Diagnosis of deficiency in patients at risk (GI and renal disease) or who have signs of acrodermatitis enterohepatica.

Ref values
0 – 1 yr	75 – 145 μg/dl
2 – 10 yr	70 – 130 μg/dl
11 – 18 yr	65 – 125 μg/dl
Adult	60 – 120 μg/dl

*Values for serum are approx. 15% higher than for plasma.

URINE

Timed Collection (24 hr)

Although "24-hr collection" is frequently requested, and the urinary excretion of some substances (especially steroids) is subject to diurnal variation, it is seldom essential that the collection be exactly 24 hr. However, **it is essential to record accurately the start and stop times,** so the actual duration can be determined.

1. At START time: the patient voids, the time is recorded, and the urine is discarded.
2. *ALL* urine produced after this time is saved.
3. At STOP time: the patient voids, the time is recorded, and this last specimen is included.

With present methods, the patients need not be on any special diet for most of the urine collections.

(*exception:* aldosterone – Na^+ intake should be controlled; (*see* below).

Note: Organize urine collection to avoid periods during and for 6 hr after renal, bone, or gallium scans (such urine is radioactive and is hazardous to ward and biochemistry staff) and IVP (there may be interference by the contrast medium, or stress-induced changes in urine chemistry).

ALDOSTERONE
24-hr. No preservative; keep specimen cool.

Note
1. Request also: urine Na^+, plasma Na^+, and plasma K^+.
2. Urine aldosterone is less variable than plasma.
3. Avoid (where possible) drugs listed under BLOOD ALDOSTERONE, p 354. Note on requisition any drug being taken or recently discontinued.
4. Correct hypokalemia before aldosterone assay, and control Na^+ intake (see p 328).
5. At HSC, value reported as 'urine aldosterone' is 'pH 1' aldosterone (3-oxoconjugated + free – excludes tetrahydroaldosterone). Urinary aldosterone excretion cannot be equated with 'aldosterone secretion rate', because much of the aldosterone secreted is excreted as tetrahydroaldosterone.

Nomogram (p 389) relates urinary aldosterone/24 hr (corrected for surface area) to urine sodium. (See p 399 and Ped Clin N Am 25:67, 1978).

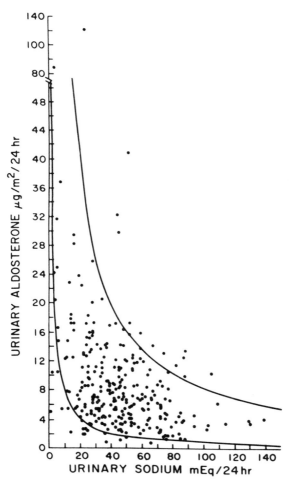

Ratio of daily aldosterone excretion to surface area is plotted against sodium excretion in 60 normal children, aged 1 mo to 17.5 yr (283 determinations). The hyperbolas indicate the 5th and 95th percentiles (*From* New, M.I., *et al.,* Am J Cardiol *37:*658, 1976, with permission.)

URINE

AMINO ACIDS, QUANTITATIVE
> 10 ml random specimen. Keep it cool.

Purpose
> Further investigation of abnormal screen. Usually less informative than blood amino acids.

Ref value
> See report form

AMINO ACIDS, SCREEN
> See METABOLIC STUDY, p 394

AMITRIPTYLINE
> See TOXICOLOGY, p 399

AMPHETAMINE
> See TOXICOLOGY, p 399

AMYLASE
> 24-hr. No preservative

Ref value
> <260 Somogyi U/hr

BARBITURATES
> See TOXICOLOGY, p 399

BILIRUBIN
> Random specimen. Assayed qualitatively with Icto-test tablets.

CADMIUM
> 24-hr; in acid-washed bottle.

**CATECHOLAMINES
(NOREPINEPHRINE + EPINEPHRINE)**
> 24-hr. Preservative: hydrochloric acid

Purpose & Comments
> As VMA (p 400) but less sensitive than VMA in the diagnosis of neuroblastoma. Also, the assay is more subject to interference than VMA or HVA.

Ref value*

<1 yr	<20 μg/24 hr
1 – 5 yr	<40 μg/24 hr
6 – 15 yr	<82 μg/24 hr
Adult	<100 μg/24 hr

*Alternative set of values, see J Pediatr 93:266, 1978.

URINE

CODEINE
See URINE TOXICOLOGY, p 399

COMPOUND 'S'
See 11-DEOXYCORTISOL, p 392

COPPER
Contact Dr A. Sass-Kortsak, ext 1753

COPROPORPHYRIN
See PORPHYRINS, p 397

CORTISOL (urine 'free' cortisol)
24-hr; no preservative

Purpose
1. To test for excess cortisol production.
2. To assess efficacy of therapy for Cushing's disease.

Note
Normally, the free (non-protein-bound) fraction of plasma cortisol is a very small part of total. This 'free' fraction passes into the glomerular filtrate; a fairly constant proportion is not re-absorbed and is excreted in the urine. When the fine control of cortisol production is disturbed, urine free cortisol increases.

Ref value*
4 mo – 10 yr
<27 μg/24 hr (35 – 176 μg/g creatinine)
11 – 20 yr: <55 μg/24 hr (<44 μg/g creatinine)
Adult: 18 – 98 μg/24 hr (13-60 μg/g creatinine)

*Alternatively,
4 – 12 yr
40 – 110 μg/g creatinine (J C E M 36:702, 1973)

CREATININE CLEARANCE
See p 35
See also BLOOD, CREATININE CLEARANCE, p 364

URINE

11-DEOXYCORTISOL
24-hr: no preservative.

Purpose
Diagnosis and follow-up of congenital adrenal hyperplasia (11-β-hydroxylase type)

Ref value
(as tetrahydro derivative)
Poorly defined in infants.
3 − 22 yr: up to 0.5 mg/m^2/24 hr

Note
Most (but not all) patients with this form of adrenal hyperplasia have hypertension. In early life, affected patients may excrete normal amounts of this steroid. ACTH stimulation for 3 days may be of value in assessing equivocal cases.

DEXAMETHASONE SUPPRESSION TEST
See p 51

DINITROPHENYL HYDRAZINE (DNPH) TEST
See METABOLIC STUDY, pp 33, 394

ETHCHLORVYNOL
See TOXICOLOGY, p 399

GLYCOSAMINOGLYCURONOGLYCANS
See MUCOPOLYSACCHARIDES, p 395

GONADOTROPINS
Not available. See BLOOD FSH (p 367) and LH (p 373)

HEMOGLOBIN
Random specimen. Qualitative (dipstick) test. If positive, concn will be determined.

URINE

HOMOVANILLIC ACID (HVA)
24-hr. Preservative: hydrochloric acid

Purpose & Note

As VMA. HVA is of little help in diagnosing pheo-chromocytoma.

Ref value*

<1 yr	<35 mg/g creatinine
1 – 2 yr	<23 mg/g creatinine
2 – 5 yr	<14 mg/g creatinine
5 – 10 yr	<9 mg/g creatinine
10 – 15 yr	<12 mg/g creatinine
Adult	<9 mg/g creatinine

*Alternative ref value, see J Pediatr 93:266, 1978.

17-HYDROXYSTEROIDS
24-hr, no preservative

Purpose

Investigation of adrenal hyperfunction – 17-hydroxysteroids are urinary metabolites of glucocorticoids. For dexamethasone-suppression test, see p 51.

Note

1. Test is of no value in patient receiving steroids other than dexamethasone.
2. In 11-hydroxylase deficiency (rare form of congenital adrenal hyperplasia) and in cases of adrenal tumor, other steroids may contribute to the 17-hydroxysteroid fraction.
3. Obese individuals may excrete excess 17-hydroxysteroids.
4. This test is less satisfactory than urine free cortisol in detection of Cushing's disease.

Ref value

0 – 1 yr	<2.0 mg/24 hr
1 – 2 yr	0.5 – 2.5 mg/24 hr
2 – 4 yr	1.0 – 4.0 mg/24 hr
4 – 6 yr	1.0 – 4.8 mg/24 hr
6 – 8 yr	1.0 – 5.6 mg/24 hr
8 – 10 yr	1.0 – 7.0 mg/24 hr
10 – 12 yr	1.5 – 8.0 mg/24 hr
>12 yr	2.0 – 10.0 mg/24 hr

KETONES
Qualitative test only

URINE

17-KETOSTEROIDS
24-hr; no preservative

Purpose
Investigation of precocious puberty, virilization, hirsutism. 17-ketosteroids are urinary metabolites of adrenal androgens (in adult males, as much as 33% of total ketosteroids may be from the testis).

Ref value

0 – 14 days	<2.5 mg/24 hr
14 days – 2 yr	<0.5 mg/24 hr
2 – 3 yr	<1 mg/24 hr
3 – 8 yr	<2 mg/24 hr

Then, gradual increase to adult values.

Adult male 9 – 22 *Adult female* 6 – 15 mg/24 hr

For values after dexamethasone-suppression test, see p 51

LEAD
Use blood-lead value to diagnose lead toxicity. Urine-lead of diagnostic value only after administration of chelating agent to patient with borderline blood lead.

MERCURY
24-hr collection preferred. Specimen must be collect-ted in acid-washed bottle.
Toxicity: 24-hr, >80 μg/24 hr
Random specimen, >80 μg/liter
Normally, much lower than this, but dental fillings may elevate value to this level.

METABOLIC STUDY
Random specimen of urine

Purpose
The following screening tests are performed to detect metabolic disease:

1. Two-dimensional amino acid chromatography
   Aminoaciduria

2. Cyanide nitroprusside test
   Cystinuria, homocystinuria, glutathionemia, certain defects of tubule-transport

3. DNPH test
   Detects ketoacids in cases of PKU, MSUD, methionine malabsorption, tyrosinemia.

   Note. Also detects ketones found in normal subjects after prolonged fast.

394

URINE

METANEPHRINES
(METANEPHRINE + NORMETANEPHRINE)
24-hr. Preservative: hydrochloric acid

Purpose
>   Adjunct to VMA test in diagnosis of pheochromo-
>   cytoma. See VMA, p 400

Ref value

<2 yr	<4.6 mg/g creatinine
2 – 10 yr	<3 mg/g creatinine
10 – 15 yr	<2 mg/g creatinine
Adult	<1 mg/g creatinine

METHADONE
>   See TOXICOLOGY, p 399

METHAMPHETAMINE
>   See TOXICOLOGY, p 399

MORPHINE
>   See TOXICOLOGY, p 399

MUCOPOLYSACCHARIDES
(MPS: GLYCOSAMINOGLYCURONOGLYCANS)
24-hr

Ref value
>   Up to 20 mg/24 hr (expressed as hexuronic acid).

Note
>   A normal result does *not* rule out *all* mucopolysac-
>   charidoses.

MYOGLOBIN
>   Random specimen.
>   Rarely indicated.
>   Reacts like Hb by dipstick. If positive, confirmation
>   (differentiation from Hb) and quantification are
>   available.

NITROPRUSSIDE TEST
>   See METABOLIC STUDY, p 394

ORGANIC ACIDS
>   Random specimen; ideally, collected when child is
>   most ill. Keep specimen cool.

Purpose
>   Further investigation when abnormal results of
>   metabolic study.

URINE

OSMOLALITY
Random specimen.

Ref value
Infant
50 – 600 mOsm/kg water
Child & adult: maximum (dehydration):
800 – 1400 mOsm/kg water
Child & adult: minimum (water diuresis):
40 – 80 mOsm/kg water

OXALATE
24-hr. Preservative: hydrochloric acid

Purpose
Diagnosis of primary oxaluria; monitoring excess oxalate excretion in disease of terminal ileum.

Ref value
Adults: up to 50 mg/24 hr

PBG SCREEN
See PORPHYRINS, p 397

PHENCYCLIDINE
PHENOTHIAZINE } See TOXICOLOGY, p 399

PHOSPHOETHANOLAMINE
24-hr

Purpose
Adjunct in diagnosis of hypophosphatasia.

Ref value
See report form

URINE

PORPHYRINS
1. Random **fresh** specimen (20 ml) for screening tests for porphobilinogen (PBG) and porphyrins.
2. 24-hr collection (kept cool in dark) for quantifying PBG.
3. 24-hr collection (sodium carbonate preservative) for quantifying uro-, proto-, and coproporphyrins.

Purpose
Diagnosis of hepatic porphyrias.

Note
1. Screening tests are of value *only during acute attack.*
2. If result of screening abnormal: 24-hr collection for appropriate quantification.
3. Acute intermittent porphyria: urine PBG, by quantification, may be increased between *(as well as during)* attacks.
4. Porphyrias characterized by acute episodes: attacks usually precipitated by drugs (e.g., barbiturates, estrogens, sulfonamides).
5. Porphyrinuria may occur in lead poisoning, liver disease, and conditions of increased erythropoiesis.
6. *See also* PORPHYRINS in BLOOD (p 376) and FECES (402)

Ref value
In adults (ranges poorly defined in children)

Coproporphyrin	$0 - 250 \ \mu g/24$ hr
Protoporphyrin	not detected
Uroporphyrin	$0 - 30 \ \mu g/24$ hr
Porphobilinogen (PBG)	$0 - 3000 \ \mu g/24$ hr

POTASSIUM
Varies widely, depending upon intake.

URINE

PREGNANETRIOL
24-hr; no preservative

Purpose
Diagnosis and management of congenital adrenal hyperplasia (21-hydroxylase deficiency). Urinary metabolite of 17-hydroxyprogesterone.

Note
Test unhelpful in first week(s) of life, because of immature hepatic metabolism of 17-hydroxyprogesterone (Pediatrics 49:198, 1972).

Ref value
3 wk – 6 yr	<0.5 mg/24 hr
6 – 16 yr	<1.1 mg/24 hr
Adult	<3.5 mg/24 hr

PRE-OP URINE
Random specimen

Purpose
Qualitative (dipstick) test for protein, glucose, blood, pH, and ketones.

PROPOXYPHENE
See TOXICOLOGY, p 399

PROTEIN (QUANTITATIVE)
24-hr or other timed sample.

Ref value (approx.)
Over 1 yr <100 mg/m²/24 hr

PROTOPORPHYRIN
See PORPHYRINS, p 397

REDUCING SUBSTANCES
Random specimen.
Qualitative test (Clinitest tablet): detects reducing substances (e.g., glucose, galactose, fructose, lactose, pentoses, homogentisic acid), most of which are not detected by glucose-specific dipsticks (e.g., Clinistix).

ROUTINE URINE
Random specimen (**NOT** available *stat*).

Purpose
As pre-op (above); also, microscopy for casts, cells, crystals, bacteria, and mucin.

URINE

SODIUM
24 hr; no preservative.

Ref value

Infant: $6 - 10$ mEq/m² of body surface
(approx. $0.3 - 3.5$ mEq/24 hr)
Child: $40 - 180$ mEq/24 hr
Adult: $80 - 200$ mEq/24 hr

Urinary Na⁺ excretion should be appropriate in relation to serum Na⁺ level.

SPECIFIC GRAVITY
Random specimen. Assayed by refractometry.

Ref value

After fluid-deprivation: Children >6 mo & adults: >1.020

TOXICOLOGY (DRUG SCREEN)
Random specimen, 50 ml
See TOXICOLOGY (BLOOD), p 383

Screen: amphetamine, barbiturates, codeine, methadone, methamphetamine, morphine, phenothiazine

Special request: amitriptyline, ethchlorvynol, phencyclidine, propoxyphene

UROBILIN
Random specimen
(oxidation product of urobilinogen)

UROBILINOGEN
Random fresh specimen (urobilinogen is unstable).

Purpose

Qualitative test.
1. Absent in complete biliary obstruction.
2. Increased in severe hemolytic jaundice and some liver disorders.

UROPORPHYRIN
See PORPHYRINS, p 397

URINE

VANILMANDELIC ACID (VMA)
24 hr. Preservative: hydrochloric acid

Purpose
Diagnosis and management of patients with neural-crest tumors (neuroblastoma, pheochromocytoma)

Note
1. Neuroblastoma: 80% of patients have VMA values 2 – 10 times normal.
2. VMA may be nonspecifically elevated (occasionally to more than twice normal) in fever, asthma, chronic anemia, or after surgery.
3. Method at HSC is unaffected by diet, but (if possible) patient should be off all drugs — especially methyldopa — 4 days before and during urine collection.

Ref value*

Up to 1 mo	$<180\ \mu g/kg/24\ hr$
1 mo – 2 yr	$<230\ \mu g/kg/24\ hr$
over 2 yr	$<150\ \mu g/kg/24\ hr$

*Alternative set of values; see J Pediatr 93:266, 1978.

FECES

CHYMOTRYPSIN

Random specimen, minimum approx. 10 g. Keep specimen cool. May also be part of collection for fecal fat (*below*)

Purpose

Crude guide to pancreatic function: e.g., in cystic fibrosis.

Ref value (37°C ATEE substrate) 30 − 750 U/g

COPROPORPHYRIN

See PORPHYRINS, p 402

FAT

Complete 3- or 5-day collection, with patient eating diet of known fat content.

Purpose

Assessment of fat absorption.

Ref values	Fecal fat
Premature infants	<20% of intake
Term infants	<15% of intake
>3 mo	<10% of intake

OCCULT BLOOD

Random specimen

FECES

PORPHYRINS

Random specimen, *minimum* 20 g. Keep specimen cool.

Purpose

Diagnosis of porphyrias (Practitioner 221:219, 1978; Lancet 2:1036, 1977).

Normal in acute intermittent porphyria or cutaneous hepatic porphyria (cutanea tarda, or acquired type).

Most useful diagnostically in porphyria variegata (protocoproporphyria, or 'South African type') or hereditary coproporphyria: both may present with skin photosensitivity or acute abdominal pain and/or neurologic symptoms.

Unless there are strong indications for quantification, only a screening test will be performed; if abnormal result, sample will be quantified.

See also PORPHYRINS in BLOOD (p 376) and URINE (p 397).

Ref values

(in adults — poorly defined in children)

Coproporphyrin $<700 \mu g/100$ g *wet* weight
Protoporphyrin $<1500 \mu g/100$ g *wet* weight

Note. Fecal porphyrin may be elevated after upper GI bleeding.
Coproporphyria: Q J Med 46:229, 1977
Variegata: Am J Med 65:80, 1978
Erythropoietic protoporphyria: N Eng J Med 297:98, 1977

PROTOPORPHYRIN

See PORPHYRINS, above

TRYPSIN

Enzyme unstable. Test not available.

UROPORPHYRIN

See PORPHYRINS, above

CEREBROSPINAL FLUID

CHLORIDE
Of no diagnostic value — merely reflects plasma Cl

GLUCOSE
0.1 ml fresh CSF

Purpose
Adjunct to bacteriologic investigation of CSF.
Glucose decreased if metabolized by leukocytes, bacteria or cancer cells in CSF.
Normal in meningitis or encephalitis due to viruses.

Ref value
When blood glucose is normal: 37 – 64 mg/dl

IMMUNOGLOBULIN G (IgG)
See PROTEIN (*below*)

PROTEIN
0.3 ml CSF

Purpose
1. Adjunct to bacteriologic investigation of CSF. Protein increased if blood or pus present and in nonpurulent cerebral inflammation (e.g., tuberculous or syphilitic meningitis, multiple sclerosis, polyneuritis). Usually very high (>500 mg/dl) if spinal canal blocked.
2. CSF protein electrophoresis is of little diagnostic value. CSF IgG may be of value in diagnosing multiple sclerosis, etc. (Neurology 28:988, 1978).

Ref values

	CSF Total Protein	CSF IgG
Premature neonate	15 – 130 mg/dl	Normal = <10% of CSF total protein
Term neonate	40 – 120 mg/dl	
Up to 1 mo	20 – 70 mg/dl	
>1 mo	15 – 40 mg/dl	

GASTRIC CONTENTS

TOXICOLOGY
See TOXICOLOGY, URINE (p 399) for tests available.

PANCREATIC FLUID

PANCREATIC STIMULATION TEST (p 44)
See report form

SWEAT

SWEAT CHLORIDE
Determined in Chemistry by appointment.

Purpose
Diagnosis of cystic fibrosis.

Policy at HSC
1. Stimulate sweating by pilocarpine; measure by chloride-specific electrode.
2. If Cl^- <30 mEq/liter: result is normal and no further test is performed.
3. If Cl^- >30 mEq/liter: a second test is performed, with sweat collected after urocholine injection, and Cl^- is accurately quantified.

Ref values
Test result unreliable in first few days of life.
3 days – 20 yr: value consistently >60 mEq/liter is virtually diagnostic of CF.

Note
1. If strong clinical suspicion of CF, repeat testing is recommended.
2. Sweat chloride may be erroneously elevated in other conditions (e.g., malnutrition, edema, diabetes insipidus, glucose-6-phosphatase deficiency, adrenal insufficiency, ectodermal dysplasia, and hypothyroidism).
3. Cloxacillin falsely lowers sweat Cl.

PHARMACOPEIA

Notes to Prescribers

All prescriptions should be written clearly in INK, using the metric system and approved abbreviations only. The use of apothecary symbols is not permitted in this hospital.

Calculations

The most reliable method to calculate a therapeutic dose is according to body surface area (mg/m^2), but this is not always convenient or easily calculated. Catzel's percentage method correlates age and weight to a percentage of the adult dose. The accompanying table, adapted from Catzel's method, can be applied when the adult dose is known — **do not use for newborn infants.**

Age	Average Weight (kg)	Dose as Percentage of Adult Dose
2 wk +	3.2	12
4 mo	6.5	20
1 yr	10	25
3 yr	15	33
7 yr	23	50
12 yr	37	75
Adult	66	100

IMPORTANT: Remember that fat plays little part in drug metabolism; so, in the obese, avoid overdosage of required medication.

MAXIMAL DOSE IS GIVEN IN RED

ANTIBIOTIC AND CHEMOTHERAPEUTIC AGENTS

PENICILLINS (General Notes)

1. There is cross allergenicity among all the penicillins.
2. A maximum of 0.5 g/kg/day (750,000 U/kg/day) should rarely be exceeded.
3. About 2.5 mEq of Na or K (5.2 mEq with ticarcillin) is contained in each gram or 1.5 mega units of the corresponding salt of the penicillin used.
4. The intrathecal dose is 7 mg daily (10,000 units) – rarely necessary.
5. Probenecid (20 mg/kg stat, then 10 mg/kg q6h) usually prolongs levels for 2 hr and increases levels 1½ to 5 times.
6. Doses in brackets are the usual therapeutic ones but may be exceeded when special concentration barriers must be overcome; e.g., in meningitis.

Drug	po	im	iv	Notes
benzyl penicillin (G) aqueous soln of Na salt	–	25,000 to 50,000 U/kg/day divided q4 to q6h. 600,000 U/kg/day	As for im. Use Na salt (K salt is toxic in high dosage)	For extremely high dosage use Na salt (1 μg = approx 1.5 U).
procaine penicillin	–	25,000 to 50,000 U/kg/day divided q12 to 24h	–	Low prolonged level. Adequate for very sensitive bacteria only. Caution – not iv (procaine sensitivity)

MAXIMAL DOSAGES ARE PRINTED IN RED

Drug	po	im	iv	Notes
benzathine penicillin	—	600,000 U q12 days 1,200,000 U q28 days	—	Low prolonged level. Adequate, especially for prophylaxis v highly sensitive bacteria.
phenoxymethyl penicillin (V)	10 mg/kg/dose q4h or 15 mg/kg/dose q6h	—		Absorption variable (but better than absorption of penicillin G). Give ½ hr before food.
ampicillin	—	100 to 400 mg/kg/day divided q6h	100 to 400 mg/kg/day divided q6h	Same Gram-positive but more Gram-negative activity than penicillin G, especially v *Haemophilus influenzae*. Inactive v penicillin-resistant staphylococci.

MAXIMAL DOSAGES ARE PRINTED IN RED

Drug	po	im	iv	Notes
amoxycillin	50 to 100 mg/kg/day divided q6 to 8h	–	–	Well absorbed orally. Ampicillin spectrum.
ticarcillin	–	–	150 to 300 mg/kg/day divided q6h	Contains 5.2 mEq Na/g. Active v *Pseudomonas aeruginosa*. Caution – Inhibition of platelet aggregation may result in prolonged bleeding time.
cloxacillin	50–100 mg/kg/day divided q6h	100–200 mg/kg/day divided q6h	100–200 mg/kg/day divided q6h	Oral penicillin active v penicillin-resistant staphylococci. iv 5% aqueous solution slowly into tubing – not bottle.

MAXIMAL DOSAGES ARE PRINTED IN RED

Drug	po	im	iv	Notes
methicillin	—	100 to 300 mg/kg/day divided q6h	100 to 300 mg/kg/day divided q4 to 6h	Active v penicillin-resistant staphylo-cocci. Unstable in acid solution iv – 1 g/20 ml distilled water, slowly into iv tubing – not bottle. High dose for major staphylo-coccal disease. Low dose for premature infants, neonates. High doses may cause hematuria.
nafcillin			100 to 200 mg/kg/day divided q4 to q6h	Active v penicillin-resistant staphylo-cocci. Metabolized by the liver.
ticarcillin, see p 408				

MAXIMAL DOSAGES ARE PRINTED IN RED

CEPHALOSPORINS (General Notes)

1. A few children allergic to penicillins are allergic to cephalosporins also.
2. Cephalosporins are active against penicillin-resistant staphylococci.

Drug	po	im	iv	Notes
cephalothin	—	50 to 200 mg/kg/day divided q6h	50 to 200 mg/kg/day divided q6h	May cause false positive test for proteinuria. Painful by im route.
cephalexin	25 (50) to 100 mg/kg/day divided q6h	—	—	—
cefazolin	—	50 to 100 mg/kg/day divided q6h. 150 mg/kg/day	50 to 100 mg/kg/day divided q6h. 150 mg/kg/day	—

MAXIMAL DOSAGES ARE PRINTED IN RED

Drug	po	im	iv	Notes
OTHER ANTIBIOTIC AGENTS				
chloramphenicol	50 to 100 mg/kg/day divided q6 – 8h. (base) 4 g/day	—	50 to 100 mg/kg/day divided q8h. (succinate salt) 4 g/day	Watch WBC count. Dose for premature infants not above 25 mg/kg/day; for neonates not above 50 mg/kg/day.
clindamycin	15 mg/kg/day	25 to 50 mg/kg/day divided q6 – 8h	As for im	For im/iv, use phosphate salt. Watch for diarrhea (colitis).
erythromycin estolate	30 to (40) to 80 mg/kg/day divided q6h	—	—	Oral – best before meals.

MAXIMAL DOSAGES ARE PRINTED IN RED

Drug	po	im	iv	Notes
gentamicin	—	5 to (7.5) to 10 mg/ kg/day divided q8 to 12h. 250 mg/day	5 to (7.5) to 10 mg/kg/day divided q8 to q12h. 250 mg/day	iv – infuse each dose in not less than 30 min. Use high doses for meningitis. Monitor serum levels where indicated, especially in premature infants and newborns.
nitrofurantoin	6 to 10 mg/kg/day divided q6h. 0.4 g/day	—	—	Give with food or milk (nausea). Drug rash. Watch WBC count. Avoid in oliguria and renal failure (renal damage). Acid urine best. Pulmonary hypersensitivity.

MAXIMAL DOSAGES ARE PRINTED IN RED

Drug	po	im	iv	Notes
neomycin	100 mg/kg/day divided q4 to 8h for 3 days (not absorbed). 3 g/day	Not advised	—	Some absorption.
rifampin	20 mg/kg/day divided q12h for 2 days	—	—	Turns urine orange-red. Meningococcal contacts.
sulfonamides (sulfisoxazole)	120 mg/kg/day divided q6h. 4.0 g/day	—	120 mg/kg/day divided q4 to 6h. 4.0 g/day	Initial loading dose may be 60 mg/kg. For iv – up to 25 mg/ml of soln. Alkalinize urine and give adequate fluids Watch urine. Watch WBC count.

MAXIMAL DOSAGES ARE PRINTED IN RED

413

Drug	po	im	iv	Notes
trimethoprim/ sulfamethoxazole	8 mg trimethoprim 40 mg sulfamethoxazole divided q12h } /kg/day	—	—	Higher doses needed for *Pneumocystis carinii* infection and meningitis. Prolonged therapy with high doses may depress bone marrow. Folinic acid will prevent or reverse this. Monitor WBC count.
tetracycline (many preparations)	20 to 40 mg/kg/day divided q6h. 2 g/day	10 to 12 to 20 mg/kg/day divided q12h. 1 g/day	10 to 12 to 20 mg/kg/day divided q12h. 1 g/day	Administration in first decade may stain permanent teeth. Alternative preparations offer minimal advantages.
vancomycin	—	—	40 mg/kg/day divided q12h. 2 g/day	Dilute to 0.5% soln or less, in 5% glucose or isotonic saline. Inject in 20 min. Phlebitis, occasional rash. Caution in impaired renal function (deafness).

MAXIMAL DOSAGES ARE PRINTED IN RED

Drug	po	im	iv	Notes
metronidazole	10 mg/kg/day divided q8h	—	—	Avoid alcohol. Peripheral neuropathy with prolonged and high doses.
	ANTI-FUNGAL AGENTS			
nystatin	500,000 Uq6 – 8h (not absorbed)	—	—	—
griseofulvin	15 to 25 mg/kg/day q6 to 24h. 1 g/day	—	—	Prolonged therapy
5-fluorocytosine	100 – 200 mg/kg/day divided q6h	—	—	Caution – Reduce dose in impaired renal function.

MAXIMAL DOSAGES ARE PRINTED IN RED

Drug	po	im	iv	Notes
amphotericin B	—	—	0.25 to 1.0 mg/kg/day, 1.5 mg/kg/day	Use only where indications and conditions well-controlled. Dose adjusted gradually step-wise to maximum permissible. Toxicity – headache, nausea, fever, low K^+, rise in NPN and BUN. Prepare a 5 mg/ml solution with distilled water. Dilute further to final concentration of 0.1 mg/ml in 500 ml using 5% dextrose (or 5% buffered dextrose if pH of dextrose soln is below 4.2).

ANTITUBERCULOUS AGENTS, see p 183

MAXIMAL DOSAGES ARE PRINTED IN RED

FORMULARY

DRUG	DOSAGE	SUPPLIED	
acetaminophen			
Tempra	Under 1 yr	27 mg (0.3 ml) q8h	Drops	54 mg/0.6 ml
			Syrup	108 mg/5 ml
Tylenol	1 to 3 yr	60 to 120 mg/dose	Tablets	325 mg
	3 to 6 yr	120 mg/dose	Drops	60 mg/0.6 ml
	6 to 12 yr	240 mg/dose	Elixir	120 mg/5 ml
	Over 12 yr	325 mg/dose		
	Single dose: repeat q4-6h			

MAXIMAL DOSAGES ARE PRINTED IN RED

acetazolamide

Diamox	Diuretic (single daily dose):	Capsules, slow-release	500 mg
	po or im, 5 mg/kg/24h	Tablets	250 mg
	Epilepsy or glaucoma:	Vials	500 mg
	po, 8 to 30 mg/kg/24h in divided doses		
acetylsalicylic acid (A.S.A.; Aspirin)	po: 65 mg/kg/24h in divided doses q4 to 6h	Tablets	75, 300 mg
	pr: 105 mg q6h	Enteric-coated tabs	300, 600 mg
	Avoid overdosage	Suppositories	105 mg (infants)
	Salicylate intoxication		320 mg (adults)
	Rheumatic fever		

MAXIMAL DOSAGES ARE PRINTED IN RED

Adrenalin (p 440)

adrenocorticotropic hormone

(ACTH)	1 U = 1 mg. im or iv 1.6 U/kg/24h in divided doses	Ampules (aqueous)	25 U
Cortrosyn (short-acting) synthetic	im or iv	Vials	0.25 mg as powder (and diluent)
Duracton (long-acting)	im or subcutaneously 0.8 U/kg/24h as single dose	Vials	40 U/ml
Aldactone (p 461)			
Aldomet (p 449)			
aluminum hydroxide			
Amphogel	5-10 ml, or ½ to 1 tablet, 5 or 6 times daily and at bedtime	Suspension	300 mg/5 ml
		Tablets	600 mg

MAXIMAL DOSAGES ARE PRINTED IN RED

419

allopurinol			
Zyloprim	po: 10-15 mg/kg/day in 3 divided doses	Tablets	100 mg
Alupent (p 452)			
amethopterin			
Methotrexate (p 212)		Tablets	2.5 mg
		Vials	5 , 50 mg
aminophylline (p 187)			
	Slow infusion over at least 20 min.	Ampules	250 mg/10 ml
	iv: 4-7 mg/kg/dose q6h	Tablets	100 mg
	po: 5-7 mg/kg/dose q6h		

MAXIMAL DOSAGES ARE PRINTED IN RED

amobarbitone and
amobarbital sodium

Amytal and Sodium amytal	po: 6 mg/kg/24h divided q8h	Capsules	60, 200 mg
		Ampules	250, 500 mg
		Tablets	15, 30, 50, 100 mg

APL (p 430)

Apresoline (p 443)

AquaMephyton (p 455)

MAXIMAL DOSAGES ARE PRINTED IN RED

ascorbic acid	Daily requirement = 35 mg	Ampules	100 mg/ml
			250 mg/ml
		Tablets	100 mg
			500 mg
Atabrine (p 160)			
Atarax (p 444)			
atropine sulfate (p 493)		Ampules	0.3, 0.4, 0.6 mg/ml
		Tablets	0.3, 0.4, 0.6 mg
azathioprine			
Imuran	po: initial dose: 2 to 5 mg/kg/24h	Tablets	50 mg
	Maintenance dose based on clinical	Vials	50 mg
	response: 1-2 mg/kg/24h		

MAXIMAL DOSAGES ARE PRINTED IN RED

Azulfidine (p 460)

BAL (pp 437, 493)

Benadryl (p 437)

benztropine mesylate

Cogentin	Stat: im, 0.05 to 0.1 mg/kg/24h	Ampules	2 mg/2 ml
	Followed by: po, 0.04 mg/kg/24h,	Tablets	2 mg
	divided q8 to 12h, prn		

MAXIMAL DOSAGES ARE PRINTED IN RED

bethanidine

Esbaloid   Initial dose: Tablets   10, 25 mg

1 to 7 yr   5 to 10 mg/24h

7 to 12 yr   20 mg/24h

po, in 2 divided doses.

Maintenance: increase according to response.
Maximum: 20 times initial dose

betamethasone   Tablets   0.5 mg

Betnelan

Betnesol

Betnovate   Cream

                                            Lotion   available as

                                         Ointment   0.05% and 0.1%

MAXIMAL DOSAGES ARE PRINTED IN RED

bisacodyl

Dulcolax	po and pr: 0.3 mg/kg/single dose.	Suppositories	5, 10 mg
		Tablets	5 mg
	Caution: tablets are not to be chewed. Contraindicated with rectal fissures and ulceration		

brompheniramine maleate

Dimetane	0.5 mg/kg/24h divided q6 to 8h	Syrup	2 mg/5 ml
		Slow-release tablets	8, 12 mg
		Tablets	4 mg

brompheniramine and **phenylephrine compound**

Dimetapp	0.5 mg/kg/24h divided q6 to 8h	Syrup	4 mg/5 ml
		Extentabs	12 mg
		Tablets	4 mg

MAXIMAL DOSAGES ARE PRINTED IN RED

425

calcium gluconate

	Ampules	10%
	Tablets	300, 600 mg

calcium gluconogalacto gluconate

Calcium Sandoz	po: 0.5 g/kg/24h in divided doses	Ampules	10%, 20%
		Syrup	110 mg Ca^{++}/5 ml
		Strongly effervescent tablets (1 g = 90 mg Ca^{++})	500 mg Ca^{++}

calcium lactate

	po: 0.5 g/kg/24h in divided doses	Tablets	300, 600 mg
	(1 g = 130 mg Ca^{++})		

Calcium Versenate (p 438)

MAXIMAL DOSAGES ARE PRINTED IN RED

camphorated tincture of opium (paregoric)	For diarrhea: po 0.025-0.05 ml/kg/dose of HSC mixture. Maximum, 5 doses	Contains morphine 0.4 mg/ml HSC mixture supplied in 2 strengths (contains chalk suspension): 0.3 ml/5 ml 0.6 ml/5 ml

carbamylcholine chloride

Carbachol	sc: 0.25-0.5 ml once or twice daily	Ampule	0.25 mg/ml
castor oil	Single po dose: 10-30 ml depending on age Over 10 yr: 45 ml		
charcoal	Single dose: po 10-15 g mixed with water	Fine powder	

MAXIMAL DOSAGES ARE PRINTED IN RED

chloral hydrate

Noctec — Hypnotic dose: po, 50 mg/kg/24h divided q6 to 8h
Sedative dose = ½ hypnotic dose
Maximum: 1 g daily

Capsules — 500 mg
Syrup — 500 mg/5 ml

chlordiazepoxide

Librium ⎫
Solium ⎭ — Children over 6 yr: po, im, 0.5 mg/kg/24h in divided doses

Capsules — 5, 10, 25 mg
Injection — 100 mg + solvent
Tablets — 5, 10, 25 mg

chloroquine phosphate

Aralen — po: 10 mg base/kg/1st dose at 0 hr
5 mg base/kg/2nd dose at 6 hr
5 mg base/kg/3rd dose at 18 hr
5 mg base/kg/4th dose at 24 hr

Tablets — 250 mg = 150 mg chloroquine base

MAXIMAL DOSAGES ARE PRINTED IN RED

428

chlorothiazide

| Diuril | po: 20 mg/kg/24h divided into 2 doses | Tablets | 250, 500 mg |
| | | HSC suspension | 50 mg/ml |

chlorpheniramine maleate

Chlor-Tripolon	po, sc: 0.35 mg/kg/24h divided q6h	Ampules	10 mg/ml
		Syrup	2.5 mg/5 ml
		Tablets	4 mg
		Slow-release tablets	8, 12 mg

MAXIMAL DOSAGES ARE PRINTED IN RED

chlorpromazine

Largactil

General dose: po, 2 mg/kg/24h

divided q4 to 8h.

Chorea:

po: 0.5 mg/kg q4 to 6h

im: 0.5 mg/kg q6 to 8h

pr: 2 mg/kg/dose

Maximum: up to 5 yr, 40 mg/day
5-12 yr, 75 mg/day

Ampules	im:	25 mg/2 ml
	iv:	25 mg/5 ml
Syrup		25 mg/5 ml
Suppositories		25, 100 mg
Tablets		10, 25, 50, 100 mg

Chlor-Tripolon (p 429)

chorionic gonadotropin

APL

For dosage schedule see package insert

Vials   10 ml (1000 U/ml)

MAXIMAL DOSAGES ARE PRINTED IN RED

cholestyramine resin

Questran   240 mg/kg/24h in 3 divided doses with water or concentrated fruit juice   Powder   1 measure = 4 g

citrate solutions

Formula A:

Na citrate	100 g
Citric acid	60 g
Water to	1000 g

Provides 1021 mEq of Na/liter

Formula B:

Na citrate	50 g
K citrate	50 g
Citric acid	60 g
Water to	1000 g

Provides 510 mEq of Na and 462 of K/liter

Initial dose: 15 ml, 4 times daily
Maintenance: increase dose as tolerated

MAXIMAL DOSAGES ARE PRINTED IN RED

431

CORTISONE

Type	Relative Dose for Anti-inflammatory Effect	Preparations	
cortisone	25.0 mg	Tablets	5, 25 mg
		Vials (susp; im)	25, 50 mg/ml
hydrocortisone	20.0 mg	Tablets	5, 10, 20 mg
		Vials (susp; im)	25 or 50 mg/ml
hydrocortisone sodium succinate	20.0 mg	Vials (aqueous; iv, im)	100, 250, 500, 1000 mg
prednisone	5.0 mg	Tablets	1, 5, 50 mg
methylprednisolone	4.0 mg	Tablets	2, 4, 16 mg
methylprednisolone sodium succinate	4.0 mg	Vials (iv, im)	40, 125, 250, 1000 mg
triamcinolone	4.0 mg	Tablets	1, 2, 4, 8 mg
triamcinolone acetonide	4.0 mg	Vials (susp; iv, im)	40 mg/ml
dexamethasone	0.75 mg	Tablets	0.5, 0.75 mg

MAXIMAL DOSAGES ARE PRINTED IN RED

432

CORTISONE (cont'd)

Type	Relative Dose for Anti-inflammatory Effect	Preparations	
dexamethasone sodium phosphate	0.75 mg	Vials (aqueous) iv, im	4 mg/ml
betamethasone	0.5 mg	Tablets	0.5 mg
betamethasone disodium phosphate	0.5 mg	Tablets	0.5 mg

DRUG	DOSAGE	SUPPLIED	
codeine phosphate	For pain: stat dose 1.0-1.5 mg/kg po or sc, 3 mg/kg/24h in divided doses. For cough: 1/3 to 1/2 analgesic dose.	Ampules Syrup Tablets	30, 60 mg/ml 25 mg/5 ml 15, 30, 60 mg

MAXIMAL DOSAGES ARE PRINTED IN RED

Cogentin (p 423)

Colace (p 437)

cortisone acetate

Cortone	Replacement dose – 15-25 mg/m²	Tablets Vials (susp)	5, 25 mg 50 mg/ml
Cotazym (p 453)			
Cuprex (p 268)			
Cuprimine (p 453)			
cyclophosphamide (p 213)			
Procytox		Tablets (coated) Vials	25, 50 mg 200, 1000 mg
cytosine arabinoside (p 213)			
Cytosar		Vials	100, 500 mg
cytotoxic drugs (p 212)			
Daraprim (p 459)			
Darvon (p 458)			

MAXIMAL DOSAGES ARE PRINTED IN RED

434

Decadron (pp 136, 432)

deferoxamine mesylate

Desferal	Vials	500 mg

Stat: iv, 10 to 15 mg/kg/hr in 5% glucose/water as continuous drip over 8 hr.
Followed by: im, 600-1200 mg/day divided in 2 or 3 doses.
Maximum dose: 80 mg/kg/24h

Demerol (p 454)

desoxycorticosterone acetate

Percorten	Implants	125 mg
	Vials	5 mg/ml in oil

Single dose: im, 1 to 5 mg/24h

dexamethasone

Decadron (see above)

Diamox (p 418)

MAXIMAL DOSAGES ARE PRINTED IN RED

435

diazepam

Valium | po: 0.12 to 0.8 mg/kg/24h in divided doses | Ampules | 5 mg/ml
 | im (single dose) or iv (infusion): | Syrup | 5 mg/5 ml
 | 0.04 to 0.2 mg/kg. Maximum 5 mg. | Tablets | 2, 5, 10 mg
 | **Special precaution:** Protect iv from light. | |

digoxin

Lanoxin | | Pediatric elixir | 0.05 mg/ml
 | | Adult ampule | 0.25 mg/ml
 | | Pediat. ampule | 0.05 mg/ml
 | | Tablets | 0.125, 0.25, 0.5 mg

Dilantin (p 437)

dimenhydrinate

Gravol }
Dramamine } | po, im, pr: 5 mg/kg/24h in divided doses. | Ampules | 50 mg/ml
 | Maximum: 300 mg/24h | Liquid (Gravol) | 15 mg/5 ml
 | | Suppositories | 50, 100 mg
 | | Tablets | 50 mg

MAXIMAL DOSAGES ARE PRINTED IN RED

dimercaprol

BAL	im: 2.5 mg/kg q4h for 1st day	Ampules	10% in oil (100 mg/ml)
	2.5 mg/kg q6h for 1 day		
	2.5 mg/kg q12h for 10 days		

dioctyl sodium
sulfosuccinate

Colace	po: 5 mg/kg/24h divided q6 or q8h	Capsules	100 mg
		Drops	10 mg/ml
		Syrup	20 mg/5 ml

diphenhydramine HCl

Benadryl	po, im: 5 mg/kg/24h divided q6h	Ampules	50 mg/ml
	Maximum 300 mg/24h	Capsules	25, 50 mg
	Antidote to tranquilizers	Elixir	12.5 mg/5 ml

diphenylhydantoin

Dilantin	4 to 6 mg/kg/24h,	Ampules	100 mg/2 ml,
	po divided into 2 doses, or given iv		250 mg/5 ml
		Capsules	30, 100 mg
		Infantabs	50 mg
		Suspension	30, 125 mg/5 ml

MAXIMAL DOSAGES ARE PRINTED IN RED

disodium cromoglycate

Intal | For older children only: 1 capsule, 2 to 4 times daily by inhalation | Spincaps for inhalation 20 mg each

edathamil (EDTA) calcium

Calcium Versenate | iv: 75 mg/kg/24h in 2 to 4 doses. Each dose is diluted in 75-150 ml 5% dextrose/water and given over 1 hr. Give 1 to 3 courses of 5-7 days, with treatment-free intervals of 7-14 days. | Ampules | 1 g/5 ml

MAXIMAL DOSAGES ARE PRINTED IN RED

edrophonium chloride

Tensilon — Vials — 10 mg/ml

Myasthenia gravis test:
iv, 0.2 mg/kg as single dose; give 1/5 of dose slowly in 1 min; if tolerated, give remainder.
Premature infants:
im or sc, 1 mg as single dose
Warning: When testing, keep atropine sulfate syringe ready; use with caution in bronchial asthma and cardiac dysrhythmias.
Caution: May cause cholinergic reactions.

ephedrine HCl — Tablets — 15, 30, 60 mg

po: 1 mg/kg/dose, q6 to 8h.
Maximum single dose is 25 mg

MAXIMAL DOSAGES ARE PRINTED IN RED

439

epinephrine

Adrenalin chloride	sc:	1:1000 (aqueous soln), 0.01-0.025 mg/kg; maximum, 0.5 ml. Repeat q4h.	Ampule (aqueous)	1 mg/ml (1:1000)
	im:	(in oil): 0.01-0.02 mg/kg, daily or q12h.	Ampule (in oil)	2 mg/ml (1:500)
			Topical soln	1/1000

ethosuximide

Zarontin	Initial dose (po), divided into 2 doses: under 6 yr, 250 mg/24h over 6 yr, 500 mg/24h	Capsules	250 mg
		Syrup	250 mg/5 ml
	Increase dose by 250 mg/day every 4 to 7 days until control is achieved without side-effects.		

ferrous sulfate (p 445)

fludrocortisone

| Florinef | po: 0.05-0.2 mg daily | Tablets | 0.1 mg |

MAXIMAL DOSAGES ARE PRINTED IN RED

440

furosemide

Lasix

po:
Infants, 5 to 10 mg/dose/day
Children, 20 mg/dose/day
Over 7 yr, 40 mg/dose/day
im: ½ oral dose
iv: ¼ oral dose

Adverse reactions: Enhances the nephrotoxicity of cephalosporins and cardiotoxicity of digoxin. Watch for hypokalemia.

Ampules   10 mg/ml
Tablets   40 mg

Furadantin (p 412)

glucagon

sc, im, or iv: 0.025 mg/kg as single dose

Vials   1 mg, 10 mg

Gravol (p 436)

MAXIMAL DOSAGES ARE PRINTED IN RED

441

guanethidine

Ismelin

po: 0.2 mg/kg/24h as single dose
Increase every 7 days by 0.2 mg/kg to
maximal effect

Contraindications: Pheochromocytoma;
monoamine oxidase inhibitors

Tablets — 10, 25 mg

haloperidol

Haldol

po: 0.5-1.0 mg q12h; can be increased
cautiously: watch for side-effects as
dose approaches 10 mg/day
Do not give to infants under 3 yr.

Tablets — 0.5, 1, 2, 5 mg

heparin sodium

1 mg = 120 U;
iv infusion: dilute heparin to 10 U/ml
Initial dose: 50 U/kg
Maintenance: 100 U/kg q4h
Monitor with clotting time

Ampules — 1000, 10,000 U/ml

MAXIMAL DOSAGES ARE PRINTED IN RED

hydralazine

Apresoline

Initial po dose: 0.75 mg/kg/24h divided q6h; increase to 7.5 mg/kg/24h over 3 wk if necessary.

If given alone iv or im: 1.7 to 3.5 mg/kg/24h divided q6h

If given with reserpine: 0.15 mg/kg/day (single dose)

Ampules   20 mg/ml
Tablets   10, 25, 50 mg

hydrochlorothiazide

HydroDiuril

2 mg/kg/24h in 2 divided doses

Tablets   25, 50 mg
HSC suspension   1 mg/ml

hydrocortisone acetate

Cortef

im or po

Injection (susp)   50 mg/ml
Tablets   10, 20 mg

MAXIMAL DOSAGES ARE PRINTED IN RED

443

hydrocortisone sodium succinate			
Solu-Cortef	iv or im	Vials	100, 250, 500 mg and 1 g
hydroxyzine			
Atarax	po: 2 mg/kg/24h divided q6h	Ampules Capsules Syrup	50 mg/ml 10, 25, 50 mg 10 mg/5 ml
imipramine			
Tofranil	For enuresis: 6-14 yr Initially, 10 mg at suppertime. Increase x 10 mg every 2 wk until 50% improvement. Maximum: 6- 8 yr, 50 mg 8-10 yr, 60 mg 10-14 yr, 75 mg	Tablets	10, 25, 50 mg

Inderal (p 457)

Intal (p 438)

MAXIMAL DOSAGES ARE PRINTED IN RED

ipecac syrup

Emetic dose:
6 to 12 mo: 10 ml
1 to 10 yr: 15 ml
10 yr and over: 30 ml

Followed by water; repeat ipecac only once after 20 min if needed.

Single unit dose of syrup
15, 30 ml

IRON PREPARATIONS

elemental iron (Fe^{++})

Prophylactic dose: 1 mg Fe^{++}/kg/24h

Therapeutic dose: 6 mg Fe^{++}/kg/24h divided q8h

ferrous gluconate (Fergon)
- Elixir — 300 mg/5 ml
- Tablets — 300 mg (36 mg Fe^{++})

ferrous sulfate (Fer-in-Sol)
- Drops — 75 mg/0.6 ml (15 mg Fe^{++})
- Tablets — 300 mg (60 mg Fe^{++})

iron dextran injection

Imferon
- Ampules — 2 ml (50 mg Fe^{++}/ml)

[see package insert]

MAXIMAL DOSAGES ARE PRINTED IN RED

isoniazid [INH]

Rimifon	Tablets	50, 100, 300 mg

po: 10 mg/kg/day in 2 doses
Maximum: do not exceed 300 mg/day

isoprenaline)
(isoprenaline)

Isuprel	Ampules	1, 5 ml (1:5000)
	Tablets (sub-lingual)	10 mg
	Elixir	[see label]

po: 3-7 yr, ½ tablet
over 7 yr, 1 tablet
iv: see package insert

Konakion (p 455)

Lasix (p 441)

Levophed (p 452)

Librium (p 428)

magnesium-aluminum hydroxide

Maalox	Suspension	400 mg/5 ml
	Tablets	800 mg

po: 10-20 ml/dose 20 min after meals and at bedtime

MAXIMAL DOSAGES ARE PRINTED IN RED

446

magnesium hydroxide

Milk of Magnesia	po: 0.5 ml/kg/dose	Suspension	300 mg/5 ml
		Tablets	300 mg

magnesium sulfate

(Epsom salts)	For hypertension: iv: 1% solution at 1 to 2 ml/min	Ampules	50% 2 ml
	Caution: Keep calcium gluconate available in case of respiratory depression.		
	Cathartic dose: po: 250 mg/kg/single dose	Crystals	

Mandelamine (p 449)

mannitol, see p 136

	Ampules	25% 50 ml

MAXIMAL DOSAGES ARE PRINTED IN RED

mebendazole

Vermox   100 mg bid   Tablets   100 mg

Mellaril (p 462)

menadiol sodium diphosphate

Synkavite (p 464)

meperidine HC1 (p 454)

meprobamate

Equanil   po: 25 mg/kg/24h divided q8 to q12h   Tablets   400 mg

          Caution: drug dependency

mercaptopurine (p 212)

Purinethol   Tablets   50 mg

MAXIMAL DOSAGES ARE PRINTED IN RED

methimazole

    Tapazole — Initial dose: 0.4 mg/kg/24h, divided q8h, up to 15 mg/24h; Maintenance: 50% initial dose — Tablets — 5 mg

methenamine mandelate

    Mandelamine — Initial dose: 0.1 mg/kg/24h increase by 0.05 mg/kg/24h to: maximum 3g/24h divided q8h — Suspension / Strong susp / Tablets — 250 mg/5 ml / 500 mg/5 ml / 250, 500 mg, 1 g

Methotrexate (p 212)

methyldopa

    Aldomet — po: 10 mg/kg/24h. Can increase to 65 mg/kg/24h divided q8 to 12h. iv: 20 to 40 mg/kg/24h divided q6h — Ampules / Tablets — 250 mg/5 ml / 125, 250, 500 mg

methylene blue (p 450)

MAXIMAL DOSAGES ARE PRINTED IN RED

methylphenidate

Ritalin   po: 6 yr or older: 5-10 mg, 2 or 3 x day. Increase by 5-10 mg/wk.
Maximum, 60 mg/day   Tablets   10, 20 mg

methylprednisolone

Medrol   Tablets   2, 4, 6 mg
Slow-release capsules   2, 4 mg

methylprednisolone sodium succinate

Solu-Medrol   Mix-O-Vial   40, 125, 500 mg
Vials   1 g

methylthionine chloride (methylene blue)   iv: 1 to 2 mg/kg/dose
Dilute solution to 1% before use   Ampules   50 mg/ml (5%)

metronidazole

Flagyl   10 mg/kg/24h divided q8h   Tablets   250 mg

MAXIMAL DOSAGES ARE PRINTED IN RED

mineral oil – liquid petrolatum	po: 0.5 ml/kg/dose	
morphine sulfate	im: 0.1 to 0.2 mg/kg/dose q4-6h Maximum dose 15 mg	Ampules	8, 10, 15 mg/ml
Mysoline (p 456)		
naloxone HC1 (pp 481, 495)		
Narcan	iv: Neonates, 0.005 mg/kg as a single dose. Children, 0.01 mg/kg/dose q3 min until effective. Adolescents, 0.4 mg/dose q3 min until effective.	Ampules	0.02, 0.4 mg/ml
Nembutal (p 453)		
neostigmine		
Prostigmin	po: 2 mg/kg/24h divided q3 – 4h. Single im dose: 0.04 mg/kg. Single iv dose: 0.02 mg/kg.	Ampules Tablets	0.25, 0.5 mg/ml 15 mg

MAXIMAL DOSAGES ARE PRINTED IN RED

Drug	Dosage	Form	Strength
nitrofurantoin			
Furadantin		Tablets Suspension Vials	50, 100 mg 25 mg/5 ml 180 mg/20 ml
norepinephrine bitartrate			
Levophed	iv infusion only: 1 ml of solution in 250 ml dextrose/water Infuse at 0.5 ml/min. Titrate dose with BP.	Ampules	4 ml (0.2%)
Oncovin (p 464)		Vials	1, 5 mg
orciprenaline sulfate			
Alupent	po: 2 mg/kg/24h divided q6h inhalation: 0.01 ml/kg/dose	Aerosol-metered inhalant soln Syrup Tablets	0.75 mg/dose (50 mg/ml) 10 mg/5 ml 20 mg

MAXIMAL DOSAGES ARE PRINTED IN RED

pancreatic enzymes (p 180)

Cotazym	Capsules	
Viokase	Powder	
	Tablets	325 mg

paregoric USP (p 427)

paraldehyde	Ampules	2, 5, 10 ml

Sedative dose: po, im, pr:
0.2 ml/kg
Maximum: 10 ml/dose
iv: 0.1 ml/kg diluted to 5%
with iv soln

penicillamine

Cuprimine	Capsules	250 mg

po. Infants and young children:
250 mg single dose given in fruit juice.
po. Older children: 1 g/24h divided q6h;
can increase to 4-5 g/24h
For dosage as chelating agent see

pentobarbital sodium

Nembutal sodium	Ampules	50 mg/ml
	Capsules	50, 100 mg
	Suppositories	30, 60, 120, 200 mg

Sedative dose: po, pr: 6 mg/kg/24h
divided q8h

MAXIMAL DOSAGES ARE PRINTED IN RED

453

Percorten (p 435)

pethidine (meperidine) HCl

Demerol	pre-op: po or im, 1.0-1.5 mg/kg/dose	Ampules	100 mg, 50 mg/ml
	post-op: iv, 0.2 mg/kg/dose	Tablets	50 mg
	analgesic: im, 1.5 mg/kg stat dose		
	Maximum single dose 100 mg		

Phenergan (p 457)

phenobarbital sodium

Sedative dose: po 0.5 to 2 mg/kg/dose q4 to 6h	Ampules	50, 120 mg/ml
Maximum: 30 mg	Elixir	10, 15 mg/5 ml
Anticonvulsant dose: 3 to 6 mg/kg as single dose.	Tablets	15, 30, 60, 100 mg
Maximum: 100 to 200 mg		

phentolamine

Rogitine (p 52)	Ampules	5 mg/ml

phenylephrine; Neo-Synephrine ophthalmic soln, see p 101

MAXIMAL DOSAGES ARE PRINTED IN RED

454

phytomenadione (K$_1$)

AquaMephyton }
Konakion }

Neonates:
prophylactic dose: im 0.5 to 1.0 mg
therapeutic dose: iv 5 mg
Infants: po 2 mg
Older children: po 5 to 10 mg

Ampules
(aqueous)   10 mg/ml
Ampules   1 mg/0.5 ml

piperazine citrate (p 159)

Antepar

Syrup   500 mg/5 ml

Pitressin (p 464)

potassium chloride

K-Lyte Cl

Slow-K

Infants and children: po
sufficient to maintain serum K
at 3.6 to 5.5 mEq/liter

Ampules   20 mEq/10 ml
(Flavored mixture makes a soln
of 1 mEq K$^+$/ml)
Slow-release   600 mg (8 mEq K$^+$)
tablets

potassium iodide

Preoperatively for thyrotoxicosis
0.9 ml soln/24h divided q8h

Aqueous soln of KI
saturated = 1 g/ml

MAXIMAL DOSAGES ARE PRINTED IN RED

455

pralidoxime chloride (USP)			
Protopam	iv: 25-50 mg/kg; maximum, 2 g; as 5% soln in N saline over 10-15 min. Repeat q10-12h prn **Contraindications:** see package insert	Vials	1 g
Prednisolone		Ampules	25 mg/ml
		Tablets	1, 5 mg
Prednisone		Tablets	5, 50 mg
primaquine **phosphate**	po: 0.3 mg/kg of base daily – (maximum 15 mg) for 14 days		
primidone			
Mysoline	po: infants, 18 mg/kg/24h divided q8h Older children, up to maximum 2 g/24h divided q6 to 12h	Suspension	250 mg/5 ml
		Tablets	125, 250 mg

MAXIMAL DOSAGES ARE PRINTED IN RED

456

Pro-Banthine

probenecid (p 406)

Benemid

Procytox

promethazine HCl

Phenergan | po, pr, im: 0.5/kg/dose: | Ampules | 25 mg/ml
| For nausea and vomiting, q4-6h | Suppositories | 12.5, 25, 50 mg
| For motion sickness, q12h | Syrup | 10 mg/5 ml
| | Tablets | 10, 25, 50 mg

propranolol

Inderal | po: 1 to 2 mg/kg/day, q6h | Ampules | 1 mg/ml
| iv: 0.05 to 0.1 mg/kg over 10 min | Tablets | 10, 40 mg

propantheline bromide

Pro-Banthine | po: 1.5 mg/kg/24h in 4 divided | Ampules | 30 mg/ml
| doses after food and at bedtime | Tablets | 7.5, 15 mg
| Maximum: 30 mg 4 times daily | |

MAXIMAL DOSAGES ARE PRINTED IN RED

propoxyphene napsylate

Darvon-N	Adult dose: 100 mg q3 to 4h prn Restriction: The safety and efficiency of this drug has not been established in children under 12 yr.	Capsules	100 mg

propylthiouracil

Propyl-Thyracil	Initial dose po: 6-7 mg/kg/day divided q8h for 3-6 wk; then 3-6 mg/kg/day	Tablets	50, 100 mg

Prostigmine

protamine sulfate

	iv: infuse slowly Dose: 1 mg for each 1 mg heparin given in previous 4h, up to 50 mg q4 to 6h	Ampules	10 mg/ml (1%)

Protopam (p 456)

pseudoephedrine HCl

Sudafed	po: 4 mg/kg/24h divided q6h	Syrup Tablets	30 mg/5 ml 60 mg

MAXIMAL DOSAGES ARE PRINTED IN RED

458

Purinethol (p 212)

pyrimethamine (p 160)

Daraprim	po: 1 mg/kg/day x 4 days then 0.5 mg/kg/day x 1 month	Tablets	25 mg

pyrivinium pamoate

Vanquin	po: 5 mg/kg in 1 dose	Suspension Tablets	50 mg/ml 50 mg

quinacrine

Atabrine (p 160)		Tablets	100 mg

reserpine

Serpasil	po: 0.02 mg/kg/24h divided q12h Acute hypertension: im 0.07 mg/kg/ dose (combine with apresoline if necessary)	Ampules Tablets	2.5 mg/ml 0.1, 0.25 mg

rifampin (p 413)

Rimifon (p 446)

Ritalin (p 450)

MAXIMAL DOSAGES ARE PRINTED IN RED

459

Rogitine (p 52)

salicylazosulfapyridine

Salazopyrin
Azulfidine — Initial dose: 75 to 150 mg/kg/24h divided q4 to 6h
Maintenance: 40 mg/kg/24h divided q6h — Tablets 500 mg; Enteric-coated tablets 500 mg

secobarbital sodium

Seconal sodium — Sedation: po, pr: 6 mg/kg/24h divided q8h — Capsules 50, 100 mg

senna (standardized)

Senokot — Single po dose as needed: granules 1.5 to 6 g; syrup 2.5 to 10 ml; tablets ½ to 2 — Granules, Syrup, Tablets: 3 g = 15 mg; 5 ml = 10 mg; each = 8.6 mg of standardized senna conc.

Serpasil (p 459)

MAXIMAL DOSAGES ARE PRINTED IN RED

Solium (p 428)

spironolactone

   Aldactone   po: 1.5-3.0 mg/kg/day, in 4 doses   Tablets   25 mg

Sudafed (p 458)

sulfonamides

succinylsulfathiazole		Tablets	500 mg
sulfadiazine		Ampules	250 mg/ml
		Tablets	500 mg
sulfamethazine		Tablets	500 mg
		Suspension	500 mg/5 ml
sulfamethizole		Tablets	250, 500 mg
sulfamethoxazole	(Fixed combination – trimethoprim: sulfa, 1:5)	Adult tablets	80:400 mg
		Pediatric tablets	20:100 mg
		Pediatric susp	40:200 mg/5 ml

MAXIMAL DOSAGES ARE PRINTED IN RED

Drug	Dosage	Form	Strength
sulfisoxazole		Ampules Suspension Tablets	2 g/5 ml 500 mg/5 ml 500 mg
Synkavite (p 464)	Not recommended for neonates and infants		
Synthroid (see below)			
Tapazole (p 449)			
Tensilon (p 439)			
thioridazine			
Mellaril	po: 1 mg/kg/24h divided q6 to 8h Note: Not recommended for children under 2 yr.	Solution Suspension Tablets	30 mg/ml 10 mg/5 ml 10, 25, 50, 100 mg
L-thyroxine sodium			
Synthroid	0-6 mo: 7.5-10 µg/kg daily 6-12 mo: 5.0-7.5 µg/kg daily Over 1 yr: 2.5-5.0 µg/kg daily Maximum, 0.3 mg/day	Tablets	0.025, 0.05, 0.1, 0.15, 0.2 mg

MAXIMAL DOSAGES ARE PRINTED IN RED

Tofranil (p 444)

trimethadione

Tridione (p 174)

Valium (p 436)

Vanquin (p 459)

VASOPRESSIN PREPARATIONS

vasopressin injection (USP)

| Pitressin (aqueous) | Aqueous | im: 0.1 U/kg Maximum, 5.0 U | 20 U/ml 10 U/0.5 ml |

vasopressin tannate injection (USP)

| Pitressin tannate | Tannate in oil suspension: shake well | im: 0.2 ml/dose; increase to 1 to 2 ml. q24 to 48h Maintenance: dose can be given q24 to 72h | 5 U/ml |

MAXIMAL DOSAGES ARE PRINTED IN RED

vasopressin synthetic: desmopressin acetate (DDAVP)			
Minirin	5-20 μg intranasally once or twice daily	Intranasal soln	0.1 mg/ml
Vermox (p 448)			
Versenate calcium (p 438)			
vincristine sulfate (p 212)			
Oncovin		Vials	1, 5 mg
vitamin K preparations			
phytomenadione	For infants and young children	Ampules	1 mg/0.5 ml
		Tablets	5 mg
Synkavite	Note: not suitable for infants po: 5 to 10 mg daily iv: 1 mg daily	Ampules	5, 10 mg/ml
		Tablets	5 mg
Zarontin (p 174)			

MAXIMAL DOSAGES ARE PRINTED IN RED

EMERGENCIES

CALL FOR HELP – dial 25 to reach switchboard emergency line and state whether this is a two-five or two-three call.

1. a) *Code 25* is the code for a cardiac arrest. It alerts members of the resuscitation team (senior medical and surgical residents, and anesthetist) by special bell-boy.

      b) "Twenty-five", followed by location of the emergency, is announced over the loud-speakers to alert other staff.

2. *Code 23* preceding a page over the loud-speakers indicates an emergency other than cardiac arrest and demands immediate response from the person paged.

Poisoning: see Toxicology, p 484.

A. Airway
1. Extend the child's head.
2. Remove obvious foreign material from the airway.
3. If necessary, lift the mandible forward to open airway.

B. Breathing
1. Check air exchange: watch chest movements, and feel for air at the mouth and nose.
2. If ventilation is inadequate, begin artificial ventilation (mouth-to-mouth, mouth-to-nose, bag and mask).
3. Check gas exchange – but don't stop ventilating.
4. Start giving O_2 as soon as equipment and personnel available.
5. Continue ventilation until return of good spontaneous respiration.

C. Circulation
1. Check carotid pulse (or precordium, in infants and small children).
2. If effective circulation is absent, begin external cardiac massage (ECM).

a) ECM = compression of the heart between the sternum and spine. Must be continuous to be effective, and must be combined with artificial ventilation. *Rapid* institution of ventilation and ECM when required are necessary for success.

b) Place patient on a firm surface (e.g., hand, tray, spinal board).

c) *Infants:* compress at 80-100/min with 2 fingers at midsternal level.

d) *Children* up to 5 yr: compress at 80/min just below midsternum.

e) *Children* over 5 yr: compress at 60-80/min over lower third of sternum.

D. Drugs

1. *Oxygen*

2. *Establish a good iv line.*

3. *Sodium bicarbonate,* 7.5% or 8.4% (0.9 and 1.0 mEq/ml), **STAT iv,** 2-3 ml/kg.
   - If effective circulation absent, continue with 1 ml/kg q 10 min.

4. *Epinephrine* 1 in 10,000 (1 ml of 1:1,000 adrenalin, diluted up to 10 ml with N saline) 1.5 – 5 ml iv.

5. *Intracardiac drugs may be necessary* if an iv line cannot be established in the first 10 min of an arrest (e.g., if no response by then).

E. Etiology

1. Connect ECG to monitor

2. Check blood gases

3. Review history and examination for cause of emergency.

F. Further therapy under ECG control (*see also* p 205)

1. Defibrillation when required (2-5 Joules/kg)

2. Calcium chloride (or gluconate) 10%, 1 ml/5 kg body wt.

3. Isoproterenol (Isuprel), give as bolus: strength: 10 μg/ml (0.2 mg diluted to 20 ml) dose: 0.5 ml/kg up to 10 ml.

4. If heart block, give Isuprel 0.2 μg/kg/min iv by constant infusion.

5. If no cardiac response, repeat bicarb, adrenalin, Ca^{++}, q10 min.

6. Give plasma or other iv expander, 10 ml/kg.

ANAPHYLACTIC SHOCK

1. Place patient in head-low position and keep warm.
2. Epinephrine (1:1000), 0.01 ml/kg up to 0.50 ml, sc
   a) can repeat once in 5 min
   b) can inject 2/5 this amount iv slowly, by mixing it with withdrawn blood
   c) if vein cannot be entered, inject sublingually.
3. If anaphylaxis is result of an injection, place tourniquet on a limb proximal to injection site.
4. Call for resuscitation cart, and either
   - notify Anesthesia **or**
   - **call code 25 (if cardiac arrest).**
5. Inject iv (slowly) or im, either
   a) diphenylhydramine HCl (Steri-vial Benadryl HC1, 10 mg/ml) 1-2 mg/kg body wt, to a maximum of 50 mg, **or**
   b) chlorpheniramine maleate (Chlor-Tripolon), 10 mg/ml (not in infants) 10-20 mg im (max. 40 mg/24h) **or** 5-20 mg iv (inject **slowly** over 1 min) as a single dose
      i) draw the Chlor-Tripolon into a 10-ml syringe
      ii) draw 5-10 ml of the patient's blood into the syringe (the blood acts as a diluent)
      iii) inject the mixture during 1 min.
6. Inject hydrocortisone sodium succinate (Solu-Cortef) iv (p 432)
   a) 500-1000 mg in Mix-o-Vial, over at least 30 sec
   b) can add similar amount to iv fluids over next 8 hr.
7. Oxygen by mask.
8. If BP falling, treat as for shock (p 472).
9. If bronchospasm present, give aminophylline, 3.5 mg/kg iv *slowly* and then as for asthma (p 185).

ASPIRATION

1. Suction mouth and pharynx.
2. Check airway and breathing as for general emergency.
3. If child is breathing, place him semiprone, head down, and administer 100% O_2.
4. a) Have assistant call Anesthesia resident, for intubation and immediate bronchial suction.
   b) Use 2-10 ml N saline for bronchial toilet.

5. If solid particles in tracheobronchial tree are large enough to prevent oxygenation, request immediate bronchoscopy.
6. Auscultate lungs and take BP, pulse, and respirations, q 30 min.
7. Chest radiograph stat.
8. Establish an iv line and give steroid therapy and antibiotics (p 407).

Respiratory Failure: see Respirology, p 191

CONVULSIONS & COMA

Undiagnosed Coma — see Neurosurgery, p 284

Etiology
1. Anoxia
2. Febrile convulsions (see p 173)
3. Infection: see Infectious Diseases, p 130
4. Intoxication: see Toxicology, p 484
5. Congenital defect
6. Vascular
7. Metabolic: see Tests of Metabolic Function (p 55) and Metabolic Disorders (p 254)
8. Epilepsy: see Neurology, p 177
9. Trauma (p 474)
10. Other
    a) anaphylaxis (e.g., penicillin); see p 469
    b) collagen disease: lupus, polyarteritis
    c) encephalopathy: postimmunization (smallpox, pertussis); Reye's syndrome
    d) acute infantile hemiplegia
    e) hysteria
    f) tumors — neoplasia (see Hematology, p 215); tuberous sclerosis.

CONVULSIONS

Convulsions in Neonate: see Neurology, p 177

Management
A medical emergency — after 10 min, patient may suffer irreversible brain-cell damage. Especially at risk are febrile children aged 6 mo to 4 yr.
1. Ensure adequate airway — suction, O_2 if necessary

2. Anticonvulsant drugs
   a) The drug of choice is diazepam (Valium):
      0-5 yr: 1 mg per yr of age, iv slowly
      > 5 yr: total 5 mg, iv slowly (over 2 min) q3
      min x 2 or 3 until convulsion stops.
   b) **Plus either**
      i)   5% paraldehyde drip (12.5 ml paralde-
           hyde in 250 ml 2/3 − 1/3 glucose–saline
           solution) to a total of a 4 ml/kg body wt,
           over 2 hr (titrate iv as necessary to con-
           trol seizures); **or**
      ii) paraldehyde pr, 0.2 ml/kg, mixed with
           equal vol of mineral oil. Can repeat
           dose q2h prn.
   c) Phenobarbital (Luminal) 5-10 mg/kg iv or im
      (p 454), also, can be given if necessary.
3. If convulsion persists:
   a) infant 0-6 mo: intubate
   b) age 6 mo − 4 yr: have assistant call Anesthesia
      (to perform intubation) and give rapidly acting
      barbiturate.
4. Gastric suction to prevent aspiration.
5. Any child who has been convulsing more than 30
   min:
   a) start dexamethasone (Decadron) 2-10 mg stat
      iv (p 433);
   b) then give Decadron 0.5-4 mg (iv, im, or po)
      q6h.
6. Sponge to reduce fever (normothermia is ideal).
7. Take blood for
   a) Na^+, K^+, Cl^-, pH, glucose, and Ca; and
   b) alkaline phosphatase if any suspicion of tetany.
8. If hypoglycemia suspected: give trial dose of 50%
   glucose, 2-10 ml iv.
9. If tetany suspected: give trial dose of 10% Ca gluconate 5-10 ml iv.

Investigation

1. History: recent illnesses, drugs (especially failure to
   take anticonvulsants), trauma, description of seizures, family history.
2. Physical examination: temperature, BP, head measurement, transillumination, funduscopy (no cyclo-
   plegics). Auscultate skull.

3. Tests
   a) Fever but no papilledema: do LP.
      - Record pressure and cells, send CSF for sugar, protein, smear, and bacterial and viral cultures.
   b) In addition, consider:
      - urine: routine, Phenistix, heavy metals, porphyrins
      - blood: CBC, chemistries
      - EEG
      - radiographs (p 82): skull, wrist, knee
      - brain scan (p 84)
      - subdural tap (p 74).

Continuing Management: see Neurology, p 177.

SHOCK

Definition: inadequate tissue perfusion.

Diagnosis
1. *History* — blood loss, burns, trauma, acute fluid loss, sepsis, acute hypoxic episode, previous steroid administration, drug overdose.
2. *Clinical appearance* — confusion, cool extremities, progressing to grey pallor, deteriorating level of consciousness.
3. *Signs* — tachycardia, hypotension.

Etiology
1. Hypovolemia: blood loss, ECF loss, relative hypovolemia (vasodilation, capillary leak)
2. Septic
3. Cardiogenic
4. Anaphylactic (p 469)
5. Acute adrenal insufficiency (p 246)

Management of Shock

A. Establish adequate circulatory volume
B. Treat underlying cause
C. Support vital organs.

A. Establish Adequate Circulatory Volume

1. Insert central venous line to measure CVP and assess response to treatment:
   a) normal CVP = 0-10 cm H_2O
   b) if shock is present, try to maintain CVP above 6 cm H_2O.
2. Intravenous fluids: expand blood volume, to increase peripheral perfusion and cardiac output.
   a) Give boluses of 10 ml/kg q10 min until peripheral perfusion is good or CVP >12 cm H_2O.
   b) Give appropriate fluid to replace known losses (e.g., blood for blood loss); but, **initially,** give whatever fluid is quickly available (e.g., Ringer's lactate or saline soln, plasma, or whole blood).
   c) Give colloid solutions (plasma or blood) as soon as possible:
      i) crystalloid solutions (e.g., Ringer's lactate or saline) remain in the intravascular space only briefly (20 min) when CVP is low
      ii) high vol of crystalloid solution adds risk of tissue edema (lung, brain, etc.).

B. Treat Underlying Cause

1. Control blood loss.
2. Investigations
   a) CBC; platelets; PT and PTT; type and cross-match; blood for culture.
   b) Arterial blood gases (ABG), serum electrolytes, glucose, Ca, BUN.
   c) Other cultures as indicated (urine, tracheal aspirate, etc.).
   d) Defer CSF studies if indicated until shock controlled and clotting studies reported.
   e) ECG.
3. Treat sepsis if suspected (p 137).

C. Support Vital Organs

1. Administer O_2 to all patients in shock.
2. Treat acidosis: Na bicarbonate, 2 mEq/kg iv *stat* and repeat as indicated by ABG.
3. Support myocardium:
   a) adequate intravascular volume
   b) if CVP >12 cm H_2O, and peripheral perfusion still inadequate, give inotropic agents.

4. *Inotropic Agents* – give only if under continuous monitoring of CVP and arterial pressure, and preferably in intensive-care area.
   a) Dopamine – continuous infusion by pump at 4-10 μg/kg/min.
   b) Isoproterenol (Isuprel), 0.01-0.1 ng/kg/min – *contraindicated if heart rate >200/min or tachyarrhythmia present.*
   c) Digoxin – request Cardiology consult (p 201).
   d) If BP adequate but peripheral perfusion poor, consider vasodilation:
      i) steroids (hydrocortisone), 50 mg/kg *stat* iv; repeat q1h x 4 if needed; then 15 mg/kg q3h for 48 hr
      ii) chlorpromazine
      iii) sodium nitroprusside.
5. Other organs:
   a) kidney – urine catheter, to monitor urine output
   b) lung – positive pressure ventilation as indicated
   c) brain – steroids, adequate oxygenation
   d) GI tract – watch for subsequent GI bleed
   e) hemopoietic system – if clotting abnormalities exist, consult Hematology for DIC studies.

BURNS

Flame burns, and burns due to explosion, see Plastic Surgery, p 305.

TRAUMA

Priority by injury

1. Injury interfering with vital physiological functions
   – airway
   – hemorrhage
   – shock.
2. Severe injuries, but no immediate threat to life. In most instances there is time to diagnose.
3. Injuries producing occult damage. Child may require surgery, but no injury is apparent initially.

Treatment Priorities

1. Establish patent airway
   a) clear the oral cavity
   b) clear airway as necessary
   c) oral or nasal intubation.
2. Control hemorrhage — by direct pressure.
   — Tourniquet rarely indicated.
3. Control shock
   — establish an iv line (make every attempt to establish this in an upper extremity)
4. Gastric decompression.
5. Obtain history and perform physical examination. Meanwhile:
   a) splint fractures
   b) insert catheters
   c) order radiography
   d) order other relevant investigations.
6. Patient should not be taken for radiography or other investigation until:
   a) condition is stable
   b) airway is established
   c) iv and duodenal tubes inserted.

General comments

1. Essential to establish the priorities in management.
2. One doctor must be in charge.
3. Communicate frequently with the parents.
4. Head injuries rarely produce shock.
   — Shock is usually due to thoracic or abdominal injuries, and less frequently to fractures.

RESPIRATORY EMERGENCIES IN INFANTS AND YOUNG CHILDREN
Respiratory Failure: see Respirology, p 191.

1. In the newborn, respiration is mainly diaphragmatic. Because the ribs and costal cartilages are soft, paradoxical breathing results; this is marked in premature infants and significantly increased if the airway is obstructed.
2. Tension pneumothorax often severely compresses the opposite lung (due to mediastinal shift).
3. Trachea and bronchi are easily compressed, because they are relatively soft.
4. Radiographs of chest are more important than clinical examination in these cases; always order, in addition to making clinical appraisal.

Clinical Entities

Pneumothorax

1. Sudden onset of acute respiratory distress suggests tension pneumothorax.
2. Consider pneumothorax whenever traumatic injuries with respiratory distress.
3. Acute tension pneumothorax (chest tympanitic, with no air entry on auscultation): immediate aspiration, then insertion of suitable catheter, occasionally necessary before obtaining radiograph.

Staphylococcal Empyema

1. 40% of all cases in infants < 3 mo; further 40% by 2 yr.
2. Perform needle aspiration; send pus for culture.
3. Insert chest tube(s) into pleural cavity, and connect to underwater drainage.
4. Give cloxacillin iv (p 408) until culture and sensitivity known; then continue appropriate antibiotic therapy.

Pulmonary Cysts, congenital or acquired

1. Congenital cysts are bronchogenic in origin.
    a) may be closed and filled with mucinous fluid, or may communicate with bronchus and contain air
    b) surgical excision is necessary.
2. Acquired cysts are usually caused by staphylococcal pneumonia.
    a) Many are self-limiting and need no special treatment.
    b) Those that enlarge, and cause compression similar to tension pneumothorax, must be excised.

Congenital Lobar Emphysema

1. Usually in upper and middle lobes; commonly result in progressive overinflation of affected lobe.
2. Radiographic appearance can be confused with tension pneumothorax — differentiated by careful examination and identification of peripheral lung marking.
3. Do not aspirate — could cause tension pneumothorax.
4. Emergency thoracotomy, to excise the affected lobe, is mandatory.
5. Do bronchoscopy immediately before lobectomy — foreign body or inspissated mucus in the bronchus can simulate lobar emphysema.

Respiratory Distress Syndrome: *see also*
Neonatalogy, p 162.

Consult a pediatric general surgeon early in all cases of respiratory distress due to suspected or proven pneumothorax, empyema, lung cysts, lobar emphysema, diaphragmatic hernia, or chest trauma.

Chest trauma

1. Severe multiple fractures of ribs = unusual in childhood; but chest injury can result in contusion or laceration of lungs, blood vessels, or tracheobronchial tree without much evidence of external bruising.
2. Massive hemothorax or pneumothorax is common.
   a) Usually it is managed by intercostal closed-tube drainage.
   b) Persistent bleeding or massive air leak despite adequate drainage indicates more severe injury, requiring further investigation and possibly thoracotomy.

After thoracic surgery

1. Postoperative breathing exercises, under guidance of a physiotherapist (see Rehabilitation Med, p 97) are ordered pre-operatively for most patients.
2. Postoperative orders, including chest radiography, must be approved by staff surgeon.

ENDOCRINOLOGY

Diabetes Mellitus
- ketoacidosis, see p 243
- emergency surgery, see p 246

Adrenal Insufficiency, see p 246

PSYCHIATRY

Childhood Psychosis

Rare but serious

Presentation

1. Withdrawal – decreased interaction with others; decreased or distorted speech; pre-occupation, daydreaming, and rhythmic activity (rocking and head banging).
2. Hyperaggressive, uncontrolled physical violence and destructiveness, including self-destructiveness.

3. Bizarre behavior (touching, smelling, licking), phobias, irrational fears (e.g., of germs, noises, darkness).
4. Regression in habits (e.g., toilet training).
5. Adolescent more like adult (hallucinations, paranoid delusions, thought disorder, suicide attempts).

Differential Diagnosis
Mental retardation, severe emotional deprivation, minimal brain dysfunction.
— Can occur in conjunction with these.

History
1. Complete history of child and the family situation.
2. Precipitating events — loss of parent by death, separation, or illness; immigration; infection, hospitalization, surgical procedures; exhaustion; family problems, disordered family.
3. Medication history.

Examination
1. Complete, particularly neurological. State of consciousness, sensorium, alertness.
2. Orientation to person, time, and place.
3. Memory for recent and remote events.
4. Thought processes (delusions, thought disorder).
5. Affect — anxiety, inappropriate feeling states, depressions.

Management
1. Provide secure environment; quiet single room.
2. Explain procedures.
3. Reassure parents and child.
4. Preferably, keep child with parents during interview; but adolescent may prefer to be seen alone.
5. Constant surveillance and physical holding to prevent destruction of self and others. If child left alone, remove potentially harmful objects.

Medication
1. Chlorpromazine (p 430) for acute schizophrenic and some organic reactions.
2. *Caution* if patient, already sedated, is hypotonic, has liver damage, or is adolescent using street drugs.

Follow-up
Refer all children with suspected psychosis to Psychiatry.

Suicide Attempts

Presentation

1. *Young child* (<10 yr)

   Walks out in front of a car; "falls out" of a window; "accidentally" swallows ASA or cleaning agent; is "accident prone" and often comes close to being killed.

2. *Adolescent*

   Slashes wrists, takes overdose of drugs, attempts hanging, has motor-vehicle accident, or attempts other form of suicide.

Management

1. Treat medical or surgical emergency.
2. Avoid moralistic comments.

   Assess seriousness of attempt

1. How close to success?
2. Was patient alone at time of attempt?
3. Did he threaten suicide or forewarn others, and when? (e.g., was suicide note found before or after the attempt?)
4. Were there signs/symptoms of severe depression? Examples: Sudden weight change, insomnia (especially early morning wakening), increasing social isolation, inability to function in school/with peers/with family, giving away his belongings.
5. Were there previous suicide attempts? If so, how serious and in what circumstances?
6. Is the patient determined to repeat attempt when released from hospital?
7. Is patient psychotic (out of touch with reality), or in full possession of mental faculties, when seen?
8. What precipitated the attempt? — (e.g., retaliatory angry punishment of an unfaithful boyfriend; self-punishment of an adolescent who feels hopeless about himself).
9. Is the patient going back to rejecting environment, abusive parents, supporting family?
10. Will patient have help of psychiatrist or social worker in the community?

Drug Overdose (See also Toxicology, pp 491, 496)

History

1. History of visits to dr or Emergency with odd "unphysiological" pains (i.e., drug-seeking behavior or withdrawal syndrome)?

2. History of repeated attacks of nasal congestion, rhinorrhea (part of heroin-withdrawal syndrome)?

3. Try to obtain accurate description or sample of the drug taken, from the patient's friends or parents (for analysis, see Biochemistry, pp 383, 399).

4. Inquire about previous treatment for addiction.

Physical Examination

- Respiration slowed, labored (heroin, barbiturates).
- Pupils pinpoint, sluggish (heroin), or dilated (atropine).
- Nasal mucous membranes irritated (cocaine, heroin).
- Superficial vein 'tracks' and deep-vein thrombophlebitis (iv drug use).
- Fever, leukocytosis, abscess formation, local cellulitis.
- Signs of pulmonary edema (heroin overdosage).
- Signs of subacute/acute bacterial endocarditis (one of the few times when the right heart valves are involved) or of such organisms as staph, *Candida*, Gram-neg bacteria, enterococci.
- Signs of septic pulmonary embolus or pneumonia.
- Signs of acute hepatitis (many long-term drug users have chronic hepatic dysfunction unrelated to viral hepatitis).
- Signs of tetanus, sepsis.

Differential Diagnosis

COMA

Suspect opiates, barbiturates, alcohol, and — very importantly —

a) suspect COMBINED INTOXICATIONS

b) do not overlook the other medical/surgical causes of coma (metabolic and neurologic disorders; p 471), which may CO-EXIST with the acute drug overdosage.

c) Solvent sniffers may partly asphyxiate themselves, using a plastic bag, and be comatose on arrival. They usually smell of the solvent.

CONVULSIONS (p 471)

Suspect barbiturate withdrawal (morphine withdrawal in neonates), contamination of drug with strychnine (e.g., LSD and other hallucinogens), cocaine (marked pyrogenic effect in young children).

PSYCHOTIC BEHAVIOR OR MANIA

Suspect lysergic acid diethylamide (LSD), or other hallucinogens (MDA, psilocybin, PCP, mescaline), chronic amphetamine abuse, cocaine, contamination of hallucinogenic drugs with atropine.

PANIC

Suspect LSD, hashish, tetrahydrocannabinol (THC), amphetamines.

EUPHORIA

Suspect hallucinogens (LSD, MDA), amphetamines, solvents (gasoline, glue, acetone), cocaine, low-dose barbiturates, and occasionally cannabis (grass, hashish, THC).

Treatment
1. As for convulsion (p 470), coma, cardiorespiratory arrest (p 467).
2. Obtain samples of blood, urine, and stomach contents (see Biochemistry, pp 383, 399).

Opiate (heroin, morphine, codeine, methadone) poisoning (*see also* p 495)

Overdose occurs when heroin used is purer than expected.

Specific Therapy
1. Narcotic antagonist (Narcan) (p 451) the drug of choice. Dose, 0.01 mg/kg iv for child and 0.4 mg/dose for adolescent. Repeat prn up to q3 min until an effect is achieved.
2. Nalline also can be used,
   a) Dose, 0.1 mg/kg iv up to max of 5 mg/dose. Repeat q15-20 min.
   b) If no response after 2 injections:
      i) reconsider diagnosis of drug overdosage, or
      ii) suspect combined intoxication (heroin and barbiturates), or
      iii) suspect concomitant medical condition (subdural hematoma, metabolic acidosis).
   c) **Caution:** can cause respiratory depression if given in large doses.
3. Patient may respond to either drug initially, then relapse, if no further dose given.

Methadone Poisoning

1. Average dose for a heroin-user on methadone maintenance is 60-120 mg.
2. In a non-tolerant adolescent, this dose can cause respiratory depression.

3. In a child under 6 yr, this dose can cause coma and fatal respiratory depression within 1-3 hr.

Treatment: narcotic-antagonists (p 451)

Barbiturate Poisoning

1. Longer-acting agents (phenobarbital) are relatively less potent and excreted by the kidney. Therefore, forced diuresis with 2/3:1/3 iv solution can be used.
2. Shorter-acting agents (secobarbital) have greater potency and are degraded by the liver.
3. Both types are potentiated by alcohol.
4. Toxicity can occur with serum levels as low as 3 mg/dl of short-acting and 10 mg/dl of long-acting barbiturate.
5. Death may occur at even lower levels in non-tolerant individuals or children.

Treatment (see also p 491)

1. Gastric lavage if ingestion recent and to obtain a sample for analysis.
2. Observe vital signs.
3. Support circulation and maintain hydration.
4. Assisted ventilation for respiratory failure.
5. Determine blood barbiturate levels (p 383). The level may rise 6 hr after injection, due to absorption of drug not removed by lavage.
6. If intoxication severe, peritoneal dialysis.

Synthetic Nonbarbiturate Hypnotics

1. Glutethimide presents like barbiturate overdose, except respiratory function is relatively good although sudden apneic spells may occur.
2. Shock is commoner than with barbiturates.

Hallucinogens (see pp 494-5)

Lysergic acid diethylamide (LSD), LSD_{25}, or STP (2,5 dimethoxy-4-methylamphetamine). Bad reaction may be due to individual's personality, latent fears, experiences with the drug, the milieu at time of taking it, size of the dose, or adulterant (e.g., belladonna, atropine, amphetamine, strychnine).

Medical intervention **may** not be needed. The patient can be "talked down" in a quiet room by persons he knows and trusts. He should never be left alone in strange surroundings.

Caution: Phenothiazines are contraindicated — they react adversely with anticholinergic adulterants like phencyclidine or atropine.

If no improvement, give diazepam po (p 436); or, if patient is acutely toxic, give diazepam 1 mg/min iv, slowly, up to 10 mg.

Caution: diazepam in large doses given quickly may depress respiration.

This effect is potentiated by ingestion of alcohol.

"Flashbacks"

Spontaneous recurrence of a hallucinogenic experience a few days to a year after the last experience, may be triggered by use of another drug (cannabis).

Anti-anxiety agents have been used (e.g., diazepam). Reassurance, and a cautionary statement about further drug-use, are indicated.

Stimulants—Amphetamines

1. Moderate overdosage ("over-amping") can usually be handled nonmedically.
2. Severe large overdose characterized by extreme violence or paranoia: a tranquilizing agent, such as diazepam, may be indicated.
3. Chronic amphetamine abuse can cause psychotic reaction.
4. Hypertensive crises require drug therapy (p 238).

Solvents

Toluene, acetone, naphtha, Carbona, carbon tetrachloride, gasoline.

1. Treatment is usually supportive and symptomatic.
2. Tranquilizing agents, such as diazepam or chlorpromazine, may be indicated if panic is extreme.
3. Hypoxia may occur if a plastic bag is used and the patient falls asleep.
4. Chronic use of such agents can lead to liver, kidney, and bone-marrow damage.

Cannabis Derivatives — (Marihuana and Hashish)

1. Overdose, which is rare, is commoner with hashish — which contains more tetrahydrocannabinol (THC).
2. Ingestion gives more bad reactions than smoking.
3. Be alert to effect of adulterants, contaminants, and that previous bad experiences with hallucinogens may be reactivated by cannabis.

TOXICOLOGY

Prevent Absorption

INGESTED POISON

Dilute poison
1. Give water, to provide bulk and facilitate vomiting. No contraindications.
2. Can give activated charcoal (2 Tbsp in water) also.

Evacuate poison
Induce emesis

Contraindications: ingestion of corrosive or less than 30 ml hydrocarbon; convulsion or coma.
1. Syrup of ipecac (10-15 ml *stat*) – acts in about 10-20 min.
   a) Can repeat once.
   b) If not effective:
2. Trigger pharyngeal (gag) reflex.
3. *Gastric lavage* – suction out stomach contents first.
   Contraindications:
   – ingestion of corrosive or less than 30 ml hydrocarbon
   – convulsions
   – in coma, unless a cuffed endotracheal tube is in place.
4. *Activated charcoal*
   Absorptive action results in GI decontamination.
   a) Maximal effect if given within 30 min of poison ingestion.
   b) Effective against
      i) antipyretics and analgesics: ASA, sodium salicylate, acetaminophen (paracetamol), dextropropoxyphene
      ii) sedatives and hypnotics: phenobarbital, secobarbital, pentobarbital, ethchlorvynol, glutethimide
      iii) antidepressants and tranquilizers: imipramine, nortriptyline, meprobamate, chlorpromazine
      iv) other agents: chlorpheniramine, quinidine, phenylbutazone, chloroquine, digoxin, probenecid.
   c) Dose: children <5 yr = 15 g; 5-10 yr = 15-30 g and >10 yr old = 30-50 g activated charcoal (1 g = 1 cc charcoal powder)

i) Mix appropriate amount in 120-240 ml fluid (juice, soft drink, etc).

ii) Give charcoal mixture orally or by nasogastric tube.

5. **Do not give** ipecac and charcoal together. (Charcoal inactivates ipecac and prevents emetic action.)

UNKNOWN POISON

1. Ensure support of vital functions.
2. Proceed as for Ingested Poison, unless poisoning was by another route.
3. Save vomitus and lavage aspirates, and obtain blood and urine samples, for toxicologic analysis.
4. Presence of a particular symptom complex may aid in recognition of the poison absorbed (see p 496), so that specific antidote can be used.

INJECTED POISON

— **if treatment can be started within a few minutes of injection**

1. Apply tourniquet proximally and ice locally.
2. Do not release tourniquet until patient is in intensive-care area. (Shock may occur).

POISONING BY RECTAL ROUTE

Give enema.

INHALED POISON

1. Move the patient into uncontaminated air.
2. Maintain clear airway.
3. Give O_2.

POISON IN CONTACT WITH SKIN OR EYE

1. Wash with copious amounts of water.
2. Do not use chemical antidotes.
3. Contact Poison Control Center (ext 1700) for specific antidotes.

Salicylate Intoxication (see Fig, p 486)

Causes

1. Accidental ingestion by toddler — 87.5 mg of ASA per kg taken as 1 dose, or 5 ml of Oil of Wintergreen, is enough to cause intoxication.

2. Therapeutic overdosage.
3. Suicide attempt.

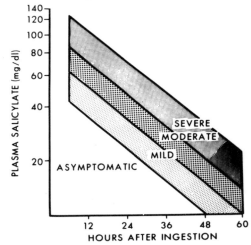

Done's nomogram of plasma salicylate levels. (Done, A. K.: Salicylate intoxication. Significance of measurements of salicylate in blood in cases of acute ingestion. Pediatrics 26:800, 1960.) (With permission)

Signs and Symptoms
1. Overbreathing, vomiting, pyrexia, dehydration.
2. More serious are convulsions, pulmonary edema.

Investigation
1. Blood for salicylate (toxic level >30 mg/dl, or lower in infants), pH, bicarbonate, Na^+, K^+, Cl^-, BUN, and blood sugar.
2. Note
   a) Infants usually have a mixed acid–base disturbance (p 167), primary metabolic acidosis, and primary respiratory alkalosis.
   b) Older children and adults usually have respiratory alkalosis.
   c) Urine often contains reducing substance and ketones – do not confuse with diabetes mellitus.

Treatment

General measures
1. Induce vomiting (p 484).
2. Prevent bleeding: give vitamin K_1 oxide, 1 mg im.
3. *Replacement therapy:* give fluids iv
   a) replace two-thirds of deficit in 24 hr
   b) maintenance therapy — give 100 ml/100 cal expended (caloric expenditure may be increased by 50%; see p 118)
   c) **Note.** Usual total fluid therapy = 150-250 ml of '2/3:1/3' soln per kg body wt:
      i) add 40 mEq KCl/liter after patient voids.
      ii) measure urine output and alter therapy accordingly.
4. Correct metabolic acidosis (p 126).

Special measures
Conditions that may need special measures are:
Clinical
a) semicoma or coma, convulsions, severe hyperventilation, oliguria
b) respiratory depression or pulmonary edema.
Biochemical
a) marked decrease in plasma HCO_3^- or in plasma pCO_2
b) high steady-state plasma salicylate, Done nomogram in 'severe' range (see fig, p 486)
c) severe azotemia
1. *Alkalinize urine*
   a) give $NaHCO_3$ 3 to 4 mEq/kg (may cause alkalemia).
   b) give acetazolamide (Diamox) 5 mg/kg im q4h x 3 (be alert for metabolic acidosis).
2. *Remove salicylate extrarenally*
   a) exchange transfusion
   b) peritoneal dialysis, with or without 5% albumin
   c) hemodialysis.

Acetaminophen Poisoning (*see Fig, p 488*)

Acetaminophen = popular analgesic/antipyretic agent without anti-inflammatory effect.
1. Usual dosage causes few side effects; overdosage can result in severe hepatic necrosis and death.
2. As with ASA, acetaminophen intoxication may be accidental, therapeutic overdosage, or suicide attempt.

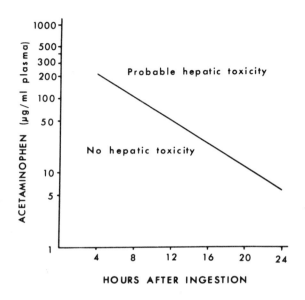

Rumack—Matthew nomogram* for acetaminophen poisoning. Semilogarithmic plot of plasma acetaminophen level in relation to time after ingestion.

Note

1. Time coordinates refer to time of ingestion.
2. Serum levels drawn before 4 hr after ingestion may not represent peak levels.
3. Use nomogram only in relation to a single acute ingestion.
4. $T_{1/2}$ exceeding 4 hr = probability of significant hepatic damage.

(*B. H. Rumack & H. Matthew: Acetaminophen poisoning and toxicity. Pediatrics 55:871-6, 1975; copyright, American Academy of Pediatrics, 1975. With permission.)

Clinical course = triphasic

1. From a few hours up to 2 days after ingestion: nausea, vomiting, anorexia, paleness, lethargy.
2. First-phase symptoms decrease, hepatic necrosis develops, liver becomes enlarged and tender.
3. Days 3-5: jaundice, coagulation defects, hypoglycemia, encephalopathy, renal failure.

Pathogenesis of hepatotoxicity

1. Rapid acetaminophen absorption; peak plasma levels 1-2 hr after ingestion.
2. Normally, is metabolized in liver by glucuronide and sulfate conjugation and excreted in urine.
3. Normally, small portion metabolized via liver microsomal cytochrome oxidase, glutathione conjugation, then excreted as mercapturic acid.
4. With overdosage, glutathione is depleted and intermediate metabolite accumulates in, binds to, and destroys liver cells.
5. Hepatotoxic dosage: in children, >140 mg/kg/dose; in adults, 10-15 g/per dose.
6. Plasma concentration accurately predicts hepatotoxicity.

Treatment

Supportive, and specific antidote.

N-acetylcysteine (Mucomyst) seems to combine with the noxious intermediate metabolite as a glutathione substitute.

1. Loading dose = 140 mg/kg, diluted in 3 vols of cola-type soft drink.
2. Followed by 70 mg acetylcysteine per kg, po q4h, for a total of 18 doses.
3. For best results, *give first dose within 12 h of the overdose ingestion.*

Ingestion of Petroleum Distillate

Guidelines for Management

1. **Stat: chest radiograph, PA and lateral, in all cases.**
2. Admit all patients whose chest films are positive.
3. All patients: repeat chest film in 12-24 hr.

GUIDELINES FOR MANAGING INGESTION OF PETROLEUM DISTILLATE

Symptoms	Amount	Contents	First Aid
None	Less than 30 ml (<6 mouthfuls)	Petroleum distillate only	None
None	More than 30 ml (>6 mouthfuls)	Petroleum distillate only	Induce emesis with syrup of ipecac
None	Any amount	Petroleum distillate with dangerous contents*	Induce emesis with syrup of ipecac
Significant symptoms: loss of gag reflex; convulsion, coma; difficulty breathing	More than 30 ml (>6 mouthfuls)	Petroleum distillate with or without dangerous contents*	Endotracheal intubation: gastric lavage

*e.g., highly toxic pesticides, or additives such as camphor, naphthalene, heavy metals, nitrobenzene, trichlorethane.

Important to Remember

1. *Emesis is contraindicated if the patient*
   a) is comatose
   b) has loss of gag reflex
   c) is convulsing
   d) has cardiac arrhythmia
   e) is in respiratory distress; **or**
   f) has ingested a product with a corrosive additive.
2. *Emesis is*
   a) *too late if* patient already symptomatic
   b) *superfluous if* vomiting has already occurred.
3. Volume of a mouthful swallowed by a child 1-3 yr old = approx. 5 ml.
4. *Emesis indicated* if patient has *ingested even a small amount* of aromatic hydrocarbons or volatile oils:
   a) *aromatic hydrocarbons such as benzene, toluene, and xylene* (used as paint thinner, paint remover, solvent for rubber and plastic cements)
      – cause CNS, pulmonary, and bone-marrow toxicity.
   b) *volatile oils such as turpentine and eucalyptus* are locally irritating as well as productive of severe systemic symptoms.

Barbiturates (p 482) and Anticonvulsants

1. Induce vomiting or do gastric lavage.
2. Give activated charcoal (pp 484-5).

Severe

1. Admit to constant nursing care.
2. Assisted ventilation may be required for respiratory failure.
3. Analeptics contraindicated in children.
4. Start iv therapy (p 118): monitor blood levels of the drug.
5. Induce alkalinization of urine – increases excretion of long-acting barbiturates (p 487).

Mild

1. Observe closely for at least 8 hr, for drowsiness, slow respiration.
2. Push oral fluids.

Tranquilizers (Phenothiazine)

1. As for barbiturates (p 491).
2. Extrapyramidal crisis: give Benadryl, 0.5 to 1.0 mg/kg/dose, iv or po (p 437).

Iron

Lethal dose of $FeSO_4$ = 0.9 g/kg body wt (elemental iron, 180 mg/kg body wt).

Signs
Vomiting, bloody diarrhea, hypotension, shock.

Treatment

Mild ingestion
1. Induce vomiting with ipecac (p 484).
2. Gastric lavage with 5% Na bicarbonate soln.
3. Give cathartic.

Excessive ingestion (>500 mg elemental iron or 2 g $FeSO_4$)
1. Radiograph of abdomen (radiopaque tablets).
2. **Stat** obtain plasma iron level (0.5 ml blood in special citrated micro tube).
3. Obtain serum iron and serum TIBC.
4. Notify director of Poison Control.

Shock or coma
1. Treatment for shock, see p 472.
2. If stat plasma iron is over 300 μg/dl:
   Consult director of Poison Control re use of deferoxamine: either
   a) deferoxamine iv, 10-15 mg/kg body wt/hr iv in 5% glucose/water as continuous infusion for 8-12 hr; **or**
   b) deferoxamine im, 600-1200 mg/day in 2 or 3 doses a day (maximum, 80 mg/kg/day).
   Note. Deferoxamine complexes with iron to form deroxamine, which is excreted by the kidneys and imparts a reddish color to the urine.

Lye (Sodium Hydroxide)

Corrosive common in drain- and oven-cleaners.

1. Esophageal burns can be present without mouth burns.
2. Emesis and gastric lavage are contraindicated.
3. Admit all patients to ENT service, including those in whom ingestion of lye is only suspected (p 109).

Insecticides

General treatment

Induce emesis and wash out stomach.

Specific treatment

Depends on product ingested.

ORGANIC PHOSPHATE

Causes nausea, headache, weakness, sweating, ataxia, tremor, disturbed vision, salivation, miosis, tearing, and muscle fasiculation.

Treatment

1. Complete atropinization; can be repeated in 15-30 min. To produce dry mouth, mydriasis, and tachycardia.
2. If product on clothes or skin, wash thoroughly.
3. Respiratory problems: treat with suction and assisted ventilation.
4. Atropine sulfate, 0.05 mg/kg im or iv (p 422)
5. Protopam chloride (PAM) 25-50 mg/kg, up to 2 g (p 456), iv *slowly* in 5% glucose/water; repeat q12h prn.
6. Notify director of Poison Control and Anesthesia.

Antimony, Arsenic, Copper, Mercury

Dimercaprol (BAL), 2-3 mg/kg, im, q4-12h (p 437).

Cyanide

1. Amyl nitrite by inhalation; and sodium nitrite 3% iv, 2-5 ml/min.
2. Stop both if BP falls.

Chlorinated Hydrocarbons
(DDT, Lindane, Chlordane)

Cause irritability, tremor, and convulsion.
Treat symptomatically.

Hallucinogens

CHEMICAL

Lysergic acid diethylamide (LSD); mescaline; dimethyltryptamine (DMT); diethyltryptamine (DET); 2,5 dimethoxy-4 methyl-amphetamine (DOM or STP); 3,4-methylenedioxyamphetamine (MDA); trimethoxylamphetamine (TMA); methoxy-methylenedioxyamphetamine (MMDA), PCP (phencyclidine).

Signs

1. Pupillary dilation, hyperreflexia, euphoria, hypertension, sweating, acute confusional and paranoid states.
2. Nausea and vomiting may occur early.

Treatment (p 482)

1. Notify Resident in Adolescent Medicine **stat.**
2. Provide physical safety.
3. Avoid frightening stimuli, such as loud noises and unnecessary procedures.
4. If necessary, give diazepam (Valium; p 436).
5. Phenothiazines contraindicated.

NATURAL HALLUCINOGENS

Notify Resident in Adolescent Medicine **stat.**

Peyote; morning-glory seeds

Signs: similar to those with chemical hallucinogens
Treatment: as for chemical hallucinogens (above)

Marihuana; hashish (pot, grass, tea, hash, etc.)

Signs

1. Moderate dilation of pupils, conjunctivitis, dryness of the mouth, increased hunger, postural hypotension.
2. Initial stimulation followed by sedation.
3. Distorted perception and paranoid ideations are frequent but usually less intense than with hallucinogens.

Treatment

1. Notify Resident in Adolescent Medicine **stat.**
2. Provide tranquil environment.
3. Give diazepam (Valium; p 436).

Narcotics

Heroin, morphine, Demerol (pethidine, meperidine), methadone, Nisentil, diphenoxylate (Lomotil), propoxyphene (Darvon).

Signs

1. Pin-point pupils, cyanosis, bradycardia, slowing of respiration.
2. Convulsions, stupor, or coma.

Treatment

1. Maintain adequate airway.
2. Give naloxone HCl (pp 451, 481).

Digitalis Products

See pp 205, 436

Lead

Source

Paints, batteries, lead toys, gasoline vapor, industrial dusts.

Signs and Symptoms

Irritability, weight loss, projectile vomiting, anorexia, abdominal pain, weakness, paralysis and encephalopathy, lead lines on gums, papilledema.

Management

Advise Poison Control *stat.*

TOXICOLOGY TESTS

Requisitions

Standard HSC Clinical Chemistry requisitions required.

Specimens

Tests on blood

1. Salicylate: send 1.5 ml heparinized or clotted blood.
2. Barbiturates: send 1.5 ml heparinized or clotted blood.
3. Stat plasma iron: send 0.5 ml of blood in a special citrated micro tube.
4. *Drug screening tests on blood and urine:* available only after consultation with and arrangement through Clinical Chemistry.

POISONING: COMMON SIGNS & SYMPTOMS

Altered Vital Signs

1. Pulse rate
   a) *slow:* digitalis, lily-of-the-valley, narcotic depressants
   b) *rapid:* alcohol, amphetamines, atropine, ephedrine
2. Respirations
   a) *depressed:* alcohol, barbiturates (late), narcotic depressants, tranquilizers
   b) *rapid:* amphetamines, barbiturates (early), carbon monoxide, methanol, petroleum distillates, salicylates
   c) *wheezing, pulmonary edema:* mushrooms (muscarinic), narcotic depressants, organic PO_4 insecticides, petroleum distillates
   d) *paralysis:* organic PO_4 insecticides, botulism
3. Temperature
   a) *pyrexia:* salicylates, mercury, phenothiazines, phenylpropanolamine, fenfluramine, atropine, benzatropine, anticholinergic agents
   b) *hypothermia:* barbiturates, methadone, insulin, tannin
4. Blood pressure
   a) *hypertension:* sympathomimetics including alupent and methylphenidate; methadone; LSD; tricyclic antidepressants combined with sympathomimetics; liquorice
   b) *hypotension:* antihistamines, phenothiazines, diazepam, narcotic depressants, thiabendazole, anticholinesterases

5. Cardiac
   a) *arrhythmias:* antihistamines, aminophylline, tricyclic antidepressants, amphetamines, phenothiazines.
   b) *heart block:* digitalis, phenothiazines

Neurologic Signs

1. **Ataxia:** alcohol, barbiturates, bromides, carbon monoxide, diphenylhydantoin, hallucinogens, heavy metals, organic solvents, tranquilizers
2. Pupils
   a) *pinpoint:* mushrooms (muscarinic), narcotic depressants (opiates), organic PO_4 insecticides
   b) *dilated:* amphetamines, antihistamines, atropine, barbiturates (coma), cocaine, ephedrine, LSD, methanol, withdrawal from narcotic depressants
   c) *nystagmus on lateral gaze:* barbiturates, minor tranquilizers (meprobamate, benzodiazepine)
3. **Convulsions, muscle twitching:** alcohol, amphetamines, antihistamines, boric acid, camphor, chlorinated hydrocarbon insecticides (DDT), cyanide, lead, organic PO_4 insecticides, plants (lily-of-the-valley, azalea, iris, water hemlock), salicylates, strychnine; withdrawal from barbiturates, benzodiazepine, meprobamate
4. **Coma/drowsiness:** ethyl alcohol, antihistamines, barbiturates and other hypnotics, carbon monoxide, narcotic depressants (opiates), salicylates, tranquilizers
5. **Paralysis:** botulism, heavy metals, plants (coniine in poison hemlock), triorthocresyl phosphate

Signs Related to the Mouth

1. **Salivation:** arsenic, corrosives, mercury, mushrooms, organic PO_4 insecticides, thallium.
2. **Dryness:** atropine, amphetamines, antihistamines, narcotic depressants.
3. **Breath odor:**
   Acetone: acetone, alcohol (methyl, isopropyl), phenol, salicylates
   Alcohol: ethyl alcohol
   Bitter almonds: cyanide
   Coal gas: carbon monoxide
   Garlic: arsenic, phosphorus, organic PO_4 insecticides, thallium
   Oil of Wintergreen: methyl salicylate
   Petroleum: petroleum distillates
   Violets: turpentine

Skin Color

1. **Cyanosis:** aniline dyes, carbon monoxide, cyanide, nitrites, strychnine.
2. **Jaundice** (hepatic or hemolytic): aniline, arsenic, carbon tetrachloride, castor bean, fava bean, mushroom, naphthalene, yellow phosphorus.
3. **Red flush:** alcohol, antihistamines, atropine, boric acid, carbon monoxide, nitrites.

Violent Emesis (in many cases, with hematemesis)

Aminophylline, bacterial food poisoning, boric acid, corrosives, fluoride, heavy metals, phenol, salicylates.

Abdominal Colic

Black-widow-spider bite, heavy metals, narcotic-depressant withdrawal.

CHILD ABUSE

('BATTERED-CHILD SYNDROME')

Definition
Physical injury and/or deprivation of nutrition, care, or affection, in circumstances indicating that such injury and/or deprivation are not accidental.

On Presentation

Immediately: notify Child Abuse Team (call locating) if you suspect child abuse.

Diagnosis
A. History
   1. Guardian: Social characteristics; family relationships.
   2. Child: Development; past and present illness; emotions.
   3. Crises: Precipitating event(s); how managed.

B. Physical
   1. Complete examination is essential.
   2. Severity ranges from normal to dead on arrival.
   3. Injuries:
      a) Obvious – none, malnutrition, cuts, bruises, fractures, burns.
      b) Hidden – psychological, intracranial, retinal hemorrhages, intra-abdominal, healed fractures.

C. Laboratory
   1. Hematology – rule out blood dyscrasia.
   2. Skeletal survey – record recent or past fractures; rule out accidental fractures and metabolic bone disease.

D. Color photography – record obvious trauma.

Management

	Immediate	*Long-term*
A. Injuries	Admit **or** send home	Clinic or family physician
B. Protection	Notify Children's Aid Society. Admit to hospital **or** send home with another guardian	social workers pediatrician psychologist psychiatrist

ABBREVIATIONS & SYMBOLS

2/3–1/3 soln	solution of 3.3% dextrose in 0.3% NaCl
ABG	arterial blood-gas measurements
ACD	acid/citrate/dextrose
ADH	antidiuretic hormone
ADP	adenosine diphosphate
AHG	antihemophilic globulin
ALL	acute lymphatic leukemia
ALT	alanine aminotransferase; *was* (serum) GPT
AMP	adenosine monophosphate
ASOT	antistreptolysin titer
AST	aspartate aminotransferase; *was* (serum) GOT
ATP	adenosine triphosphate
BEI	butanol-extractable iodine
BSP	bromsulphthalein (sulphobromophthalein)
Ca	total calcium
Ca++	ionized calcium
cc	*use for gases or volume – not liquids* (ml)
CCC	catheter cinecystogram
CDP	continuous distending pressure
CEA	carcino-embryonic antigen
CFT	complement-fixation test
CIE	counterimmune electrophoresis
C.I.U	Clinical Investigation Unit
CMV	cytomegalovirus
CNPB	continuous negative-pressure breathing
COAL	cystine, ornithine, arginine, lysine
CPAP	continuous positive airway pressure
CPD	citrate/phosphate/dextrose
CPPB/V	continuous positive-pressure breathing/ventilation
CPS	carbamyl-phosphate synthetase (carbamate kinase, EC 2.7.22)
C.S.R.	central supply room
CT	computed tomogram/tomography
CVP	central venous pressure
DIC	disseminated intravascular coagulation
DNPH	dinitrophenyl hydrazine (test for keto acids)
DOCA	deoxycorticosterone acetate

EBV	Epstein–Barr virus
ECF	extracellular fluid
ECHO	enteric cytopathic human orphan virus
ECM	external cardiac massage
EDTA	ethylenediaminetetraacetic acid
EMG	electromyogram
ETT	endotracheal tube
EUA	examination under anesthesia
FSH	follicle-stimulating hormone
GFR	glomerular filtration rate
G-6-PD	glucose-6-phosphate dehydrogenase
IDU	idoxuridine
INH	isonicotinic acid hydrazide
IPPB/V	intermittent positive-pressure breathing/ventilation
it	intrathecal(ly)
ITP	idiopathic thrombocytopenic purpura
LBW	(infant of) low birth weight
LCD	liquor carbonis detergens
LCT	long-chain triglycerides
LE	lupus erythematosus
M	(molar) moles/liter
MCT	medium-chain triglycerides
MSUD	maple-syrup-urine disease (branched-chain ketonuria)
μ	(micron) use μm
NBT	nitroblue tetrazolium (dye-reduction test)
NPS	nasopharyngeal suction
NPT	nasopharyngeal tube
N soln	Normal-strength solution
NTT	nasotracheal tube
O.C.C.C.	Ontario Crippled Children's Centre
OCT	ornithine carbamyl transferase (or OTC, q.v.)
OD	right eye
17-OH-CS	hydroxycorticosteroids
17-OHP	hydroxyprogesterone
OS	left eye
OTC	ornithine transcarbamylase (ornithine carbamoyltransferase, EC 2.1.3.3)
OU	each/both eye(s)
P.A.R.	postanesthesia (recovery) room

PAS	para-aminosalicylic acid
PEEP	positive end-expiratory pressure
PID	pelvic inflammatory disease
PKU	phenylketonuria
p-npp	p-nitrophenyl phosphate
PPD	purified protein derivative
PT	prothrombin time
PTC	plasma thromboplastin component
PTT	partial thromboplastin time
RAIU	radioactive-iodine uptake
RIA	radioimmunoassay
SGA	(infant) small for gestational age
SGOT	serum glutamic-oxaloacetic transaminase (now aspartate aminotransferase)
SGPT	serum glutamic-pyruvic transaminase (now alanine aminotransferase)
SIDS	sudden-infant-death syndrome ("crib death")
2/3–1/3 soln	solution of 3.3% dextrose in 0.3% NaCl
SSPE	subacute sclerosing panencephalitis
TBG	thyroxine-binding globulin
THAM	tris(hydroxymethyl)-aminomethane
TMP:SMX	trimethoprim–sulfamethoxazole
T(ORCH)	toxoplasmosis, other (viruses), rubella, CMV, herpes
TPI	*Treponema pallidum* immobilization test
T_3RIA	triiodothyronine radioimmunoassay
TSH	thyroid-stimulating hormone
URI	upper respiratory-tract infection
VDRL	venereal disease research laboratory (test)
VMA	vanillin mandelic acid (in urine)
WPW	Wolff–Parkinson–White syndrome
ZIG	zoster immune globulin
ZIP	zoster immune plasma

A

See **blood tests, urine tests,** and **poisons,** for specific tests/poisons

See **blood tests**, **urine tests**, and **poisons**, for specific tests/poisons

See **blood tests, urine tests,** and **poisons,** for specific tests/poisons

C

See **blood tests, urine tests,** and **poisons,** for specific
tests/poisons

See **blood tests, urine tests,** and **poisons,** for specific tests/poisons

See **blood tests, urine tests,** and **poisons,** for specific tests/poisons

See **blood tests, urine tests,** and **poisons,** for specific
tests/poisons

See **blood tests, urine tests,** and **poisons,** for specific tests/poisons

See **blood tests**, **urine tests**, and **poisons**, for specific tests/poisons

F

See **blood tests, urine tests,** and **poisons,** for specific tests/poisons

G

See **blood tests, urine tests,** and **poisons,** for specific
tests/poisons

See **blood tests, urine tests,** and **poisons,** for specific
tests/poisons

I

See **blood tests, urine tests,** and **poisons,** for specific tests/poisons

See **blood tests, urine tests,** and **poisons,** for specific tests/poisons

See **blood tests, urine tests,** and **poisons,** for specific
tests/poisons

M

See **blood tests, urine tests,** and **poisons,** for specific
tests/poisons

See **blood tests, urine tests,** and **poisons,** for specific tests/poisons

See **blood tests, urine tests,** and **poisons,** for specific tests/poisons

See **blood tests, urine tests,** and **poisons,** for specific tests/poisons

R

See **blood tests, urine tests,** and **poisons,** for specific tests/poisons

See **blood tests, urine tests,** and **poisons,** for specific
tests/poisons

See **blood tests, urine tests,** and **poisons,** for specific tests/poisons

See **blood tests, urine tests,** and **poisons,** for specific tests/poisons

See **blood tests**, **urine tests**, and **poisons**, for specific tests/poisons

V

See **blood tests**, **urine tests**, and **poisons**, for specific tests/poisons

See **blood tests**, **urine tests**, and **poisons**, for specific tests/poisons